PX/
448
JoN
③

Nurse Prescribing

FHSW

For Baillière Tindall

Senior Commissioning Editor Jacqueline Curthoys
Project Development Manager Karen Gilmour
Project Manager Jane Shanks

Nurse Prescribing

Politics to Practice

Edited by

Mark Jones MSc BSc (Hons) RN RH
Primary Care Policy Advisor
Royal College of Nursing
London, UK

Foreword by

Baroness Julia Cumberlege
House of Lords
London, UK

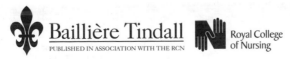

Baillière Tindall
PUBLISHED IN ASSOCIATION WITH THE RCN

Royal College
of Nursing

Edinburgh London New York Oxford Phildelphia St Louis Sydney Toronto

BAILLIÈRE TINDALL
An imprint of Elsevier Limited

First published 1999
  Reprinted 2004

ISBN 0 7020 2314 0

British Library Cataloguing in Publication Data
A catalogue record for this book is available from the British Library

Library of Congress Cataloging in Publication Data
A catalog record for this book is available from the Library of Congress

Note
Medical knowledge is constantly changing. As new information becomes
available, changes in treatment, procedures, equipment and the use of drugs
become necessary. The editors, contributors and the publishers have, as far as
it is possible, taken care to ensure that the information given in this text is
accurate and up to date. However, readers are strongly advised to confirm
that the information, especially with regard to drug usage, complies with the
latest legislation and standards of practice.

 your source for books,
journals and multimedia
in the health sciences
www.elsevierhealth.com

The
publisher's
policy is to use
paper manufactured
from sustainable forests

Typeset in Great Britain by
Phoenix Photosetting, Chatham, Kent
Printed in China
B/02

Contents

Accountability issues; Collaborative working;
Relationships with drug and appliance manufacturers;
Is nurse prescribing useful?; Conclusion; Questions for discussion;
Further reading

Contributors

Maggie Banning RGN SCM BSc(Hons) MSc PGDE
Lecturer in Life Sciences, Royal College of Nursing Institute, London, UK

Alastair R L Buxton BSc(Hons) ACPP MRPharmS
Chairman, Young Pharmacists Group/Community Pharmacist,
Birmingham, UK

Helen Caulfield LLB MA
RCN Solicitor, Royal College of Nursing, London, UK

Stephen Chapman BSc PhD MRPharmS
Professor of Prescribing Studies, Department of Medicines Management,
Keele University, Staffordshire, UK

Sultan Isam Dajani BPharm MRPharmS ACPP Diploma Comm.Pharm
Member of Council of The Royal Pharmaceutical Society, Public Relations
Officer of The Young Pharmacist's Group, Journalist, Pharmacist, and
Manager/Consultant, Hampshire, UK

Pauline Emmerson MSc RN RM HV CPT
Nurse Practitioner, Masters House, London, UK

Peter Fellows LRCP MRCS MB BS
General Medical Practitioner, Deputy Chairman, and former Chairman,
Prescribing Subcommittee of the GMSC, Lydney Health Centre,
Gloucestershire, UK

Gabby Fennessy MSc BA
Clinical Effectiveness Information Manager, Royal College of Nursing
Institute, London, UK

Elizabeth Gardiner BA(Hons)
Health Policy Analyst, formerly Parliamentary Officer at the Royal
College of Nursing, London, UK

Veronica James MA PhD RGN
Professor of Nursing Studies, University of Nottingham School of
Nursing, Medical School, Queen's Medical Centre, Nottingham, UK

Mark Jones MSc BSc(Hons) RN RHV
Primary Care Policy Advisor, Royal College of Nursing, London, UK

Jahn Dad Khan MRPharmS ACPP
Vice Chairman - The Young Pharmacists' Group, Birmingham, UK

Penny Lawson RGN DN NP Dip
Joint Manager/Nurse Practitioner, Three Boroughs Primary Health Care
Team, London, UK

Mary Mayes BA BSc RGN RSCN NPDip
Nurse Practitioner, Beacon Road Surgery, East Sussex, UK

Ann Ogilvie RGN DPSN(PN) BSc(Hons)
Practice Nurse, West Yorkshire, UK

Anne Marie Rafferty RGN DN DPhil(Oxon)
Director, Centre for Policy in Nursing Research, London School of
Hygiene and Tropical Medicine, London, UK

Eileen Shepherd RGN DipN
Independent Nurse Consultant, Nottingham, UK

Sir Roger Sims JP
Member of Parliament for Chislehurst 1974–1997, Member of the House
of Commons Select Committee on Health, and of the Royal College of
Nursing's Parliamentary Panel, Orpington, Kent, UK

Jan Towers PhD NPC CRNP
Director of Governmental Affairs, Practice and Research, American
Academy of Nurse Practitioners, Office of Health Policy, Washington DC,
USA

Fiona Winstanley BSc(Hons) DPS DN RGN
Prescribing Pilot District Nurse, now Senior Lecturer – Community
Nursing, University College Suffolk, Ipswich Hospital, UK

Foreword

Nurse prescribing is simply common sense – or so I thought in 1985. I have not changed my mind, but nearly fifteen years later I am appalled that it has taken me so long to persuade others of its merits.

The team of four, which undertook the Review of Community Nursing for England, had no doubts. Nurse prescribing was one of 14 recommendations and we saw it as the most significant. We checked out the implications. No legislation was required – simply regulations, no additional resources were necessary, and there were no professional implications. Wrong, wrong, wrong.

Perhaps it was naïve to accept this advice but it was the most authoritative available at the time. Nevertheless I never doubted the strength of the case and I have never given up. As a Regional Chair I was able to ensure that the policy for nurse prescribing became a manifesto commitment, which was to prove invaluable. Soon after taking my seat in the House of Lords I was able to collaborate with Sir Roger Sims in passing the necessary legislation. In 1992 as a Junior Health Minister with direct access to the Treasury I was able to overcome their qualms about costs so that pilot schemes could be inaugurated; then to keep the pressure on when momentum was lost. As one legislative barrier fell more appeared but I was able to influence the appointment of the wise Dr June Crown to overcome the final hurdles. In 1997, I was now in opposition, but the new Government gave me a pledge to continue the pursuit of Nurse Prescribing countrywide.

The one constant throughout this lengthy and tiring campaign has been the support of the nursing profession. Trevor Clay was an enthusiast, as has been Christine Hancock. I have had support from two Chief Nursing Officers and departmental officials who have been dogged in their determination to see this programme through. Fiona Winstanley and Anthea Clegg were the visionaries who established the Association for Nurse Prescribing. Leadership is important but the inspiration for me has come from countless nurses up and down the country. I think of those courageous pilot site nurses and the pioneers in Bolton. I think of their supportive managers and GP colleagues, but above all I think of Mark Jones.

Mark has been indefatigable in his campaigning on this issue and this impressive volume is testimony not only to his determination but to his intellect. *Nurse Prescribing – Politics and Practice* is the most remarkable record of the difficulties which have been overcome in order to implement a change in professional practice – a change that benefits patients, enhances the nursing profession, cements primary care teams and gives more time to family doctors to spend with their patients. But this book is more than that – it is an imperative to enhance practice. I unreservedly commend it to you.

Baroness Cumberlege
House of Lords
London

Introduction and overview

Mark Jones

Welcome to what has been one of the most frustrating books to compile, both for contributors and myself as editor. In the true tradition of the nurse prescribing debate, political manoeuvring – in particular the constant postponement of the Crown II Report – has meant we have had to take the best shot at finally getting something published. We know that this report is seminal to the future of nurse prescribing, and many of the authors have based their contributions on their best guess as to what it would say and others on a very last minute glimpse of the final document. I have tried to give a full critique of Crown in the final chapter, and I trust this does justice to such an important part of the nurse prescribing history.

To begin, however, with Chapter 1, which takes us back to the initial arguments in favour of the extension of prescribing rights to nurses. Here I allude to the beginnings of the political debate and examine some of the powerbases ranged for and against the concept. The chapter provides an overview of developments from the late 1970s to the present day, highlighting themes to be developed by colleagues as the book progresses.

Ever mindful of its position in the hierarchy of power within the health care sector, nursing was keen to enlist the support of medicine and pharmacy as it sought prescribing rights. In Chapters 2 and 3 we have the viewpoint of opinion leaders within these professions – by and large supporting prescribing for nurses, but not without a series of caveats and a robust defence and offensive positioning so far as their own interests are concerned. In general, the long held philosophy of 'you scratch my back and I'll scratch yours' is not lost on our doctor and pharmacist colleagues.

Roger Sims and Elizabeth Gardiner (Ch. 4), and Helen Caulfield (Ch. 5) give us two unique insights into the legal developments impinging upon the nurse's right to prescribe. Sims and Gardiner explain the complex parliamentary process which was manipulated in order to achieve statutory authority for nurses to prescribe, while Caulfield explains the quagmire of law, regulations, Acts of parliament and Statutory Instruments which have served – and still do serve – as obstacles to those nurses who feel they should be able to prescribe, or at least supply and administer medicines in the best interests of their patients. Reading Caulfield's chapter in particular, one realises the difficulties facing anyone attempting to ensure that their practice is legal and that they will not end up in court.

Having made our case for nurse prescribing, and achieved the necessary legislation to make it happen, in Chapter 6 Maggie Banning addresses the question of the required education. Her analysis is a definite 'reality check' as she points out the deficiencies of current educational provision for nurse prescribers which are portrayed as woefully inadequate. Banning challenges us to accept her hypothesis that making a case for prescribing and having the legal ability to do so is one thing, but are nurses really prepared to commit themselves to the kind of intense study which she believes is needed to make them competent prescribers?

Following Maggie Banning's grounding in reality, Anne Marie Rafferty and colleagues (Ch. 7) ponder the seemingly unthinkable question – is the quest for nurse prescribing really in the best interests of patients and clients, or in seeking these rights is nursing just trying to emulate its medical counterpart in some self-centred professional project? Well, they do not put it quite like that, but others have made this point – not least members of the nursing profession. In seeking to justify the need for nurses to prescribe, it is important that we consider this question. Surely the ability to prescribe is bound to have an effect on the status of the profession, but we must ensure that the desire to enhance the standard of care we give is the prime motivation. Rafferty, James, and Shepherd help us to do this.

Chapters 8 to 11 take us into the 'real world' of nurse prescribing. In Chapter 8, Fiona Winstanley describes her experience as a true nurse prescriber in one of the pilot sites, while Anne Ogilvie (Ch. 9), Emmerson and Lawson (Ch. 10), and Mary Mayes (Ch. 11) describe the strategies employed by practice nurses and nurse practitioners to circumvent the legal obstacles preventing them from prescribing in the truest sense – something they all consider to be a nuisance and simple inconvenience limiting their practice and denying the best possible care to their patients.

In Chapters 12 and 13, Gabby Fennessy and Stephen Chapman ask whether nurse prescribers will be able to justify and account for their prescribing practice. Fennessy explores the complexity of audit and suggests the important skills would-be prescribers need to develop so as to demonstrate their effectiveness. Chapman further challenges us to consider whether nurses are actually capable of managing the whole concept of cost and care effective prescribing, as he details the current trend toward effective medicines management'.

Jan Towers (Ch. 14) gives us some hope from America, where all 50 of the United States and the District of Columbia now have some form of nurse prescribing legislation in place. This has taken over 30 years to achieve, and frustrated as we may be in the UK, it seems that we have not done at all badly over the last 2 decades. We have yet to make the final push though, and Towers shares with us some strategies adopted by our transatlantic colleagues which we might use to make nurse prescribing the reality it should be in this country. For my sins, in the final chapter of the book I try to bring a glimpse of what the future might mean for nurse prescribing. This analysis begins with the publication of the second Crown Report and moves to suggest the forthcoming model for the extension of prescribing rights to nurses. Moving on from this, a vision for nurse prescribing for the next decade is presented – including its ups and downs, but making every effort to complete the text by leaving us on a high note!

I hope you find our thoughts and ideas useful. Please use the suggested questions for consideration to examine your own perspectives on nurse prescribing, and prepare yourself for this exciting development.

1

Nurse prescribing

The history, the waiting, the battle

Mark Jones

Key issues

♦ Overview of the arguments put forward for nurse prescribing.

♦ The tactics used by the RCN and others to place nurse prescribing on the government's agenda.

♦ How lobbying tactics were used to achieve legislative change.

♦ The significance of the two Crown reviews into prescribing.

INTRODUCTION

This account of nurse prescribing – from politics to practice – was first published as the NHS celebrated its first half century, and the health care world, along with everyone else, waited just one more year for the dawn of the new millennium. In such a climate it is suprising that something as simple as giving prescribing rights to nurses should cause so much brow furrowing and consternation among policy makers and professional groups (including some quarters of nursing itself). Yet this issue causes instant debate wherever it is mentioned, bringing out both the best and the worst of inter- and intra-professional argument concerning the development and emergence of new health care roles.

This chapter begins a book containing an account of one of (if not *the*) hardest fought battles of nursing: a battle in the seemingly constant struggle towards the victory of being recognised as an autonomous profession – whatever that might mean. The various authors elaborate on the political and professional dynamics of nurses' quest to prescribe, and 'real-life', 'on the ground' practitioners tell of the strategies adopted to circumvent what they see as the inconvenience at not being able to prescribe and of their experiences as they actually get to write a legal prescription for the first time. For its part, this introductory chapter seeks to present a chronology of the nurse prescribing quest: it sets out the initial arguments used – which still hold true today – and highlights the key turning points as the various players seek to make nurse prescribing a reality. Subsequent contributors will analyse various aspects of this over-view in detail; however, it is hoped that this introduction will assist anyone who has not yet examined in detail the concept of nurse prescribing.

EARLY DAYS

Moving back from the brink of the millennium, it still seems that the notion of giving nurses prescribing rights is a new phenomenon, perhaps dreamt up by nurse visionaries (or dreamers if you prefer) sometime within the last few years – 5 at most. But, at the time this chapter is being written, the first documented evidence available of the case for nurse prescribing being articulated is almost exactly 20 years old. On 4 September 1978, the Association of Nursing Practice (ANP) of the Royal College of Nursing (RCN) presented its parent body with a report entitled 'District nurses' dressings' (RCN, 1978). The ANP described the problems faced by district nurses as they tried to obtain dressings, equipment and aids to meet their patients' needs, yet were often hampered by poor supply departments and the laborious procedure of having to get a general practitioner (GP) to prescribe the items which the nurses knew were needed.

The trouble in obtaining a simple sterile dressing pack, for example, was frustratingly reported:

> Where district nurses have to rely on dressing packs obtained on the authority of FP10, signed by a doctor, there is a particular problem in that these dressing packs contain no forceps or gallipots. If these are required for the dressing procedure they must be sterilised by boiling in the patient's own home. It would appear that some GPs are reluctant to prescribe dressings from a pre-heated pack because of the expense. The district nurse, in these circumstances, is packing tins of dressings and baking them in the oven in the patient's home. (RCN, 1978)

The author is aware he is keen to stress the longevity of the nurse prescribing debate, but is it not somewhat ridiculous that just 20 years ago district nurses were driven to such anachronistic activity simply because they did not have the authority to prescribe the kind of dressing pack they needed to meet their patients' assessed needs?

The problem was not confined to dressing packs: district nurses were well aware that, on a daily basis, they were making decisions on particular dressings or appliances, or adjustments to medication required by patients, but had to find GPs to sanction these decisions and to prescribe the items needed. GPs simply endorsed the nurses' decision without question. In many cases the district nurse was simply frustrated at having to spend time making seemingly unnecessary trips between the patient's home and the GP practice. As if this inconvenience were not bad enough, other groups of nurses came forward with reports that patients actually suffered as a result of nurses having to seek medical endorsement of their decisions: for example specialist community nurses with responsibility for palliative care described situations where they could not increase the dose of an analgesic, or administer it before the exact time for which it was prescribed because, technically, to do so would be to act in breach of prevailing legislation by prescribing a prescription only medicine. Patients were left in pain with their relatives watching the clock while nurses tried to contact a doctor to authorise the medication change (Jones and Gough, 1997).

The essential tenets of the nurse prescribing case 20 years ago, therefore, were much the same as today. Nurses – at least in many specialist areas – have a knowledge base commensurate with being able to make accurate decisions as to the kind of prescribable products their patients require in order to meet their assessed need for nursing care. This includes the ability to vary the dose of a drug prescribed by someone else within agreed parameters, and to prescribe a drug for the first time for any given patient. Compounding the case was the obvious time and effort district nurses in particular were taking to obtain prescriptions from GPs once they had seen patients at home and determined their needs. Given these facts, was it not logical to at least consider giving some nurses some prescribing rights?

Although such an analysis seems straightforward in the present climate, in the early 1980s, when nurses first began to explore the potential for prescribing certain items, this was radical thinking. These two arguments (of the nurse having the specialist knowledge base to make prescribing decisions yet having to find a GP to action that decision – leading to time-wasting on the part of both nurse and doctor – plus the more serious factor of denial of immediate care to patients) went on to be the key points in the campaign to extend prescribing rights to nurses.

First hope: the Cumberlege Report

Fortuitously, just as the awareness of this whole issue was growing within the nursing profession, the government commissioned a review of community nursing provision by a team of health experts and economists under the chairmanship of Julia Cumberlege. The review team were asked to consider community nursing provision in England, and make recommendations for the future of that provision. The Royal College of Nursing saw this as an excellent opportunity to bring forward the arguments for amending legislation to allow nurses to prescribe (Jones and Gough, 1997).

The final report of the Cumberlege review team acknowledged all of the arguments for nurse prescribing. Cumberlege readily accepted the point that experienced district nurses were wasting their time and that of both patients and doctors, and recommended that qualified community nurses should be able to prescribe from a limited range of medicines, appliances and dressings (DHSS, 1986). The Cumberlege Report was positively received by government, and in 1987 the House of Commons Social Services Select Committee supported the specific call for prescribing rights for community nurses (House of Commons Social Services Committee, 1987). Buoyed up by their success at achieving recognition of the prescribing issue, the Royal College of Nursing began to gather support for putting the Cumberlege and select committee recommendations into practice (Jones and Gough, 1997). The RCN took its case and arguments for nurse prescribing along to the bodies it considered to be at one and the same time potential allies and opponents – the British Medical Association (BMA) and the Royal Pharmaceutical Society of Great Britain (RPSoGB).

Better the enemy you know?

The RCN did not consider the BMA and RPSoGB to be true 'enemies', but if any opposition to nurse prescribing were going to arise, it was likely that these bodies would have some influence. In May 1988, 10 years after its district nursing membership voiced the initial concerns about reliance on GP prescribing for items they needed to deliver care, the RCN presented the BMA with a discussion paper which laid out the 'criteria determining prescribing activity by nurses' (RCN and BMA, 1988). In the paper, the college envisaged the extension of prescribing rights to district nurses, health visitors, practice nurses, family planning nurses, school nurses, and specialist nurses including diabetes specialists, stoma care nurses, and nurses for the terminally ill. The RCN stressed the need for nurse prescribers to work in partnership with 'relevant GPs and local pharmacists' with an agreed approach to diagnosis and identification of minor disorders for which nurses would prescribe. The paper also emphasised the need for comprehensive training for nurse prescribers, and suggested that any confusion over what had been prescribed could be reduced by the use of patient held prescribing records.

Similar overtures were made by the RCN to the pharmacists. A series of meetings with the RPSoGB throughout 1987 and early 1988 sought to reduce any anxiety that allowing nurses to prescribe would be fraught with difficulty. The college advanced similar arguments to those it had presented to the BMA, emphasising that nurse prescriptions should be traded through the pharmacist and that this professional would remain the final checking point of all nurse prescribable items.

After much initial opposition and a good deal of negotiation, a tacit agreement between nursing, medicine, and the pharmacists was reached in late 1988. The case for nurse prescribing was seen to be justifiable and sustainable, and it was agreed the government should be petitioned to sanction this initiative (RCN and BMA, 1988). The RCN then began a concerted push for the implementation of the Cumberlege recommendations. In particular, it campaigned for the right of community nurses to be able to prescribe any medicines they might need to deliver nursing care and draw up agreements with doctors (later to be known as 'protocols') under which they could supply and administer a range of prescription only medicines.

THE CROWN REPORT

With support from the BMA and the RPSoGB, the RCN were successful in persuading the government to take their case for extending prescribing rights to nurses seriously, and Dr June Crown was asked to lead an advisory group, to report by 1 October 1987. The group was given the responsibility of:

> *advising the secretary of state, after consultation with the Standing Medical Advisory Committee, the Standing Nursing and Midwifery Committee and the Standing Pharmaceutical Committee, how arrangements for the supply of drugs, dressings, appliances and chemical reagents to patients as part of their nursing care in the community might be improved by enabling such items to be prescribed by a nurse, taking into account where necessary current practice and likely developments in other areas of nursing practice. (DoH, 1989, p. 3)*

Clearly the RCN was correct in forming an alliance with pharmacists and doctors, given that together these three professional interest groups were to be the focus of Crown's consultation process. The terms of reference went on further to reflect much of the case that had already been made by the College for nurse prescribing to become a reality. The Crown group were specifically asked to make recommendations on:

> i.   *the circumstances in which nurses might prescribe, order or supply drugs, dressings, appliances and chemical reagents, taking account of such professional and ethical issues as responsibility and inter-professional communication;*
>
> ii. *the categories of items which might properly be prescribed, ordered or supplied by nurses and the arrangements which would be needed for drawing up and maintaining a list of such items;*
>
> iii. *the methods by which drugs, dressings, appliances and chemical reagents might be prescribed, ordered or supplied by nurses, having regard to current guidance on the safe and secure handling of medicines. (DoH, 1989, p. 3)*

It is noteworthy that in the context of prescribing per se, the Crown review's scope was not limited to any particular grouping of community nurses (i.e. any notion that district nurses and health visitors only should be considered for prescribing rights).

The remainder of the tasks set before Crown were again to consider points raised by the RCN in their initial arguments, particularly those relating to the palliative care examples discussed earlier, that is 'to make recommendations on the circumstances in which a nurse might properly vary the timing and dosage of drugs prescribed by a doctor'. Finally, all of these deliberations needed to be set in the context of cost, with the review being asked to consider implications for nurse training and to consider resource implications in general (DoH, 1989, p. 3).

In spite of a 2-month delay causing some suspicion about a negative content and requiring an 'upbeat' intervention in the form of a press release from Virginia Bottomley, the Crown team were diligent in their work, and managed to produce a report containing 32 recommendations only slightly adrift of its intended publication date. The Crown Report (DoH, 1989) was warmly welcomed by the nursing profession in general, and most definitely by the Royal College of Nursing (RCN, 1990). Essentially, everthing the college had asked for was contained within the report. Crown recommended that nurses would be able to prescribe from their own formulary of items needed for the delivery of nursing care, that doctors and nurses should collaborate in the drawing up of 'group protocols' to facilitate the easy supply of medicines to groups of patients with similar needs (e.g. immunisations) and in a similar system of protocols specific to individual patients, permitting nurses to vary the time and dosage of medicines prescribed. To cap it all, the report even gave a quite reasonable start date for all of this to happen – 1 April 1992.

Which nurses to prescribe?

All was looking good, but the question of which nurses should prescribe came to taint the response to the Crown recommendations. So far as the ability to write a prescription – what Crown termed 'initial prescribing' – was concerned, the recommendation was that, 'for the present, authority for the initial prescribing from the Nurse's Formulary should be introduced for nurses with a district nurse or health visitor qualification only' (DoH, 1989, p. 25). The basic rationale given for this decision was that health visitors and district nurses could easily be identified on the register held by the United Kingdom Central Council for Nursing, Midwifery and Health Visiting (UKCC) as having completed further education since their initial registration. Crown also indicated that other specialist community nurses were not likely to need to prescribe, as they were, by and large, hospital based and able to obtain supplies more easily and were in close proximity to prescribing doctors. Furthermore, the UKCC had yet to complete its work on defining the nature of specialist practice, and as such a suitable marker of post basic education and competence was not available. However, the door was not closed to other nursing groups, as Crown indicated that: 'Once initial prescribing by district nurses and health visitors has been introduced and evaluated, we recommend that consideration should be given to extending initial prescribing to other groups of specialist nurses' (DoH, 1989, p. 27).

Practice nurses in particular began to voice to the RCN their concerns that they still did not get a 'look in'. As the practice nurse membership base of the college was increasing exponentially (Jones, 1996), and practice nursing proponents were beginning to demand that the they should be extended the same right to prescribe as health visitors and district nurses (see for example Fullard, 1990; Jeffrey, Fry and Wagner, 1990; Carlisle, 1990), it is not suprising that their voice began to be heard also. Discussion of the Crown recommendations by the governing Council led to a position statement that practice nurses were included within the group for whom the college would campaign for prescribing powers (RCN, 1990). The college even went so far as to get John Greenway, one of its 'parliamentary panel' of supportive MPs, to ask the Secretary of State in the Commons whether practice nurses would feature in the government's plans for nurse prescribing, with Virginia Bottomley replying positively that 'such an arrangement [introduction of nurse prescribing] would help not only practice nurses but health visitors and district nurses'.

NURSE PRESCRIBING – AT WHAT COST?

Moving back to the nurse prescribing mainstream, as was the case with much health care reform and report recommendations under the Thatcher administration, the Crown Report was not to be implemented without further consideration, and the main questions were around cost. As was required of it, the Crown review had made an attempt to consider the economic implications of its recommendations, but by its own admission, 'providing detailed estimates of the costs and benefits of nurse prescribing has proved somewhat problematic' and largely because 'there is no such service in this existence in this country, nor any comparable service overseas which we could use as models, our costings would have to be based on a variety of assumptions, none of which can at present be tested' (DoH, 1989, p. 58).

Clearly the government were not going to implement a proposal as radical as nurse prescribing without having considered cost–benefit data rather more robust and detailed than that provided by Crown; they commissioned the accountancy firm Touche Ross to undertake a more thorough analysis. Given that in order to meet the 1 April 1992 implementation date, Crown had set December 1991 as the deadline for bringing forward legislative change (Jones and Gough, 1997), the announcement of the Touche Ross cost–benefit analysis brought about suspicion as to the government's true commitment to the initiative. Encouraged by the RCN, Liberal Democrat MPs questioned Virginia Bottomley in the Commons as to whether the announcement of the analysis was in fact a delaying tactic, resulting in the reply 'I hope to disabuse the hon. gentleman of such suspicions. The cost benefit analysis is important and we hope to announce the details shortly' (Bottomley, 1991). However, the rest of the minister's response was a little more unsettling: while she reiterated government support, several points of potential delay were indicated:

> *We will certainly make all the information available [from the analysis]. However, there are other issues to be considered – such as deciding the precise formula, training, and the relationship between nurse and general practitioner prescribing. It is a complex matter, but has strong support and we shall carry forward that work.* (Bottomley, 1991)

Touche Ross eventually began its analysis, but although it adopted a more rigorous approach than the Crown team were either equipped for or asked to use, they essentially faced the same difficulties. That is, there were no direct comparisons for a nurse prescribing model to be introduced in the UK, and most of the costs could only be the subject of conjecture. Touche Ross did manage to estimate the cost of training the existing workforce of health visitors and district nurses at around £8 million, yet they also anticipated savings in nurses' and GPs' time of around £12.5 million a year (DoH and Touche Ross, 1991). This was not suprising, given the original assertion in the case for nurse prescribing that district nurses were wasting time tracking down and badgering GPs to endorse their prescribing decisions. The problem here is that the nurse and doctor cash savings were not real, given that the sums quoted were already subsumed within the NHS budget and were unlikely to be released as true savings should nurse prescribing be introduced. This was certainly the case for the millions of pounds Touche Ross estimated as potential savings to patient and carer groups should nurse prescribing be introduced – since the government does not pay patients and carers no real savings would be generated.

Not particularly bolstered by the Touche Ross data, yet still having gone on record as supporting the principle, the government dragged its feet in moving forward in any way, shape or form on the issue of nurse prescribing. Parliamentary time was certainly not set aside in order to translate the Crown recommendations into the reality of practice through the necessary legislative change, and the all-pervading power of the Treasury and its influence on key government decisions became evident. Virginia Bottomley may well have been seen to support nurse prescribing, but another agenda – the size of the NHS drugs bill – was beginning to cause concern. As Touche Ross was undertaking its analysis, the

Department of Health published a document entitled *Improving prescribing* (DoH, 1990), considering the implementation of an indicative prescribing scheme for GPs. The approach was to be a soft one, but the message was clear – spiralling drugs cost were to come under scrutiny and the government would not consider the budget to be open-ended. Practice nurses featured in this analysis, but unfortunately – due to their close relationship to and direct employment by GPs – the adverse reaction was that any extension of prescribing rights to them would blow a hole in the GP drugs budget (Jeffrey *et al.*, 1990).

This theme of cost–benefit will continue to underlie our analysis of the introduction, or otherwise, of nurse prescribing, but we move again to consider the reaction of the RCN to the lackadaisical government attitude toward the whole issue.

PARLIAMENTARY TACTICS

In Chapter 4, Sims and Gardiner give a detailed account of how the RCN used the parliamentary system in the effort to achieve legislative change to facilitate nurse prescribing. In summary, the College was not prepared to allow the government's reticence to introduce the necessary legislation to undermine the principle of nurse prescribing. Without amendments to a whole range of Acts of parliament, not least the regulations operational-ising the 1968 Medicines Act, nurses could never be recognised as prescribers. The RCN had one key weapon in their armoury – the existence of their 'parliamentary panel'. The RCN does not sponsor MPs and peers but has a 'parliamentary panel' comprising about 12 members of parliament from all parties who support the RCN in parliament, and who meet on a regular basis to discuss nursing issues. There were, until the 1997 general election, no nurses in the House of Commons, but other panel members were chosen for their interest in health, their ability to work on a cross-party basis, and their commitment to promote the interests of nurses and nursing. From late 1990 to early 1991 the RCN began a sustained lobbying activity of all MPs in the Commons, and in particular its own panel. In what could be considered to be both an ambitious and audacious move, the college was keen to capitalise on the 'private member's Bill' facility existing within the Commons. Through this facility, backbench MPs are able to introduce their own legislation, irrespective of the government's own priorities. MPs who want to put forward a Bill enter their names into a ballot held at the beginning of each session of parliament. Those who have their names picked out towards the top of the ballot have priority in the very limited amount of time allocated to backbenchers. The chance of success is generally small, and it is usually the case that only uncontroversial Bills with government support are adopted, and even then only the top six have a real chance of being a success. Nevertheless, given that the government was not exactly falling over itself in 1990 to facilitate nurse prescribing through the appropriate legislation, the RCN decided – against the odds – to press ahead with its own four-clause Bill simply entitled the Nurse Prescribing Bill. Those MPs entering the ballot, including parliamentary panel members, were written to suggesting they support the issue of nurse prescribing if they were successful. When the ballot results were out, the 20 MPs selected were written to again with a draft copy of the Bill, asking for their definite support. Unfortunately, the MPs selected high up the ballot order were already committed to other causes, but Dudley Fishburn MP, who was drawn at position nine, agreed to take the RCN Bill forward.

As had been predicted, Dudley Fishburn's Bill ran out of time in the Commons and came nowhere near reaching the statute books. However, the letter writing campaign increased awareness among MPs, and a subsequent opinion poll survey showed 69% supporting or strongly supporting nurse prescribing, with a further 28% in favour of the principle with some reservations (RCN, 1991). Although the Fishburn Bill technically failed, the public relations campaign surrounding it was a great success. The RCN continued to pressurise the government as a result, and enlisted the support of patient and carer groups to lobby William Waldegrave, the next Secretary of State to deal with the issue. Speaking at the 1991 RCN Congress in Harrogate, Waldegrave told delegates, 'we will do it [introduce legislation] unless the analysis turns up some unexpected serious problem' (Waldegrave, 1991).

Again the government fell back on the excuse of needing the Touche Ross cost–benefit analysis before moving forward. The report was ready in time for its contents to influence the parliamentary agenda as would be laid out in the Queen's Speech of November 1991. Even though the results of the analysis were not totally conclusive, there certainly was no evidence of the 'unexpected serious problem' of which William Waldegrave had been so wary. Nevertheless, nurse prescribing was indeed absent from the speech – a clear indication that the government had no intention of bringing forward the legislation required – and the Crown recommendation of April 1992 as a start date for nurse prescribing was rendered unachievable. Faced with this legislative block the RCN went back to the same strategy and attempted to use a private member's Bill to circumvent governmental intransigence. This time the outcome was far better. The Conservative MP for Chislehurst, Roger Sims, came third place in the private member's ballot and decided to introduce a Bill to support nurse prescribing. Perhaps aware of the futility in putting off the inevitable, or more probably the chance of getting the issue over with without being directly implicated, the government eventually let it be known they would support the Sims Bill. With tacit governmental assistance the Bill was drafted and put before the Commons (House of Commons, 1991).

In spite of Department of Health's reluctance to act, and a lack of overt support in the past, the Sims Bill received widespread government support in its passage through both lower and upper houses of parliament (Jones and Gough, 1997). Finally, 2 years after the publication of the Crown Report, the primary legislation permitting nurse prescribing, the Medicinal Products: Prescription by Nurses, etc. Act, was given royal assent in 1992. Although the Crown Report timetable was a year adrift, the nursing profession could rest assured that prescribing powers for nurses would at last be a reality – or would they?

But at what price?

The ogre of Treasury influence had never gone away, even if forgotten by the RCN, and not openly acknowledged by the Department of Health. Given that Virginia Bottomley had assured Dudley Fishburn across the benches of the House of Commons in May 1992 that nurse prescribing was well on course for a revised implementation date of October 1993 (Bottomley, 1992), it was thought that there was nothing to fear from her forthcoming speech concerning NHS priorities for 1993. Perhaps it should not have come as such a suprise as it did, given the concern over NHS spending levels, but in the same breath as Virginia Bottomley talked in November 1992 of a 2.5% increase in the number of patients to be treated in 1993 she also dashed the hopes of all supporters of nurse prescribing:

> *This increase in services is the result of the extra funds which have been announced today for the NHS next year and of the efficiency improvements which we expect the service to make . . . We have had to take a number of hard decisions in drawing up these spending plans. We have had to focus on priorities so that there is more to spend on essential services, and I am therefore announcing today that further steps will be taken to reduce the rate of growth in the NHS drugs bill. I have also decided reluctantly to postpone the introduction of nurse prescribing.* (DoH, 1992)

Less than 8 months after the legislation was passed permitting its introduction, nurse prescribing was on the rocks, a victim to NHS spending priorities, and although unproven, a victim of Treasury association with the increasing cost of the drugs bill.

The link between the initiative and NHS spending – in particular with the drugs budget – seemed too great to break. In March 1993 the Department of Health introduced the 'prescribing incentive scheme', intended to encourage GPs through a series of cost-shifting financial incentives to minimise their prescribing bills (DoH, 1993). The earlier soft approach envisaged in *Improving prescribing* (DoH, 1990) was clearly not working, and now the department was forced to speak to GPs in the following terms – reduce your drugs costs and financial benefits for your practice will accrue elsewhere. Nurse prescribing was almost like a small boat drifting on this sea of drug cost containment. Speaking at the Medpharm 1993 conference, Health Minister Brian Mawhinney followed through with this analogy as he put the whole issue in perspective when questioned by the author on the continual delays to nurse prescribing implementation:

> I would like to offer a personal opinion, if Ministers are allowed to have personal opinions that is. I would like to see nurse prescribing launched in a climate in which it could be properly assessed, a climate in which it would have a fair wind ... As I have said, the next twelve months are going to be tough for prescribing in general, and to launch nurse prescribing now would not do it justice. (Jones 1993)

In spite of this, the RCN was not minded to give up the fight. The nursing and health care press in general were full of positive comments about nurse prescribing, and indeed the 'lay press' also seemed to be very much in favour of the initiative. After more lobbying, a further concession was obtained from the government, one which has quite an interesting background for practice nurses.

THE PILOT PROJECT

Given the preoccupation with cost implications, the Department of Health devised a rather neat strategy of dealing with their being condemned for not implementing nurse prescribing, plus their own agenda of convincing the Treasury that the scheme would not break the prescribing budget. The idea was a nurse prescribing 'pilot scheme'. Speaking at the 1994 national conference of practice nurses, Julia Cumberlege announced the criteria for the selection of pilot sites. There would be eight selected from applications from GP fundholding practices (thought to be the most financially reliable and having computer systems able to track the nurse prescribing budget) where there was a joint commitment toward the project with community trusts (DoH, 1994).

The nurse prescribing demonstration pilots were selected to represent four fundholding practices in the north of England, and four in the south. Following selection of the sites, secondary legislation was put before parliament to come into effect on 3 October 1994 (Sowerby, 1994). This legislation actually made it legal for those nurses in the pilot sites with a district nursing or health visiting qualification, and having completed the approved prescribing training, to prescribe from a limited formulary, in addition to allowing pharmacists to dispense from a nurse prescription (House of Commons, 1994). The Nurse Formulary to be used was quite limited in content, essentially reflecting the draft prepared at the time the original legislation was passed (BMA, RPSoGB and RCN, 1992), and representing those items highlighted as being useful by district nurses way back at the beginning of the campaign for prescribing rights in the early 1980s. In fact, even though several years had passed since the primary legislation had entered the statute book, secondary legislation allowing the pilot project to operate was being written and translated into law as the whole thing was rolling out. Such was the confusion, the six prescription only medicines (POMs) scheduled for inclusion in the Nurse Formulary (bowel regulating, anti-fungal and wound care preparations) were not available to nurses at the beginning of the pilot as the law would have not permitted their prescription. Rather than see this as failing, the Department of Health 'spin doctors' managed to turn the late addition of the POMs into a 'further expansion' of the Nurse Formulary in early 1997 – some 3 months after the pilot scheme had been in operation (DoH, 1996).

Initial evaluation

The pilot sites generally evaluated well, reinforcing the case made by advocates of nurse prescribing – time saving for nurses, doctors and patients, and a high degree of patient satisfaction (Luker, 1997). Nurses were considered to have gained sufficient knowledge to prescribe items on the Nurse Formulary and were safe and competent in their practice. The real problem with the analysis of the pilots was the same as that previously faced by Crown and Touche Ross – the difficulty of obtaining an accurate economic evaluation. The pilot project was in reality too small to produce any realistic data and figures from the eight sites produced a variance of £83 000 net cost, to £159 000 net saving from the introduction of nurse prescribing. These figures included an initial 'set-up' cost ranging from £34 000 to £67 000 (Luker, 1997, pp. 17–18). With a 'range of uncertainty' in the order of £240 000, these figures were hardly likely to convince the Treasury that the introduction of nurse prescribing across the whole of the nation was a particularly good idea.

The Bolton site

Although the Department of Health was unlikely to admit that as a result of deciding to go with such a small initial pilot, the data obtained were of little use when considering nurse prescribing on a national scale, it did attempt to save face by widening the scope of the pilots – now increasingly being referred to as the 'demonstration sites' as a result of jibes concerning the continuous delays in nurse prescribing implementation. In an attempt to improve the data being gleaned from the initial pilot sites, Julia Cumberlege announced that the original pilot site in Bolton would be extended to include a further 60 practices within the boundary of the community trust, and nurse prescribing entered the second stage of piloting (DoH, 1996).

The Bolton 'second wave' site became a centre of attention, particularly for the nursing profession. Here it was likely that the case for nurse prescribing could be proven once and for all, especially as the director of operations for the community trust involved – Mary Cropper – was turning out to be extremely enthusiastic.

Community Healthcare Bolton rose to the challenge of taking the lead in the second wave of the demonstration project, and negotiated a rapid training programme with Manchester Metropolitan University. The university had already provided the ENB approved education course for nurses involved in the first wave pilots, but needed to steel themselves for the task of providing a similar course for Bolton's 100 plus potential nurse prescribers within a 10-week period. The negotiations went well, and the trust dispatched its staff – literally by the coachload – to Manchester. The four cohorts all completed the 3-day classroom based course and additional distance learning by 1 April 1996. In parallel, two seminars were arranged at a local hotel for the 80 GPs and pharmacists who would be involved in the project.

Over the year in which the Bolton second wave pilot was evaluated, the original core beliefs about the benefits of introducing nurse prescribing were proven once again. Nurse prescribing saved time, improved the care of patients, and perhaps most encouraging, actually saved the trust some money. Additionally, nurse morale was raised, and all primary health care teams and pharmacists involved reported enhanced working relationships (Community Healthcare Bolton NHS Trust and Wigan and Bolton Health Authority, 1997; Cropper, 1998).

Even though data from the second wave of pilots (the original sites plus an expanded Bolton) were yet to be fully analysed, the government further expanded the sites to have one operational in each English NHS region and subsequently two sites in Scotland. By summer 1998, no further analysis had been made available from any of the demonstration sites.

PRESCRIBING ALTERNATIVES

The pilot/demonstration project had been going on for so long that many people – certainly at the RCN – were not convinced they would ever see the day when nurse prescribing became a reality. This resignation also permeated the ranks of 'grass roots' nurses, but not all of them sat back and waited for the evaluation and introduction of initial prescribing rights for nurses. Nurses working in general practice prescribing limited had for many years adopted a system whereby they could supply and/or administer POMs to patients without a prescription being written by the GP for each individual. This system picked up on the recommendation of the 1989 Crown review that doctors and nurses should collaborate in drawing up local protocols whereby agreement could be reached that nurses could select a drug – POM or otherwise – from a pre-agreed list to use in immediate patient care.

The so-called 'group protocol' system allowed nurses to select and administer drugs to patients based upon their own assessment, without the need to obtain a prescription from a GP – thus cutting out the time-wasting element highlighted in the initial nurse prescribing case by their district nurse colleagues in 1978. Practice nurses found the group protocol arrangements to be invaluable, particularly for the administration of vaccines, and became major users of the system (Jeffrey et al., 1990). In fact the use of group protocols has probably been in existence for well over a decade, and was certainly mentioned as a possible way forward by the RCN in its early nurse prescribing negotiations with the BMA (RCN and BMA, 1988). GPs happily collaborated with nurses in the drawing up of protocols, and in fact endorsed their decisions as to what POMs should be prescribed as something of a paper exercise (RCN, 1995). The Treasury and some interest groups within the Department of Health, medicine and pharmacy were absorbed in limiting the right of nurses to prescribe, while in many instances nurses had an almost free rein in selecting POMs for their patients with minimal sanction from their doctor colleagues.

The protocol challenge

It was not just practice nurses and their patients who benefited from the use of group protocols; any nurses who believed they had sufficient expertise to make an informed and accurate decision as to the products required for their patients, and who did not feel the need for individual prescriptions to be made available for a medical practitioner developed similar systems. For example, Dicks reports how nurses in the Royal Marsden Hospital are able to supply and administer POMs from a list pre-agreed with medical colleagues in a group protocol arrangement extending across the whole hospital. The nurses involved are even referred to as 'prescribing nurses' (Dicks, 1998).

It was, however, another group of nurses who brought the use of group protocols into sharp focus. In 1996 the family planning forum of the RCN asked that body to obtain a definitive legal opinion as to the use of group protocols for the issuing of repeat supplies of the oral contraceptive pill, and the administration of the 'morning-after' pill. Even though group protocols had been accepted practice for many years, nobody had really questioned their legality. In Chapter 5, Caulfield discusses the legal dimension to group protocol use; it suffices to say here that the legal opinion sought by the RCN was not able categorically to support the use of group protocols in lieu of an individual prescription where POM items were concerned. The RCN made the Department of Health and the UKCC aware of their findings, and each of these organisations in turn received legal opinion supporting that of the college's counsel.

Given that the whole of the national immunisation programme rested on the use of group protocols, and the mass MMR immunisation campaign of 1995 would not have been possible without their use, this situation caused widespread concern. The health service union UNISON even went so far as to issue disclaimer forms to its practice nurse members, with the request that their GP employers should sign to say they accepted all responsibility should the nurse be taken to court over the use of group protocols in their practice. For its part, the RCN negotiated with the UKCC to arrive at a position where the latter went on record to say that the use of group protocols was an example of good nursing care, and that nurses using the system would not be considered to be professionally negligent on that fact alone. Yet, when pushed, and faced with their own legal opinion, the Department of Health was unwilling to confirm in writing that it supported group protocol use.

Eventually the Department of Health did see sense, especially as the RCN intimated it would have to advise all its members – practice nurses in particular – to stop using protocols. The department's solution was to ask Dr June Crown to undertake a second review of prescribing issues, this time considering both the protocol issue and the extension of prescribing rights to professional groups who do not have them already.

THE SECOND CROWN REPORT

Not suprisingly, given the chequered history of the nurse prescribing debacle, the Crown II Report did not make its publication target of October 1998. To give them their due, the review team were inundated with over 700 separate submissions of evidence, but the furore over protocols was not abating. As result, the pragmatic decision was taken to concentrate on the protocol issue, and consider the extension of prescribing rights at a later stage.

Group protocols

So far as protocols are concerned, the Crown II review produced its initial report, dealing with them specifically, in April 1998: this was entitled *Review of Prescribing, Supply and Administration of Medicines. A report on the supply and administration of medicines under group protocols* (DoH, 1998). At last an accepted position as to the use of group protocols was agreed, as laid out in the report (DoH, 1998).

The report agreed that the use of protocols represents good practice and should continue; however, it acknowledges that the law underpinning their use is unclear and should be revised. Furthermore, there is recognition that the standard of existing protocols is variable, with some being little more than a couple of lines on a sheet of paper. The report addresses this issue by setting out guidance in three key areas:

- The content of a group protocol
- The development of group protocols
- The implementation of group protocols.

Content

Content should firstly address the clinical condition to which the protocol applies, defining the situation and criteria for its use and which patients can, or cannot be treated under it. Secondly, the staff authorised to supply or administer medicines under the protocol should be detailed, including qualifications required and acceptance of competence to use the drugs concerned, and the need to update training and education as required. Next, treatment available under the protocol should be specified – the details of drugs involved including dose and method of administration. Finally, the need to 'manage' and monitor protocols is specified, with content including the names of the professionals drawing up the protocol, the 'professional advisory groups' which have approved the protocol (including the local drugs and therapeutics committee). The protocol should also be dated and provided with a review date after which it is no longer valid.

Development

The report recommended that the development of protocols should be facilitated by an inter-disciplinary group including a doctor, a pharmacist and a named representative of each of the professionals likely to contribute to care under the protocol. All group protocols should be approved by the relevant local professional committees, and approved by local clinical managers, with the employer giving final approval.

Implementation

Implementation of the protocol is said to require approval of the professional managers of those using it, with all participants in care under the protocol signing a copy, and with a copy being available in the clinical setting in which it is being used.

Clearly these provisos were far more directive than anything currently in place so far as protocol development and use is concerned and would take some time to achieve, particularly as it was unclear what certain aspects meant – who were the 'relevant professional advisory committees' for example? Furthermore, how many protocols had actually been drawn up with real doctor–nurse input, let alone that of a pharmacist and all the sanctions proposed in the report? The health service circular of 21 April relating to the report insisted that its recipients – health authorities, NHS trusts, regional advisers in general practice, and chief pharmacists in NHS trusts – act to ensure all group protocols comply with the above criteria and that all current protocols be reviewed immediately in the light of these criteria (NHSE, 1998).

THE CASE REVISITED?

In addition to presenting evidence to Crown concerning the use of group protocols, the RCN took the opportunity to re-state and update its case for the extension of prescribing rights to nurses. The same 20-year-old points held true – nurse prescribing would save time and money and improve patient care – but this time round the college decided to really push the issues of the nature of the Nurse Formulary and the restricted number of nurses who would be permitted to prescribe.

The RCN's basic premise

In its evidence, the RCN set out a 'basic premise' to its submission, as follows:

> The RCN is concerned that current legislation governing prescribing powers for nurses is piecemeal and unhelpful in enabling nurses to meet the health care needs of the patients across the board of care settings. Similarly, the constraints of the Nurse Formulary have hindered nurses' efforts to provide a holistic, coherent package of care to patients, which, if this constraint were removed, they would be able to do both competently and effectively.
>
> In this submission therefore the RCN sets out a rational and coherent framework for the future which enshrines three simple principles:
> - The identification of a marker of competence to which prescribing powers may be attached. This marker must reflect a knowledge base and level of practice which is appropriate to the high level skill which prescribing represents;
> - The dismantling of a separate formulary for nurses which could never keep pace with the range of medications which nurses would need to require to respond to patient need in each area of specialist practice; and
> - The use of the infrastructure governing maintenance of registration with the UKCC to make prescribing knowledge and skills the focus for updating linked to renewal of registration every three years. (RCN, 1997)

The RCN's argument was essentially that the Nurse Formulary is outdated, reflecting nursing practice of 15 years ago, with many of the items contained within it no longer in current use. Secondly, the restriction of prescribing rights to those nurses with a district nursing or health visiting qualification is seen to be similarly anachronistic, given that the UKCC and the nursing profession as a whole had embraced the concept of 'specialist practice'. The RCN was also at pains to point out that the paranoia around the likelihood of nurse prescribers making mistakes was unfounded, with UKCC data in particular showing the numbers of cases reaching professional conduct hearings in connection with drug errors to be negligible (South, 1998).

Rather than create some complex quasi-legal regulatory structure, with only certain nurses being able to prescribe, the RCN's evidence suggested that any specialist nurse – that is someone who had moved forward academically and experientially since their initial training and who had completed a prescribing course – should be able to prescribe from the British National Formulary within the boundaries of their individual competence. The College was suggesting that specialist nurses will not prescribe outwith their field of expertise, but within it will make effective and safe prescribing decisions. This particular vision of the future of nurse prescribing is considered further in the final chapter of this book.

WHY NOT GO WITH WHAT WORKS?

As the Crown II review engaged in its deliberations, the evidence from the demonstration project was seen by many to offer irrefutable proof that the model of nurse prescribing in that project worked and met all the criteria for safety and cost-effectiveness laid down by government. As Karen Luker (author of a major part of the Department of Health commissioned evaluation) put it: 'If we believe at all in evidence based health care the government should roll out nurse prescribing' (Luker, 1998). This comment from Luker came after her analysis of data from the eight original pilot sites, 157 patient diaries pre-prescribing, 148 post, and 58 nurse question-naires, plus focus groups and interviews, and a further 56 interviews with key informants. To say that the evidence for the roll out of the health visitor/district nurse and limited formulary model was mounting would be something of an understatement.

The conference at which Karen Luker made the above comments – that of the Association of Nurse Prescribing (ANP) held in Manchester on 8 March 1998 – proved to be something of a turning point in the roll out debate. In her opening address as chair, Julia Cumberlege insisted, 'we must ensure that nurse prescribing is not for trading' and gave her view of the real problem:

> *It is annoying that every conceivable argument has been put up [against nurse prescribing] – in reality these are just a smokescreen to cover the real question of cost ... nurse prescribing does not grab the headlines – it is a quiet revolution, but it is a revolution ... I am not going to give up until a nurse with a prescription pad is the norm.* (Cumberlege, 1998a)

It was perhaps fortuitous that representatives of the Community Practi-tioners and Health Visitors Association (CPHVA) and RCN were scheduled to speak at the conference, as Baroness Cumberlege issued the challenge that if something was not done nurse prescribing was likely to 'wither on the vine'. Whether they had previously been committed to working together before that point or not, these representatives had little option but to agree to unite forces with the ANP, and a meeting of all three organisations (ANP, CPHVA, RCN), to be chaired by Baroness Cumberledge, was scheduled for the following week.

The meeting came up with two new demands of the government. First that all health visitors and district nurses should be able to prescribe from the Nurse Formulary by the year 2000. This was based on the sole premise that this form of nurse prescribing had been proven beyond doubt. All the organisations concerned had a much wider vision than this, but there was no reason why this limited form of prescribing should not come into being with almost immediate effect. The 2000 timescale would permit the education and training of the almost 20 000 eligible practitioners. The second new demand was that all specialist nurses should be able to prescribe from 2005. The basis for this was the RCN argument that specialist nurses who had completed prescribing training would be able to prescribe safely and competently within their field of practice. Again, a 2005 timescale would permit identification of a level of 'specialist practice' in all nursing groups and would allow the necessary training to take place. These demands were notified to the Department of Health and considered widely by the nursing press.

A GLIMPSE OF THE FUTURE

The group were only too well aware that the secretary of state for health, Frank Dobson, was scheduled to make a speech at the opening of the RCN Congress just a few weeks after their new demands had been made. The RCN parliamentary team worked hard to ensure these messages were constantly in the minds of those advisers at the Department of Health who were working to compile Dobson's speech. Just one week before Congress was scheduled, advisers to Baroness Jay, minister of health, contacted the author for more detail behind the demand for a roll out of the current nurse prescribing model, in particular what the cost would be if the government were to agree. Some hasty calculations offered the rough estimate of £14 million to cover the training costs of around 20 000 health visitors and district nurses, including 'cover' should it be required whilst they take their courses. The minister's office merely thanked the RCN for their assistance, and even the night before Dobson's speech had given no hint as to what would be said concerning nurse prescribing. On Monday 20 April, however, the secretary of state announced to RCN Congress that £14 million would be provided to roll out the current model of nurse prescribing, with a further commitment to examining the possibility of expanding the concept to other specialist nurses and widening the Nurse Formulary once the deliberations of the Crown II review were known.

As Dobson concluded his speech, Baroness Cumberlege had her moment in the Lords as she asked Baroness Jay what the government's policy was on the roll out of nurse prescribing. Jay confirmed what Dobson had said to Congress, stating that the government was committed to a 'national programme of nurse prescribing'. As perhaps the arch supporter of nurse prescribing since her 1986 review reported, Baroness Cumberlege was overjoyed as her speech continued: 'My Lords, is the noble Baroness aware that I am going to go out right now and crack open a bottle of champagne? I am absolutely thrilled to bits. For 12 years, with the nursing organisations, I have fought for this to happen and it is a great day for me.' The first part of the new demands had been met by the government, but Cumberlege went on to question her colleague about extension beyond health visitors and district nurses. Perhaps predictably, Baroness Jay replied that the government needed to await the outcome of the Crown review (Cumberlege, 1998b). A well briefed Earl Howe asked particularly about expanding the Nurse Formulary to the wider British National Formulary (BNF) and again Baroness Jay replied that Crown was looking at this and the issue would be a longer term objective.

So, the target of rolling out the existing model of nurse prescribing had all but been met – once again due to a coordinated lobbying action spurred on by Lady Cumberlege. It was clear though that the outcome of the deliberations of the Crown II review would bring the real answers to the future of nurse prescribing. During the summer of 1998, the nursing profession waited patiently for the outcome of that review, a mere 20 years after the quest for nurse prescribing rights had begun. The future of nurse prescribing was still undecided, and the review team's work seemed more watertight than any previous health care review – no leaks, no speculation. So secretive was the work of the review group that completing this book was a nightmare of deadlines to be pushed back yet again, as each time the final Crown Report was delayed. To find out what the final episode in the history of nurse prescribing might look like, you will have to begin with a look at the future in Chapter 15.

QUESTIONS FOR DISCUSSION

- Which groups were instrumental in bringing forward the nurse prescribing debate and what was their motivation?
- What rationale was offered for the extension of prescribing rights to nurses?
- Is the quest for nurse prescribing really justified in terms of benefit to patients, or are the RCN and others just concerned about enhancing the status of nursing?

• What alternative strategies could have been adopted to facilitate the introduction of nurse prescribing?

REFERENCES

Bottomley, V. (1991) Nurse prescribing. Oral answer to Rt Hon. Archie Kirkwood MP. *Hansard*. 5 Feb.

Bottomley, V. (1992) Nurse prescribing. Oral answer to Rt Hon. Dudley Fishburn MP. *Hansard*. 3 May.

British Medical Association, Royal Pharmaceutical Society of Great Britain & Royal College of Nursing (1992) *Draft Nurse Prescribers' Formulary*. London: British Medical Association, Royal Pharmaceutical Society of Great Britain.

Carlisle (1990) Who prescribes? *Nursing Standard*, **86(9)**, 16–17.

Community Healthcare Bolton NHS Trust & Wigan and Bolton Health Authority (1997) *Evaluation of Nurse Prescribing in Bolton, 1996–1997. A pilot conducted by Community Healthcare Bolton NHS Trust and Wigan and Bolton Health Authority, funded by the Department of Health*. Bolton: Community Healthcare Bolton NHS Trust & Wigan and Bolton Health Authority.

Cropper, M. (1998) *The Progress of the Nurse Prescribing Scheme*. Paper presented to the Association of Nurse Prescribing Conference, Manchester, 18 March.

Cumberlege, J. (1998a) *Chair's Opening Remarks*. Association of Nurse Prescribers Conference, Manchester, 18 March.

Cumberlege, J. (1998b) *Nurse Prescribing. Parliamentary answer and debate*. House of Lords 20.

Department of Health and Social Security (1986) *Neighbourhood Nursing – a Focus for Care*. (Cumberlege Report.) London: HMSO.

Department of Health (1989) *Report of the Advisory Group on Nurse Prescribing*. (Crown Report.) London: HMSO.

Department of Health (1990) *Improving Prescribing*. London: Department of Health.

Department of Health (1992) *NHS to Treat Record Numbers of Patients as Spending Rises to Highest Levels Ever*. From fax transmission of press release sent by Parliamentary News Service on 13 November.

Department of Health (1993) *Prescribing Incentive Scheme 'Will benefit patients' says Dr. Brian Mawhinney*. Press Release H93/620, 11 March. London: Department of Health.

Department of Health (1994) *Nurse Prescribing – One Step Nearer*. Press Release 94/147, 24 March. London: Department of Health.

Department of Health (1996) *Lady Cumberlege Announces Extension to Nurse Prescribing*. Press Release 96/13. London: Department of Health.

Department of Health (1998) *Review of Prescribing, Supply and Administration of Medicines. A report on the supply and administration of medicines under group protocols*. London: Department of Health.

Department of Health & Touche Ross (1991) *Nurse Prescribing – Final Report: a cost benefit study*. London: Department of Health and Touche Ross.

Dicks, B. (1998) *How has Protocolised Nurse Prescribing in Hospital Changed the NHS?* Abstract and paper presented to Association of Nurse Prescribing Conference, Manchester, 18 March. London: EMAP Healthcare.

Fullard, E. (1990) Report of the Advisory Group on Nurse Prescribing. Unpublished memorandum to Terry Brown, Associate General Manager Kensington, Chelsea and Westminster FPC, 16 March. Copied to Mark Jones, Community Health Adviser, Royal College of Nursing. Unpublished memorandum. Copy held in RCN archives.

House of Commons (1991) *A Bill to Amend the Medicines Act 1968, the National Health Services Act 1977 and the National Health Service (Scotland) Act 1978 in Respect of Pharmaceutical Services, to Make Provision for Registered Nurses to Prescribe Medicinal Products in Certain Circumstances, and for Connected Purposes*. London: HMSO.

House of Commons (1994) *Medicinal Products: Prescription by Nurses, etc Act 1992*. (Commencement No. 1) Order 1994. Statutory Instrument 2408 (C.48). London: HMSO.

House of Commons Social Services Committee (1987) *Primary Health Care. First report of the committee, 1986–87*. HC 37. London: HMSO.

Jeffrey, P., Fry, J. & Wagner, V. (1990) Prescribing and the practice nurse. *Practice Nurse*, **March**, 443–446

Jones, M. (1993) *Brian Mawhinney and Nurse Prescribing*. Unpublished memo to Derek Dean, Director of Nursing Policy and Practice, RCN, describing comments made by the health minister at Medpharm 1993. Copy in RCN archives.

Jones, M. (1996) *Accountability in Practice. Guidance on professional responsibility for nurses in general practice*. Dinton: Quay Books.

Jones, M. & Gough, P. (1997) Nurse prescribing – why has it taken so long? *Nursing Standard*, **11(20)**, 39–42.

Luker, K. (1997) *Evaluation of Nurse Prescribing. Final report*. Liverpool: University of Liverpool and University of York.

Luker, K. (1998) Paper presented to the Association of Nurse Prescribing Conference, Manchester, 18 March.

National Health Service Executive (1998) *Report on the Supply and Administration of Medicines Under Group Protocols*. Health Service Circular HSC 1998/051. 21 April 1998. Leeds: NHSE.

Royal College of Nursing (1978) District nurses' dressings. Unpublished report to RCN Council from the Community Nursing Association of the RCN. Copy in RCN archives.

Royal College of Nursing (1990) Comments on the advisory group on nurse prescribing. Unpublished report to RCN Council, RCN/90/38. Copy in RCN archives.

Royal College of Nursing (1991) *RCN Poll Shows MPs Back Nurse Prescribing*. Press and Public Relations Department Diary Note Series, No. 3891, 11 April. London: RCN.

Royal College of Nursing (1995) *Whose Prescription?* London: RCN.

Royal College of Nursing (1997) Review of prescribing, supply and administration of medicines. Update on the evidence submitted by the Royal College of Nursing. Unpublished evidence to Crown II review.

Royal College of Nursing & British Medical Association (1988) Meeting on nurse prescribing – a discussion paper. Unpublished discussion paper, RCN-BMA2 CNAEXECMEET, May 1988. Copy in RCN archives.

South, L. (1998) Statistics. Letter to Jo Dilloway, Royal College of Nursing, from Lesley South, Department Manager, Professional Conduct, UKCC, in response to request for information on drug related charges before the Professional Conduct Committee. Unpublished. Copy in RCN records.

Sowerby, M. (1994) Nurse prescribing. Unpublished letter from Mike Sowerby, Project Manager, Nurse Prescribing NHS Executive, to Mark Jones, Community Health Adviser, Royal College of Nursing. 21 September.

Waldegrave, W. (1991) Speech addressing RCN Congress, Harrogate.

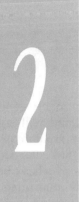

Nurse prescribing

The medical opinion

Peter Fellows

Key issues

♦ Nursing roles in the primary care team and the place of nurse prescribing.

♦ The increasing importance of the nursing role in primary care.

♦ Nurse prescribing as a logical development of the expanded role of nurses.

♦ Why doctors will or will not support nurse prescribing.

INTRODUCTION

The traditional roles of general practitioner, nurse and pharmacist are rapidly changing and will have to adapt to meet increasing demands for health care, coupled with increasing pressures on available resources. Most professionals feel threatened by the pace of change, by increasing public information on health matters, by more stringent needs for accreditation/reaccreditation, and by increasing risks of criticism and litigation. Politicians demand more and more from professionals who are already working way beyond tolerable, and therefore safe, capacity. Public sector pay levels have been held back. As a result, job satisfaction is suffering, and there are growing recruitment crises in all three professions. Medicine tends to be a conservative profession. New ideas are often viewed with caution, and changes to established practice are therefore often slow to evolve. That is no bad thing. In medicine the latest fashion often fails to live up to expectation.

ISSUES IN NURSE PRESCRIBING

Managing expenditure

It is not surprising that in such a time of uncertainty, many general practitioners will defend their traditional responsibilities, and will argue that nurses should not be allowed to prescribe. The 'internal market' developed by the Conservative government from 1990 has sharpened awareness of costs both for managers and for many doctors who have been involved in the purchasing process. There can be considerable financial benefits for practices who manage prescribing expenditure efficiently. There is concern from some doctors and from many senior health service managers that nurses do not as yet have the same awareness of the cost of things, and are likely to be susceptible to pressure sales techniques from pharmaceutical representatives. There is a perception that nurses tend to want to use the latest and most expensive dressings. Representatives often now ask to see primary care nurses, reflecting the increasing role nurses play in primary care, and their increasing economic importance to manufacturers of health products.

Pilot studies of nurse prescribing have now demonstrated cost-effectiveness (Coopers and Lybrand, 1996). In spite of this, in informal meetings which are held on a regular basis between the medical profession and Department of Health to discuss wide-ranging prescribing issues, I have heard senior health civil servants and doctors express concerns that when the close observation of such prescribing is relaxed, then prescribing costs will rise. That is probably true. Current political pressures on the civil servants of the Health Department to contain public expenditure are enormous, and this seems to be their overriding concern (Secretaries of State for Health, 1989; Panton 1993). Fears of cost escalation are no doubt behind the then government's decision in its White Paper *Delivering the Future* (DoH, 1996) to extend pilot studies and defer general introduction of community nurse prescribing for a further year. There has as yet been no move to extend the proposed nurse prescribing to include accredited practice nurses. The BMA has asked that practice nurses should be included in the group accredited to prescribe, and has welcomed the continued commitment to nurse prescribing.

Drug budgets

General practitioners could be threatened by the development of nurse practitioners as the government seeks novel ways to cope with the under-funding and doctor shortages in primary care. Some fear that such moves could threaten general practitioners' chances of ever regaining satisfactory pay levels. If nurse prescribing is widely introduced, there is concern that practice drug budgets, which many doctors have worked hard to contain, may be threatened and could escape control. In theory these budgets are merely 'indicative' targets, but the BMA has constantly been resisting moves towards fixed budgets, and there is firm pressure on each health authority to live within its allocated budget at that level (Secretaries of State for Health, 1989). There is a central reserve fund, but so far it has never been called upon. The BMA's argument that a fixed drug budget is not consistent with open access to primary care services by patients has prevailed. Trusts, however, do have fixed budgets. This has led to inappropriate 'dumping' of prescribing costs onto primary care. Community nurse prescribing might increase scope for such cost shifting. There is a very grey area here as in order to protect general practitioners from the incessant shift of work from secondary to primary care without any shift of resources (Crump *et al.*, 1995), the General Medical Services Committee (GPs' committee) of the BMA has now defined the 'core services' which GPs can be expected to provide under their contracts (BMA, 1996). This policy is an attempt to draw a line in the sand. Many of the tasks which a community nurse is involved with are 'non-core' tasks for which those GPs who are prepared to undertake the work will in future expect separate contracts and payment. Postoperative care is one example: wound care in the community following early discharge from hospital after surgery will be a non-core task for the GP. If a community nurse prescribes dressings for such a patient, who will then accept budgetary responsibility?

The budget has often seemed to be the main concern of trust managers. 'Clinical advisers' are sometimes appointed with more of a cost remit than an interest in the quality of care. For example, many trusts now employ continence advisers. Potentially they have a very useful clinical role, particularly supporting other community nursing staff. However, some managers seem to view their principal function as that of policing the district nurses' ability to issue incontinence pads. Rumour has it that some patients were lagging their lofts with them before management started employing advisers!

CLINICAL RESPONSIBILITY AND PROFESSIONAL INDEMNITY

There is a risk that as nurse prescribing becomes generalised, some GPs who are under pressure may expect nurses, who are not completely happy to accept the clinical responsibility, to prescribe. Consultants have not been averse to applying similar pressure on the GP (Harris, 1996; Crump *et al.*, 1995). There must be an explicit understanding that nurses, and indeed doctors, should never be expected to take responsibility for prescribing unless they feel happy and competent to accept the clinical responsibility involved.

Much prejudice must be overcome before generalised nurse prescribing is accepted. The professions need to work closely together so that change can be introduced without threat to any particular group. Managers need to understand that they are not in charge of the health service: they have a complementary role, through administration and organisation, in facilitating the work of the clinical professionals, but it is the professional who determines what, if anything, is wrong with the individual patient, what could be done about it, what must be done about it, and when it should be done, given resources and priorities. Managers must be reminded of the need to have respect for professional time as the most important economic resource within the NHS. Inevitably a change of attitude will take time, as professional and management demarcation is deeply entrenched, and the 'partnership principle', on the basis of which the professions agreed to form the NHS, was rejected by the last Conservative government. Since 1990, managers have been encouraged in the ethos of the 'industrial management pyramid', which most doctors believe is inappropriate for a service industry driven from the 'shop floor'. Many doctors are, as a consequence, very wary of managers' motives, and such suspicion contributes to their sense of caution about nurses' aspirations to prescribe.

In common with most doctors, as a young houseman I learnt much of my practical prescribing from experienced staff nurses and sisters on the hospital wards. I knew the theory, but their approach was founded on experience and common sense. They were not always right but their advice was often helpful. It was a nurse who taught me never to give any injection without checking it personally, even if it was the matron herself who handed me the ready-loaded syringe. That has been such an important lesson.

Prescribing required a similar discipline. The wise houseman always listened to the experienced nurse, digested the information, learnt from it, but then made up his own mind and double checked anything he was not sure of. Such is the responsibility of the prescriber (Harris, 1996). It is the signature on the prescription which matters in law: it implies an understanding of the act of prescribing, of the desired effect of what is being prescribed, and of likely unwanted effects and adverse reactions. Prescribers should be able to justify their actions not only to professional peers, but also to patients, who have a right to expect high quality care and appropriate prescription.

Nowadays patients are often remarkably well informed, particularly if something goes wrong. Patient leaflets which are being developed under European Union leaflet and labelling regulations (EEC, 1992) are often written more with the medico-legal protection of the pharmaceutical company in mind than with the real interests of the patient or prescriber at heart. Soon all medicines will have to be dispensed with these detailed leaflets, which often list rare side-effects and interactions that may stretch the knowledge of the doctor, let alone the nurse, if queried by a patient.

The medico-legal implications of nurse prescribing must not be over-looked or underestimated; GPs cannot be expected to continue to carry the responsibility once nurses have the right to prescribe in their own right. The issues of professional indemnity must be clarified.

CHALLENGING TRADITIONAL CONCEPTS

A short time ago there was a great media hullabaloo when a theatre sister at Treliske Hospital, Cornwall, was allowed to carry out an appendectomy with the surgeon assisting her. All of us who have worked in general surgery will appreciate that many experienced theatre sisters are likely to be far more competent to carry out such a procedure than the average surgical houseman. It is just such a problem of challenging traditional concepts of professional role which must be overcome in considering nurse prescribing (DoH, 1989).

According to the traditional role model, patients expect the doctor to prescribe. General practice registrars are taught that they should educate patients that doctors do not necessarily always need to prescribe. In the days before the NHS, pharmacists prescribed medicines, and were regarded by many as 'the poor man's doctor', although they were not permitted to charge fees for this aspect of their work. In fact they still do 'prescribe' many basic medicines which the patient must then pay for, but they cannot prescribe at NHS expense. In a throwback to a bygone era, the Society of Apothecaries of London still runs a qualifying examination for medical practitioners. Nurses are not generally perceived as professionals who prescribe, and yet their traditional role clearly involves the use of medications, enemas and dressings which the public would not expect the nurse to have to obtain via a doctor.

DEREGULATION AND MARKETING OF DRUGS

There is an increasing trend for drugs to be deregulated. Many drugs which were until recently prescription only medicines (POMs) are now available from the pharmacy without a doctor's prescription (RPSoGB, 1996). Others have been moved to the general sales list (GSL), and do not even require the sanction of the pharmacist.

Political, and also commercial, enthusiasm to encourage self-medication, with consequent cost savings for the NHS and increased profits for the drug companies, must be carefully moderated. Price deregulation could even threaten the public with loss-leaders on the latest headache brands from the local supermarket. Both the British Medical Association, and the Royal Pharmaceutical Society of Great Britain (RPSoGB), have stressed that medicines should be regarded as special products, not in the same category as soap powders. Patients should not be encouraged by sales techniques to buy medicines they do not need, or in larger quantities than they need. It is preferable that appropriate professional advice is available to patients when they obtain medicines which are potentially harmful. The key issue about advice from accredited health professionals – be they pharmacist, dentist, nurse or doctor – is that they will have been trained to know the limitations of their own knowledge, and will know when to refer patients for more specialist advice. Reliance on leaflets and media advertising is a poor substitute.

Drug labelling and dispensing

In the UK, as a consequence of European Union law, it has been agreed between the medical and pharmacy professions, government and the pharmaceutical industry that by the end of 1999 all licenced medicines will be produced in appropriate packs which will carry the required labelling and enclose the required detailed manufacturer's leaflet (Association of the British Pharmaceutical Industry, forthcoming). Patient packs, as they are called, which individually seal tablets, and contain either a complete course of treatment or 28 days' supply, will therefore soon become the norm for dispensing. They are to be phased in from the autumn of 1997. Pharmacists feel threatened because their traditional role in dispensing medicines is changing (RPSoGB, 1996).

The role of the computer in prescribing

Increasingly, prescribing is computer assisted, and this will probably also be true for most nurse prescriptions. The fact that the computer flags up potential interactions and other warnings diminishes arguments for having a second check on the prescription by the pharmacist at the dispensing stage. However, reliance on computer warnings could present problems for nurses because a fairly high degree of medical and pharmacological knowledge is required in order to decide whether to ignore a warning, which may well in reality be theoretical or of minor relevance. Most computer systems will attempt to grade warnings in significance (e.g. one, two or three stars). Nevertheless, nurses may have medico-legal difficulties if any such warning is overridden. Computer prescribing software might need to be developed specifically to cater for nurse prescribing. The Department of Health is developing a computer prescribing support system (known as Prodigy) which gives more background and clinical information relevant to the prescription, and which doctors have found useful in pilot studies (University of Newcastle, 1996). It is feasible that a version of Prodigy could be produced as a specific support for the Nurse Prescribers' Formulary.

GROUP PROTOCOLS

At the time of writing the government had just set up a working group chaired by Dr June Crown – *a Review of Prescribing, Supply and Administration of Medicines* – with wide ranging responsibilities, and which will undoubtedly lead to changes in prescribing legislation. One problem which this review group has been asked to resolve as a priority is the issue of group protocols for nurse prescribing. Existing law is at least 30 years out of date. It is difficult to see, for example, how general practice could now function without practice and community nurses being able to administer influenza immunisation, childhood immunisations and tetanus vaccine under an agreed 'group protocol'. If the doctor had to sanction and prescribe for each individual procedure, then the system just could not cope with the volume of work.

THE ROLE OF THE NURSE

In the midst of all this change in the way medicines are handled and distributed, it is surely appropriate to review the role which the nurse will carry forward into the next millennium.

Dressings

Many items which nurses use and have particular knowledge about are not drugs but appliances and dressings which are prescribable at NHS expense. Doctors rarely apply dressings, and their attempts to do so usually reveal only too obviously their lack of practical skill in this area. They understand the basic principles and the basic types of dressings, but most doctors' knowledge is fairly rudimentary. They usually have difficulty even remembering which size of Tubigrip is appropriate for which bit of the anatomy. Any doctor wanting to know more about a particular dressing will not ask another doctor, whose knowledge is unlikely to be any greater, but will ask a practice or community nurse. It is not surprising that nurses are so knowledgeable, since much of their working day is spent applying dressings of one sort or another. Many postgraduate nursing education lectures involve updates on dressings, and new dressings now can be quite complex in their functions. The pharmaceutical representatives who have the latest dressings to demonstrate do not want to see the doctor, they want to discuss their wares with the practice nurses, or the district nurse. Representatives undoubtedly do influence prescribing, or the pharmaceutical companies would not employ them. It is therefore hardly surprising that some doctors perceive nurses as always wanting to try the latest and more expensive dressings. Training of nurses will in future have to emphasise the need for critical appraisal of claims made for new products. Critical appraisal of scientific papers relating to drug treatments is now very much a part of medical training, and is vital for good prescribing (Edwards and Bligh, 1994). Nevertheless, doctors are also susceptible to the subtle salesmanship of the rep.

The doctor's responsibility where dressings are concerned is usually to decide on the basic principles. What is the pathology? Is the circulation compromised? Does the dressing require pressure? How often should the dressing be disturbed? Is infection a problem? What about exudate? Is there likely to be an allergic problem? The detail of the dressing is usually left to the nurse, and most doctors will trust their nurse's judgement. The dressing is usually only one part of the wider picture which the doctor is concerned with. The nurse is much more likely to know how to get something to stay put on an ear or on a big toe. At one time, not so long ago, medicine had relatively little to offer in the way of effective treatments and high technology. Then medical students spent a lot of time as 'dressers', learning the arts of fish-tail bandaging, plastering, etc. Times have moved on, and other professionals routinely now do many things which were previously the province of the doctor.

NURSE TRAINING

There is one major reservation which concerns me. Doctors, in my experience, have great respect for traditionally trained nursing staff. They are less happy about Project 2000, and about the reduction in emphasis on practical skills and hands-on experience in favour of academic achievements, and now the move to degree or diploma based courses in nursing. It is true that the traditional apprentice based training left much to be desired: it was abused through lack of supervision and excessive responsibility being foisted onto student nurses. However, the end result of such a tough training was a highly competent, caring nurse, whose judgement and common sense could be relied upon by doctors because of the broad ranging practical experience with real patients. It is doubtful that we will have another generation of nurses with the same qualities. Nursing may well move down the road of high specialisation, with marked consequences for primary care nursing which as a discipline demands very wide-ranging skills. It will also have consequences in terms of nurse prescribing, as we may well see specialised nurse practitioners developing who have high level skills in a narrow sphere, and who may be competent to prescribe to quite a high level in their own specialist field, but would not be competent to prescribe more basic things in another sphere of nursing. Developments in nurse prescribing must match the evolution of nurse training, but the tail must not be allowed to wag the dog, and those involved in nurse training must carefully consider and meet the wider needs of primary care. There may need to be different formularies for nurses of differing specialities to use as their prescribing base, though we are having enough difficulty at present arriving at consensus over a basic formulary for our traditionally trained nurses (BMA and RPSoGB, 1994).

There is a danger that we will see the demise of the general community and practice nurse accelerated by enthusiasts from within the nursing profession whose objective is for specialist nurse practitioner status. I believe it is the unique generalist structure of primary care in this country which is the vital ingredient for a successful National Health Service. Our secondary care services can be matched by many others in the Western world. Health care systems which have specialists rather than generalists as the first point of patient contact and the basis for community care are not efficient or cost-effective, and do not function well.

Evolution of nurse prescribing is sensible, and must recognise changes to working patterns and skills; nevertheless, nurses are not doctors, and I am more concerned to promote nurse prescribing for the basic materials of the generalist nurse than for the specialist nurse practitioner. The two professions must remain complementary, and practical nursing skills in personal care are those which doctors (and I suspect patients) value above all other nursing skills. Those of us who deal with patients as they are discharged from hospital, both doctors and community nurses, are increasingly aware that one consequence of the pressures on nurses in the secondary care sector is a rapid decline in those skills of personal caring for basic physical, emotional and mental needs. The professions must carefully consider the essential priorities, and whether there is spare capacity, before nurses take on additional new roles.

COST-EFFECTIVENESS

The legacy which a Conservative government leaves behind for the NHS is an all-embracing emphasis on market forces, and on cost. Unfortunately to know the cost is not necessarily to know the value. As the 'internal market' is refined, and outcomes begin to count for more, then cost-effectiveness may be seen to be more important (DoH, 1996). With luck, caring will once again be seen to have tangible value and will be brought back into the equation. Longer term gains may be seen to justify shorter term expenditure (ABPI, 1996). Such an enlightened attitude is not prevalent with politicians today, of whatever hue. They may mouth platitudes about cost-effectiveness, but their behaviour indicates that their concern is largely the immediate cost, and how cuts can be achieved. Nurses who are trained to a higher standard, and who are accredited to prescribe, could argue that they should be paid more for bearing the extra responsibility. Paring costs to the bone is more important to politicians than moving forward with the concept of nurse prescribing. They will not relish paying nurses more money to do what doctors are already doing within a cash limited income pool with open ended responsibility.

Who pays?

There are bound to be some cost implications with nurse prescribing and in the short term costs may well increase. It is not only absolute cost that is relevant, but which parcel of money will be eaten into. General practitioners have prescribing budgets which are hardening year on year (NHS Executive, 1996). Incentive schemes under which practices may retain a proportion of savings based on targets for prescribing in order to benefit other patient services within the practice are fiercely defended and important to practice developments. Practices may well be reluctant to delegate an element of control over such finances to, say, their district nurses.

Most trusts are already causing district nursing staff difficulties by refusing to supply basic items from stock if they can be obtained on prescription, and the costs thereby shifted onto general practitioner budgets. The cost to the NHS in terms of dispensing fees etc. is considerably more than the cost of direct stock purchase by the trust, but it is the particular budget which is affected that matters to trust managers, not the cost to the NHS. The hapless patient may have to arrange to get a prescription for a dressing, catheter or enema from the doctor, then get the item from the pharmacy, assuming it is in stock. An unlucky district nurse may end up as messenger and carrier between the patient, the doctor's surgery and the pharmacy. Prescription charges may also be involved, with the nurse handling money for the patient, an undesirable state of affairs since it puts nursing staff at risk of accusation. The inefficiency in terms of professional time, travelling time and patient care is enormous. The answer must surely lie in a separate budget for nurse prescribing, and a common sense approach to stock items.

Convenience for patients and professional staff, and the efficient use of professional time are the most important practical reasons for supporting nurse prescribing. Managers, financial auditors, and politicians, must take heed! Nurse prescribing should not be yet another issue determined solely by money. It should be viewed as a moral and professional issue, with an understanding that it is likely to cost a bit more, but that it will be more efficient for professionals and patients and will therefore improve the quality of service.

THE NURSE PRESCRIBERS' FORMULARY

Most of the arguments about costs fall if consideration is given to the prescribing formulary for nurses. It was never envisaged that nurses would have free rein to prescribe at will (DoH, 1989). There is a fairly limited list, no doubt of best-buy items, which the nurses can choose from. More expensive and unusual items still require a doctor's prescription. The development of a suitable formulary is continuing, and it is now published as an addendum in the British National Formulary. Generic prescribing has been emphasised by the Department of Health, but while there are points in favour, there are also many points against, and a more balanced approach is desirable. Until recently there has been insistence that all items on the Nurse Prescribers' Formulary should be generically written. If hormone replacement therapy (HRT) and contraceptive pills are ever included, it will be farcical if there is insistence on generic prescription. Consider the generic equivalent for 'Prempak-C' for example. The Joint Formulary Committee is currently considering whether to add 'water for injections' to the Nurse Prescribers' Formulary. Officials from the Department of Health have been reluctant to accept this, and the decision has been deferred. This attitude seems to defy common sense. The alternative diluent of normal saline is known to cause pain at the injection site where hypertonic solution remains after the dilution. Community nurses often need to use 'water for injections' when they are setting up syringe drivers, often out of hours. As a new member of the Joint Formulary Committee, I was concerned at the obvious obstacles which block further additions to the Nurse Prescribers' Formulary. Simple analgesics, some general sale list medicines, laxatives, suppositories, enemas, dressings, catheters, stoma appliances, incontinence devices, iron and folic acid preparations, treatments for head lice, worms and scabies are all items which nurses or midwives could sensibly prescribe (DoH, 1996). Many nurses already run, or assist in the running of well-woman and family planning clinics. I believe that suitably trained nurses could accept responsibility for prescribing HRT and contraception.

PROTOCOLS

One of the professional differences between doctors and nurses, consequent on their training, is that nurses seem better able to work to defined protocols. I have been very impressed by the way in which my own practice nurses work accurately and consistently to detailed protocols in our diabetic and asthma clinics. We are now developing protocols for hypertension and ischaemic heart disease monitoring. GPs in particular often develop short cuts and do not feel comfortable working to rigid guidelines. Much of a general practitioner's training involves learning basic techniques to help deal with the workload effectively in the short time which is available for each consultation (Balint and Norrell, 1973). For some conditions the ready acceptance of protocols might well mean that the quality and consistency of prescribing by nurses could exceed that of prescribing by doctors.

We should pause to think what actually happens now. There are diabetic liaison sisters working in the community who recommend and adjust insulin dosages; community psychiatric nurses (CPNs) will recommend and adjust dosage of antipsychotic medication, and antidepressants; Macmillan nurses recommend adjustments to drug treatments including opiate analgesics for the terminally ill; and many practice nurses have been trained to a high level to run asthma clinics (Barnes, 1997). Nurses often recommend changes to treatment regimes, and often run well-woman clinics and supervise HRT. Some run contraception clinics where they advise on the contraceptive pill, fit caps, etc. If the community nurse or practice nurse wants a dressing, enema or catheter, the prescription is usually written out and simply presented to the doctor for signature, often between patients in a busy surgery. Doctors should ask themselves how often they challenge such prescriptions. The truth is not very often, if at all.

NURSE GRADES

I am aware that significant numbers of general practitioners feel their own role could be threatened by the development of the 'nurse practitioner'. My own concern, however, is that the grading system together with nursing cost ceilings will lead to the loss of the senior generalist nurse. The higher grades will become the preserve of nurse managers and the emerging specialist nurse practitioner. Nurse grading is a mixed blessing, subject to manipulation by managers for financial reasons. Skillmix and Grademix are not synonymous, and traditional hands-on nursing must continue to offer an attractive career structure. Practice nurses employed by general practitioners, who then have a proportion of the cost reimbursed, are not exempt. Many general practitioners who have deemed a practice nurse to be worthy of G or H grade have been subjected to financial pressure from the health authority to downgrade. More practices are now being given fixed staff budgets rather than a proportion of the actual salary costs of a defined maximum number of staff. More staff can be employed by keeping grades low, and justification for higher expenditure on nurses will only be found if there is a saving in doctor costs. A nurse practitioner may well be cheaper than an additional part-time partner.

There is a serious shortage of nurses developing, as well as a shortage of general practitioners, and the number of nurses in training is falling dramatically. My own analysis is that there is no hidden army waiting to poach doctors work.

TEAMWORK

Twenty-four years ago, as a student, I spent some time at a go-ahead practice in Sonning Common. One of the innovations which had been introduced then by John Hasler, a very forward thinking GP, was the concept of a nurse practitioner. The community nursing sisters carried out some of the 'first visits' for the doctors. The scheme was reasonably successful, and was accepted well by patients. It is a shame that there has been little progress since that time. The GP's workload is intolerable at present. It is difficult to understand those doctors who complain so much about pressure of work and yet take fright at the thought that someone else may take some of that work from their shoulders: there is more than enough work to go around.

In primary care it is the concept of the coordinated team which must be developed if we are ever to meet the challenges of caring for an ageing population (DoH, 1996). Pharmacists will need to become part of that team, and increasingly in the future I believe they will work with us from common premises (RPSoGB, 1996). Such an arrangement may well in the longer term supersede doctor dispensing except in the most rural areas. The in-house pharmacy could take over the whole range of central stores and supply functions for community nursing staff, and care in the community requirements. Management of nurses will increasingly devolve from trusts to the primary care team management. Budgets will be unified under one umbrella. It may well be that all team members will ultimately be salaried. Practice based contracts evolving from Primary Care Act pilots (PCAPs) spearhead this sort of change. The pharmacist will have an important role supporting prescribing within the team, both for doctors and for nurse prescribers. Perhaps pharmacists should also be able to prescribe simple (non-POM) remedies themselves at NHS expense when it is appropriate, rather than just sell medicines and dispense for others.

We cannot stand in the way of progress, but a feeling of trust between the different professions, and between the professions and government will be required if there is to be a smooth passage for nurse prescribing. I think we are a long way yet from that point. Professionals in the NHS all feel undervalued, insecure, and threatened by politicians' relative disregard of caring qualities and professional concerns in favour of trying to balance health demands against an underweight purse. There is little hope of common sense prevailing without massive reform of NHS management, involving restoration of effective professional representation at all levels of NHS management, and a willingness of government to fund the NHS properly and pay professional staff properly for their skills.

Together the professions can provide effective health care. I feel confident about the ability of a well trained nurse to prescribe many types of medicines, appliances and dressings safely and cost-effectively. I am sure many nurses will willingly accept the necessary responsibility for the act of prescribing within their sphere of competence.

QUESTIONS FOR DISCUSSION

- Does the medical profession support nurse prescribing out of expediency or because it really believes it is a good thing?
- What are the benefits to doctors of nurses being able to prescribe?
- Does nursing need the support of medicine to promote nurse prescribing?

REFERENCES

Association of the British Pharmaceutical Industry (1996) *Agenda for Health. Putting patients first*. London: ABPI.
Association of the British Pharmaceutical Industry (forthcoming) CASE. *The case for patient packs*. (Now being amended for current schedule of introduction.)
Balint, E. & Norrell, J.S. (1973) *Six Minutes for the Patient*. London: Tavistock Publications.
Barnes, G. (1997) Attitudes of primary care doctors towards nurse prescribing in asthma. (Abstract.) American Thoracic Society 1997 International Conference, San Francisco, California. *American Journal of Respiratory and Critical Care Medicine*, **155(A71)**, 4.
British Medical Association (1996) *Core Services: taking the initiative*. London: BMA General Medical Services Committee.
British Medical Association & Royal Pharmaceutical Society of Great Britain (1994) *British National Formulary* [including the Nurse Prescribers' Formulary]. London: BMA and RPSoGB.
Coopers and Lybrand (1996) *Nurse Practitioners: evaluation report*. London: HMSO.
Crump, B.J., Panton, R., Drummond, M.F., Marchment, M. & Hawkes, R.A. (1995) Transferring the costs of expensive treatments from secondary to primary care. *British Medical Journal*, **310**, 509–512.
Department of Health (1989). *Report of the advisory group on nurse prescribing*. (Crown Report.) London: Department of Health.
Department of Health (1996) *Primary Care: delivering the future*. London: HMSO.
Edwards, R.T. & Bligh, J. (1994) Economic evaluation of drugs: Helping GPs to interpret the evidence for themselves. *Education for General Practice*, **51**, 4–8.
European Economic Community (1994) Council Directive 92/97/EEC of 31 March 1992 on the labelling of medicinal products for human use and on package leaflets. (Also the Medicines for Human Use (Marketing Authorisations etc.) Regulations 1994).
Harris, C. (1996) *Prescribing in General Practice*. Oxford: Radcliffe Medical Press.
National Health Service Executive (1996) *Prescribing Expenditure: guidance on allocations and budget setting for 1997/98*. EL (96) 107. Leeds: NHSE.
Panton, R. (1993) FHSAs and prescribing. *British Medical Journal*, **306**, 310–314.
Royal Pharmaceutical Society of Great Britain (1996) *Pharmacy in a New Age – the New Horizon*. London: RPSoGB.
Secretaries of State for Health England, Wales, Northern Ireland and Scotland (1989) *Working for Patients: indicative prescribing budgets for general medical practitioners*. London: HMSO.
University of Newcastle (1996) *Prodigy Interim Report*. Newcastle: Sowerby Unit for Primary Care Informatics, University of Newcastle.

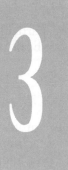

3

Nurse prescribing
What the pharmacists think

Jahn Dad Khan   Alastair Buxton
Sultan Dajani

Key issues

♦ Should the doctor's exclusive right to prescribe be challenged and if so, how?

♦ How can pharmacists challenge the nurses' continuing battle to prescribe?

♦ What is the legitimate claim to prescribing rights for pharmacists?

♦ How does nurse prescribing fit into:
  – Traditional pharmacy practice?
  – 'New' pharmacy roles?

INTRODUCTION

This chapter puts across an opinion of nurse prescribing from the viewpoint of the pharmacy profession. It encompasses the views of members of the Young Pharmacists' Group (YPG), a proactive group within the profession of pharmacy which exists to foster debate and progression within the profession.

The concept of 'medicines management' is currently a popular area of professional development among the major organisations within pharmacy. The practice of medicines management is seen to incorporate 'pharmacist prescribing'. The definition of prescribing recently used by the Crown review into prescribing is 'Authorising in writing the supply of a medicine (usually but not necessarily a Prescription Only Medicine) for a named patient'. This chapter will address the reasons that pharmacists feel that it is their right to prescribe alongside their fellow professionals in medicine and nursing. It will explain why pharmacists are particularly suited to be the profession who 'manages medicines' within our health care system.

PRESCRIBING: A PHARMACY PERSPECTIVE

The YPG was one of the first organisations within the pharmacy profession to promote pharmacist prescribing and prescribing by other practitioners such as nurses, where it was perceived to be in the patient's best interest. With this area of common interest, the YPG has enjoyed a fruitful relationship with the Royal College of Nursing (RCN). In 1995 the YPG acted as one of the catalysts for the initiation of a strategic planning project by the professional body, the Royal Pharmaceutical Society of Great Britain (RPSGB). The project was named 'Pharmacy in a New Age' (PIANA) and involved massive consultations, both inter- and intra-professionally, to develop a vision to take the pharmacy profession into the 21st century. In 1996 the Young Pharmacists Group submitted to the RPSGB a comprehensive blueprint for the future of the profession, *A Sense of Purpose: putting the patient first* (YPG, 1996). This included the concepts of 'medicines management' and 'gatekeeper to health care' as future roles for pharmacists. The RPSGB summarised the findings of the consultation in *Building the Future: a strategy for 21st century pharmaceutical service* (RPSGB, 1997), which was launched at the British Pharmaceutical Conference in 1997. The document summarised possible future roles for pharmacists under five headings:

1. The management of prescribed medicines (calls for pharmacists prescribing within agreed guidelines).
2. The management of long term conditions (monitoring medication and changing treatment where appropriate).
3. The management of common ailments (pharmacists are already experienced in this field).
4. Advice and support for other health care professionals (advising other health care professionals on medications).
5. Promotion and support of healthy lifestyles (health promotion with other health care professionals).

The profession is united behind the view that pharmacists should be involved in all aspects of medicine management, with the right to prescribe as a central tenet of that role.

PRESCRIBING: AN NHS PERSPECTIVE

In the summer of 1997 the Department of Health initiated an important review of prescribing, chaired by Dr June Crown, entitled *Review of*

Prescribing, Supply and Administration of Medicines. The review panel received submissions from many different organisations involved in health care. The first part of the report (DoH, 1998) centered on the supply and administration of medicines under group protocols. The full report examines the entire issue of prescribing and in particular the roles of different health care practitioners in relation to the prescribing of medicines. The findings of the report are of great importance to both pharmacist and nurse prescribing and it seems inevitable as the report favours prescribing by other health care professionals, then legislative changes will follow in due course.

THE HISTORY AND ROLE OF PHARMACY, AND PERCEPTIONS OF OTHER HEALTH CARE PROFESSIONALS

Looking at the history of pharmacy is a useful precursor to examining pharmacists' present and future roles. For those who wish to read further, the history of pharmacy is well documented in *Social Pharmacy: innovation and development* (Harding, Nettleton and Taylor, 1994).

Pharmacists have a long history as health advisers to the public, dating as far back as the 12th century and progressing through the middle ages and onwards. In the 19th century, it was apothecaries who generally treated ailments; physicians were employed only by the gentry or for severe illnesses (Matthews, 1967; Trease, 1964). In 1841 the Pharmaceutical Society was formed to represent three groups of people:

* Druggists (retailers or suppliers of medicines)
* Dispensing chemists
* Apothecaries (who would counter prescribe and make their own medicinal preparations and also perform minor surgical operations such as drawing teeth, lancing boils, etc.) (Burnby, 1983).

Sharp (1985) writes about his experiences working in his father's pharmacy in the early 20th century and describes how he gained an 'impressive reputation for curing ills'. He states that counter prescribing was an important role for most pharmacists, especially in the poorer areas where people could not afford to see a doctor before the introduction of the National Health Service (NHS). In the mid-20th century, enormous developments in medicine and technology began to revolutionise health care delivery. These developments had implications for the professional roles of all health care personnel and the British government, like many other governments, acknowledged these developments with a greater emphasis on primary care and health promotion. The traditional role of counter prescribing by pharmacists for the management of minor ailments has continued through all the changes in health care and during the development of the NHS and the role has been welcomed both within the profession and by government (Harding *et al.*, 1994).

What do pharmacists do?

Some of the current roles of pharmacists are listed in Box 3.1; Box 3.2 lists some of the ways that patients use pharmacists. Box 3.3 examines the future role of the pharmacist. Harding *et al.* envisage that in the future pharmacists will give advice to clients and negotiate about medications and therapies with other health care professionals, leading to a more cost-effective NHS. Examining this concept of liaison with other health care professionals, it has been demonstrated that physicians are more likely to accept product related information from pharmacists than therapeutic information from other sources. In health centre pharmacies, and where

---

Box 3.1 Areas of activity in primary care
(adapted with permission from Harding, Nettleton and Taylor, 1994)

✦ Home nursing and remedies (e.g. treatment of cuts and grazes)

✦ Over the counter (OTC) remedies (e.g. cough medicines and analgesics)

✦ Professional help, especially in paediatrics, where patients don't want to bother the GP

✦ Dispensing prescriptions

✦ Diagnostic services (e.g. pregnancy tests)

Box 3.2 How patients use pharmacists
(adapted with permission from Harding, Nettleton and Taylor, 1994)

✦ For over the counter (OTC) purchases

✦ As 'stepping stones' to doctors

✦ As alternative professional to doctor to consult, especially for minor ailments, with the benefit of accessibility

✦ As 'expert' on medicines and perceived as better than the doctor in this area

> **Box 3.3** The future role of the pharmacist
> (adapted with permission from Harding, Nettleton and Taylor, 1994)
>
> ♦ Health educator
>
> ♦ Gatekeeper to health care
>
> ♦ Referral agent
>
> ♦ Problem solver
>
> ♦ Coordinator of health care services

GPs and pharmacists have collaborated in therapeutic reviews, a resultant decrease in prescribing costs and more rational prescribing have been noted (Harding *et al.*, 1994).

How do other health care professionals perceive pharmacists?

The GP's perspective

There are many misconceptions about pharmacists' training and roles. Community pharmacists are cynically seen by some GPs as 'glorified shop-keepers' who make profits from dispensing prescriptions and the selling of OTC medicines, alongside ordinary articles of commerce. However, more enlightened GPs may see the pharmacist as an adviser on medicines – to the public and to health care professionals alike. Some GPs may perceive that pharmacists only have a role in cutting the costs of prescribing. However, many GP practices – as in pilots in Scotland, Nottingham and Walsall – have recognised the wide ranging benefits of employing pharmacists. For example there are pharmacists working within medical practices who have been involved in formulary development, in analysing PACT data and in running various clinics (e.g. Warfarin clinics). There are also pilot projects taking place using community pharmacists to manage repeat prescribing, an area of practice which accounts for a major part of the NHS drugs bill. These pilots are to be welcomed as they are beginning to utilise the true capabilities and competences of pharmacists and they are changing the attitudes of GPs to the role pharmacists can play in the health care team.

Pharmacists in the hospital sector enjoy a much closer working relationship with doctors and other health care professionals in the hospital service. This pattern of working is seen by many as a template for the progression of teamworking between community pharmacy and other professionals. Hospital pharmacists have for a long time been involved in prescribing, albeit in an 'indirect' manner, where pharmacists are very active in advising on appropriate therapies and indeed monitoring treatment. In some hospitals, pharmacists have, for example, roles in the running of anticoagulant clinics, nebuliser clinics and osteoporosis clinics. Some hospitals are also employing 'seamless care' pharmacists who ensure a smooth transition of patients between primary and secondary care, as well as monitoring patient compliance and concordance with therapies. The role can also encompass developing formularies for primary and secondary care as well as acting as the liaison point for patients and professionals.

The nurse's perspective

Compared to GPs, community nurses, health visitors and practice nurses working in a medical practice generally have a closer working relationship with community pharmacists. Nurses on the whole exhibit a better understanding of pharmacists' roles, but yet again there are many community nurses unaware of the pharmacist's possible contribution to their patients' health care. In general, nurses are more ready to enlist community pharmacists' assistance with medication related problems than their medical colleagues. In the hospital sector good professional relationships exist between all health care professionals. The relationship between pharmacists and nurses has been illustrated by George in an article entitled 'How nurses view ward pharmacy' (George, 1994), which finds that nurses have some understanding of what ward pharmacists do. The literature on this subject and experience from practice does suggest that there is still a need to educate nurses further on the roles of pharmacists.

Pharmacists, nurses, health visitors and general practitioners are all developing roles in disease prevention and health promotion. Interprofessional collaboration is essential to enable coordination of these roles (e.g. advising the public about treating head lice infestations). Harding *et al.* (1994) state that as district nurses respond to the needs of individual clients, especially the elderly, they share many clients with pharmacists. Partnerships between the two professions could bring health benefits to shared clients and their lay carers, utilising the nurses' understanding of local health problems and the pharmacists' unique knowledge of medicinal products.

The pilot projects of nurse prescribing have produced opportunities for collaboration between nursing and pharmacy. The nurses' independent prescribing role confers more autonomous responsibility for patient care, but within their management decisions nurses will need to be aware of the uses and contraindications of the drugs they prescribe as well as those of other drugs the client may be taking. Nurses need to make decisions about the severity of the symptoms the client is experiencing and how they should be managed. Any service or contribution that makes the decision-making process easier, with successful outcomes, should be sought and welcomed. Community pharmacists are well placed to meet this challenge (Harding *et al.*, 1994).

THE VIEWS OF PHARMACISTS
Should the doctors exclusive right to prescribe be challenged and if so, how?

The profession of pharmacy is in agreement with the need to challenge the exclusive right of doctors to prescribe. This section now explores the views of pharmacists when asked this question and attempts to address how this right can be challenged. The following points were raised in discussion:

- Prescribing by doctors is often seen as a 'stamping exercise' of secondary care recommendations or a repeat prescription initiated elsewhere.
- Prescribing by doctors is not considered as the best use of medicinal knowledge (i.e. pharmacists were considered the most suitable professional to prescribe due to their unique training and medicinal knowledge).
- Doctors are not the most cost-effective of prescribers.
- Doctor prescribing will not normally provide patients with choice, ease of access or the chance of increased self-responsibility for their health.
- Diagnoses should appear on all prescriptions to ensure the patient gets the most appropriate treatment.
- The success of pharmacists counter prescribing for minor ailments is surely a precursor to pharmacists being awarded full prescribing rights.
- Pharmacists are already 'indirectly' prescribing through their inter-actions with patients and doctors, in particular in hospital pharmacy practice.
- Pharmacists expertise should be utilised in formulary development, treatment selection and monitoring of treatments.
- With the development of evidence based medicine, it is necessary for the most appropriate treatment based upon the best clinical evidence available to be prescribed. Pharmacists have a major role to play in selecting that treatment, due to their knowledge of medicines.
- In the event of an adverse outcome on patient health resulting from an inappropriate medication or dose being administered, the pharmacist is considered more at fault than the prescribing doctor. In previous cases of litigation, fault has been apportioned 40% to the doctor and 60% to the pharmacist, yet it is the doctor who has exclusive prescribing rights.
- GPs currently find it increasingly difficult to manage prescribing alongside diagnosis, minor surgery and other roles. Some would welcome other health care professionals taking on part of the prescribing role in order to give them more time to spend on other aspects of their patients' care.

- The deregulation of more prescription only medicines to pharmacy medicine status means pharmacists are already recommending products for minor ailments which were once only prescribed by doctors.
- A lot of primary care pharmacists based at GP surgeries are already taking on some of the prescribing roles from GPs.
- Health care is based on a teamworking concept and prescribing should not be excluded from this idea.
- GPs have limited knowledge of wound management products, stoma appliances, etc., and in effect nurses often write the prescription but have to wait for a doctor to authorise its issue.

Discussion

Analysis of GP practices' prescribing habits up and down the country have shown that GPs who have employed pharmacists as prescribing advisers have saved money from their prescribing budgets. It could therefore be suggested that GPs do not always prescribe to optimal standards. Britten *et al.* (1995) have illustrated that there is often prescribing of inappropriate treatments and also a lack of review of long term treatments, especially within repeat prescribing systems. Britton and Lurvey (1991) demonstrate that medication review by a clinical pharmacist reduced both the number and cost of drugs prescribed for patients receiving five or more medication items. Expenditure on drugs is a major focus within the NHS and GPs are being actively encouraged to evaluate their prescribing and make changes to improve quality of care and cost-effectiveness. Pharmacists are obviously well placed to assist doctors with this kind of review, but they would also be appropriate practitioners to take over the prescribing role from doctors.

Patient needs

At present patients have to go to their GP when they require a prescription medicine. In many cases there is a long delay before a patient can be seen by a GP, frequently around 2–3 days; even then GPs often do not have enough time to spend with patients. All these factors make the prescribing process inaccessible for patients.

Diagnoses on prescriptions

Even if prescribing rights are not afforded to other health care professionals, it is imperative that in order to give the best patient care, diagnoses need to appear on the prescription. This is necessary to facilitate the shared care of patients by different health care workers, especially pharmacists. It allows the pharmacist to ensure that the patient gets the most appropriate treatment and the most cost-effective treatment for the health service. In the community, pharmacists currently have to guess the patients diagnosis, thus preventing the total review of prescribing at the time of dispensing. Experiences in hospital pharmacies, where prescribers list the diagnoses on the prescription form, suggest that by this practce the risk of errors is minimised and drug therapy is optimised.

Liability

In recent cases of prescribing errors involving litigation, mostly in America, judges have ruled that pharmacists are 'medicine experts' whereas the doctor is merely following guidelines. The apportionment of blame is usually 60–70% pharmacist fault and 30–40% GP fault. Hence it could be argued that pharmacists are experts on medicines and therefore they must prescribe and take 100% blame should a misadventure happen. Does case law suggest that the wrong health care professional is prescribing?

Increased workload of the GP

Recent research confirms that 70% of all GP consultations are for minor ailments that can be safely managed by community pharmacists and nurses. In many cases medicines are prescribed both indiscriminately and inappropriately just to keep the patient away from the GP surgery (e.g. prescribing antibiotics for the common cold). The workload of these 'inappropriate' consultations can prevent the GP from providing the level of health care that society increasingly demands and obviously reduces the time that the GP can spend with patients who have complex medical problems.

POM to P deregulation

Pharmacists have shown competence in OTC prescribing, contrary to the claims by some consumer organisations. Various audit results demonstrate this, such as the Royal Pharmaceutical Society's national audit of OTC sales of sleeping aids or the North West Regional Pharmacy audit of OTC sales of terfenadine. As more and more potent medicines are being deregulated from POM control, the role of the pharmacist is being consolidated and pharmacists can claim to be the 'experts' in treating minor ailments.

Teamwork

In areas such as wound care and stoma care where nurses have demonstrated superior knowledge compared to GPs, then they should have prescribing rights. In all other therapeutic areas the primary care pharmacist model should be utilised. It should be the role of these practice based pharmacists to manage medicines within the patient population, including the prescribing and monitoring of therapies. GPs should practice within their area of expertise, the diagnosis of illness, minor surgery, and the overall management of patients' health care.

How can pharmacists challenge the nurses continuing battle to prescribe?

This question was approached from three different angles:

• Patient viewpoint
• NHS viewpoint
• Pharmacist viewpoint.

In discussion:

Patient

• It was generally considered that nurses lacked the competence in therapeutics to prescribe.
• Queries relating to concurrent drug therapies would not be within the nurses' scope of competence and could hence remain unanswered, leading to fragmentation of care.
• Potential lack of access to medical notes was perceived to be a problem; however, in general nurses have more access to notes than pharmacists.
• The concept of multidisciplinary working in health care systems should include using the most appropriate professional from the team to carry out a task. If nurses were afforded full or greater prescribing rights this concept was not being followed.
• In our increasingly litigious society, the issue of professional liability for nurse prescribing has not been fully addressed. The responsibilities of the medical and pharmaceutical professions have been clearly demonstrated by case law.
• The issues of convenience for patients within the prescribing process would often be as problematic as is currently the case with doctor prescribing.

NHS

• Nurse prescribing could cost the NHS drugs budget more than prescribing by the medical profession.
• There is currently no quality assurance of nurse prescribing.
• Nurses lack the competence to prescribe in all conditions and they would require substantial training and accreditation before being granted full prescribing rights.

Pharmacist

- Pharmacists already possess the necessary skills and expertise to take on the prescribing role, with the knowledge to ensure appropriate patient outcomes and cost-effective prescribing.
- Pharmacists receive the most pharmacology training at undergraduate level (see Box 3.4) and thus are surely the most appropriate professionals to prescribe.
- Pharmacists were considered to be a more accessible health care professional than nurses.
- The patient's doctor should take overall responsibility for patient care; however, the prescriber should take responsibility for individual prescribing and in the majority of cases that should be the pharmacist.
- Community pharmacists would need to focus on their professional roles rather than ancillary roles (e.g. retailing), which could be delegated to business managers.

Discussion

Over a decade ago the nursing profession proposed a vision for nurse prescribing. The profession has developed the role of a number of specialist nurses (e.g. stoma care nurses and the role of nurse practitioners). The profession has increasingly been able to make an active contribution to the management of various chronic conditions such as diabetes and we have seen pilot projects of nurse prescribing within the community. These pilot projects have allowed the prescribing of wound management products and a small number of systemic drugs. The projects have had the support of the pharmacy profession. Most pharmacists would agree that nurses are the most appropriate health care team member to prescribe wound management products, as they are normally the professional most involved in the care of wounds. Nurses will wish to see these pilot projects extended to the whole profession and many may wish to increase the range of medicines that nurses can prescribe.

Box 3.4 Training in pharmacology	
Profession	**Undergraduate pharmacology course content (hours)**
Nursing	25
Medicine	500
Pharmacy	800

The pharmacy profession has been slow to call for a role in prescribing for itself. However, the example of nurse prescribing helps to legitimise the call for pharmacist prescribing, as pharmacists have a far greater knowledge of drugs than do nurses. The pharmacy profession now believes that its call for prescribing rights could improve the quality and access to health care services for patients. Pharmacists also consider that they are the appropriate profession to treat minor ailments, as pharmacists up and down the country are fulfilling this role every day. It has been estimated that 1 million people visit pharmacies every day to ask for health care advice. Smith (1993) found that one sixth of all pharmacy consultations concern children, of which more than a quarter are for children under 2 years of age.

It is critical for the future development of health care that the professions should work together synergistically rather than compete with each other for roles.

What is the legitimate claim to prescribing rights for pharmacists?

• Pharmacists are the 'first port of call' and sometimes the only health care professional to be consulted for patients' health care needs.

• The network of community pharmacies nationwide, on High Streets and in neighborhoods, makes pharmacists the most accessible members of the health care team for patients.

• Pharmacists are the only professionals who can ensure accuracy and safe supply of prescribed medicines to a satisfactory standard; they can also aid patient compliance and concordance to treatment regimens.

• Pharmacists are used to providing information on medicines both to fellow health professionals and to patients, in a language that each group can comprehend.

• Pharmacists have a very thorough understanding of the pharmacological, pharmacodynamic and pharmacokinetic properties of medicines; their knowledge on this subject is more extensive than that of other health care professionals.

• Community pharmacists are already able to provide patients with 'emergency supplies' of prescription only medications, an indirect form of prescribing.

• Pharmacists are already involved in advising physicians on the prescribing of the most clinically effective medicines and the monitoring of drug regimens in hospital and in the community.

• Improved access and patient convenience could be achieved if pharmacists were given the right to prescribe and manage repeat prescribing in chronic conditions.

- If pharmacists were given prescribing rights there could be a significant decrease in hospital admissions due to iatrogenic disease.
- Pharmacists could contribute greatly to cost-effective prescribing.

Discussion

Are GPs the most appropriate practitioners to prescribe medications? In his chapter in *Social Pharmacy: innovation and development*, by Harding and colleagues (1994), Peter Davis answers this question by stating that the significance of prescribing is threefold:

1. Doctors are essentially gatekeepers to treatment (Christense and Bush, 1981)
2. Up to 80% of all health care costs are attributed to them (Eisenberg and Williams, 1981)
3. Widespread variability raises important issues regarding the quality and motives of certain prescribing decisions (Carrin, 1987).

Davis goes on to claim that the 'thinking process' that leads to a prescribing decision is a complex one, which is based upon a number of key elements. These being the sources of available information, their feasibility and their interpretation. However, Davis maintains that the conclusions of the 'thinking process' are often made hurriedly, under conditions of clinical uncertainty. Furthermore, a considerable amount of work on interventions within prescribing, needs to be investigated with a view to changing the prescribing process (Wyatt *et al.*, 1992).

Soumarai *et al.* (1990) claim that 'Simple administrative remedies are at best blunt instruments' which potentially result in more harm than good (Soumarai *et al.*, 1991). They suggest that the most successful interventions are those involving individual instructions that relate to the clinical experience of the practitioner. The authors conclude that there are opportunities for successful working relationships between doctors and pharmacists, for example in such areas as the rationalising of prescribing patterns (Harding *et al.*, 1994).

WHAT EVIDENCE IS THERE TO SUPPORT PHARMACIST PRESCRIBING?

The American experience

Most of the literature to support pharmacist prescribing stems from work undertaken by pharmacists in America. The best known study to date is the Hepler and Strand model of 'pharmaceutical care' which is defined as the 'the responsible provision of drug therapy for the purpose of achieving outcomes that improve a patient's quality of life' (Pharmaceutical Journal,

1997a). This definition is based on the premise that pharmaceutical care is a practice in which practitioners take responsibility for patients' drug related needs and hold themselves accountable. The practicalities involve the pharmacist investigating what medicines patients are taking, what they are taking them for, and whether they need to be on them in the first place. The pharmacist will then formulate a 'care plan' which involves regularly monitoring and auditing a patient's progress.

Increasingly, many pharmacists in America are gaining the reputation of being prescribers (Flanagan, 1995) as the expansion of the clinical pharmacist's role to include prescribing has facilitated the realisation of pharmaceutical care. In California, in the 1960s, schools of pharmacy proposed a limited list of drugs considered professionally appropriate for pharmacists to prescribe. However, it was not until the 1970s that changes occurred through the Health Manpower pilot project (HMPP) (Stimmel, 1981). This looked at the feasibility of non-physician prescribing roles for a number of health care professionals; the resulting legislation led to pharmacist prescribing in 1977. The progress of pharmacist prescribing was monitored and was found to be so successful that that it led to pharmacists prescribing in other states. However, because the legislation in each state is different, the prescribing roles of pharmacists vary widely, ranging from repeat prescribing to initiating and modifying therapy (Farrell, Northeurs and Cross, 1997). Part of this pioneering success can be attributed to pharmacists marketing themselves as 'drug experts' to both patients and other health care professionals. Fortunately pharmacists are being increasingly recognised as possessing the most appropriate skills required to provide pharmaceutical care. For example, the involvement of pharmacists in medication review clinics and collaborative drug management projects has resulted in marked increases in the improvement of patient compliance and significant decreases in drug related hospital admissions. Other studies have demonstrated more limited prescribing roles, notably in three therapeutic areas: topical pediculicides (Lindane shampoo), oral analgesics and over the counter (OTC) analgesics (Eng and McCormick, 1990).

Stimmel (1983) strongly supports pharmacist prescribing and lists the following arguments in favour:

• In America, current practice pharmacist consultations have evolved into prescribing ones.
• There is an urgent need for pharmacist prescribing.
• In many American states, nurse practitioners and physicians' assistants are taught clinical pharmacology by pharmacists (analogy in the UK of pilots of nurse prescribing). Since they have the authority to prescribe, it seems a natural progression to allow pharmacists to prescribe too.
• As the need for the formulation role of pharmacists decreases and

mechanical dispensing is delegated to trained staff, new roles need to be evolved for pharmacy which will also progress health care development.

• When it comes to prescribing, pilot studies have shown pharmacists to be more acutely aware than physicians (Stimmel, 1983).

Many of these points can be applied to the situation in the UK.

Stimmel (1983) also highlights some of the negative aspects regarding pharmacist prescribing:

• Not all pharmacists are competent to prescribe
• Pharmacists are only trained in minor complaint diagnosis
• Physicians oppose it
• Patient care costs could potentially increase
• Pharmacists' access to patient information is not adequate for competent prescribing.

In order to address the above points and to strengthen the case for pharmacist prescribing, the author proposes:

• Certification to prescribe to be based upon demonstrable competence
• Pharmacists who prescribe must have access to medical notes
• Pharmacists must prescribe within an environment where there are established working relationships with physicians
• Pharmacist prescribing should be limited to long term therapy for chronic conditions and therapy for acute self-limiting illnesses that are not diagnostically complex.

These limitations have been incorporated within Californian law and legislation is pending which will allow pharmacists (within specified guidelines) to initiate drug treatment.

PHARMACIST PRESCRIBING: A UK PERSPECTIVE
Hospital pharmacists

An interesting debate at the Medicine Management Conference organised by the *Hospital Pharmacist* journal in October 1997 raised the issue of pharmacist prescribing. The findings were reported in a special feature (Hospital Pharmacist, 1997) and were accepted by an overwhelming majority of hospital pharmacists, who agreed with the new and future roles proposed. Christine Clark (former Chief Pharmacist, Salford Royal Hospitals NHS Trust) claimed that current medicine management was about pharmacists delivering pharmaceutical care; she stressed that future changes in medicine management would be brought about by changes in the political, economical, social and technological environments. Furthermore, pharmacists in hospitals had 'reached out' by being involved in:

- Providing advice to doctors
- Monitoring and assessing patient care
- Health education and promotion
- Discharge planning
- The production of treatment protocols and guidelines.

Diane Kennard defined medicine management, from a Department of Health perspective, as 'facilitating the maximum benefit and minimum risk from medicines for individual patients'.

Other references in the literature have supported the extended roles of pharmacists in the prescribing of medicines in secondary care; a pilot conducted in a hospital pharmacy looked at the perceived advantages of using a pharmacist in a role that is traditionally performed by a junior doctor (Culshaw and Davies, 1998). The study showed that the pharmacist saved the junior doctor a lot of time and that there was an improvement in the efficiency, quality and delivery of care. The senior house officer involved in the study described the results as encouraging and commented that this was to form a 'quality control' on prescribing.

Another article that supports the extension of the hospital pharmacist's role was written by Siobhan Cotter (1995), who believes the traditional roles of hospital pharmacy to be:

- Monitoring patients' drug therapy on the wards
- Creating, implementing and monitoring drug policies that aim to ensure that prescribing is cost-effective and of an acceptable clinical standard
- Contributions on the drugs and therapeutics committees on drug policy
- Advising clinical directorates, auditing policies and revising them.

Further roles postulated include:

- Inclusion as part of the multidisciplinary care teams (e.g. nutrition, cytotoxic chemotherapy, pain control teams)
- Training roles (patients, pharmacy staff, nurses and other health care professionals).

A paper by Carol Paton (1998) shows how pharmacists keeping medication histories can make major contributions to clarifying treatment plans for the long term mentally ill.

These studies, and others, suggest that there is a strong case for pharmacist prescribing, provided certain criteria are met. Issues such as continuous professional development and protocols need to addressed.

An original paper submitted by Jayne Wood and Dawn Bell (1997) looked at evaluating pharmacists' involvement in drug therapy decisions. They found that pharmacists had more chance of being involved in and influencing the outcome of drug therapy decisions if they spent more time interacting with patients and other health care professionals at ward level.

Already there are various initiatives being developed by hospitals employing 'seamless care pharmacists', who act as the interface between primary and secondary care.

Pharmacists in primary care

A conference organised by the industrial, community and hospital pharmacists groups of the RPSGB, in September 1997, discussed the 'extended roles' of pharmacists in primary care. One of the speakers was Claire Mackie, the then chairman of the primary care special interest group, and a member of the panel advising Dr June Crown. She claimed that 'the pursuit of clinical effectiveness was best achieved through the delivery of pharmaceutical care' (Pharmaceutical Journal, 1997b) and that this is dependent upon the following factors:

- Patient registration with pharmacists
- Multidisciplinary teamwork
- Audits
- Development of a single, integrated patient record
- A commitment by both patients and pharmacists.

Encouragingly, it was claimed that pharmacists in primary care had the potential to improve outcomes by educating both the patients and health care professionals on the clinical effectiveness of drug treatment and, in the future, by prescribing. Some of the roles that pharmacists in primary care had already become involved in included:

- Interpreting prescribing data
- Formulary development and prescribing systems
- Providing drug information
- Developing treatment protocols
- Education, training and clinical audit
- Pharmacist run clinics (e.g. anticoagulant clinic)
- Repeat prescribing and medication review.

Mackie also described how pharmacists could become more involved in prescribing, by reference to the prescribing model of 'Marinker and Reilley', which describes the prescribing process in five stages:

1. Assessing the problem
2. Deciding whether drug therapy is appropriate
3. Selecting the drug therapy
4. Communicating with the patient
5. Follow-up to ensure the desired outcome was achieved.

Pharmacists could make a contribution to all of these stages. Three models for pharmacist prescrbing were proposed:

1. Pharmacists acting as an independent prescribers (as currently practised with over the counter medicines)
2. Pharmacists taking on a dependent prescriber role following on from the physician's diagnosis and decision to treat
3. Pharmacists modifying dosage and directions after the physician had selected the individual therapy.

In the context of evidence based medicine, the second of the above models seems to be the most appropriate for the current time. It is interesting to note the crossover of these models with the models proposed in the USA examined earlier in this chapter, where the American authorities use some of the above models as a means of accrediting pharmacists for prescribing purposes.

John Thompson (Head of Pharmacy and Prescribing, NHS Executive) claims that pharmacists have a significant role to play in reducing the NHS drugs bill and he also emphasises that pharmacists must focus more on direct patient care.

One area where community pharmacists already have a major impact is within the provision of prescribing advice to nursing and residential home patients. This has been demonstrated by Janet Corbett (1997), who found that a practice based audit of repeat prescribing by community pharmacists was acceptable to GPs and, more importantly, led to an improvement in quality and cost-effectiveness of prescribing. Another study, conducted by Britten *et al.* (1995), looked at how pharmacists could address the inappropriate prescribing of drugs and the importance of reviewing repeat medication prescriptions. A study conducted in South Africa by Gilbert (1997) looked at the perceptions of other health care professionals with regard to community pharmacists becoming members of the primary health care team. It was found that although pharmacists are eager to be part of the primary health care team, doctors and nurses are wary, and anxious to protect their authority; parallels can be drawn with the situation in the UK.

Kay Wood (a consultant pharmacist) and her team found that a therapeutic advisory service provided by pharmacists also improved the standard of prescribing in UK general practice (Wood, 1997). Further extensive research to support pharmacists prescribing originates from the pilot projects of primary care pharmacists working in GP surgeries, either as consultants or employees.

The work of the primary care pharmacist

Doran (1997) looked at the role of pharmacists in a general practice team and described the success of a project in Doncaster where six pharmacists were employed in several practices. He argued that although doctors expressed a willingness to address prescribing issues, they bemoaned the lack of time and resources to do it. However, their concerns were allayed by having 'prescribing specialists' at hand who could comply with outpatient clinic recommendations drawn up by the secondary care sector. He felt that, from the results of this pilot study, pharmacists had a role in primary care prescribing.

In addition to advising doctors about cost-effective prescribing, primary care pharmacists can also help practice nurses in the prescribing of dressings for which they have limited prescribing rights. An article by Ros Anderson (1997), in *The Prescriber*, addresses the issue of prescribing dressings. Although primary care wound management prescribing may be 'hospital led', some hospital trusts have developed wound care protocols in conjunction with primary care which can be incorporated into a practice formulary. Her study reports that pharmacists have 'expert' knowledge to recommend the most appropriate and cost-effective dressings for patients.

Another area that the primary care pharmacists have been shown to have a huge impact on is prescribing for the elderly. Sheena Macgregor has demonstrated an extension of the primary care pharmacist model into the management of various clinics within primary care (described in Agnew, 1998). Anticoagulant clinics were initially developed and the success of these lead to the setting up of a clinic reviewing patients' eligibility to take ACE inhibitors, with the aim of reducing hospital admissions. Another successfully operated clinic was set up in Wales to detect *H. pylori* in patients suspected of suffering from stomach ulcers. Unfortunately many good ideas and clinics have been met with a great deal of resistance from GPs, but once the benefits become apparent this initial hurdle is overcome.

One of the most recent publications to give credence to pharmacist prescribing is an article entitled 'Who should accredit?' (Mackie, 1998). The article suggests that only suitably accredited pharmacists should be allowed to prescribe. Furthermore, it adds that transferring the treatment of minor ailments to pharmacists (one of the areas where pharmacists have consistently shown expertise) would have a dual effect: it would enhance the professional role of the pharmacist and it would allow doctors to spend time on more serious conditions and health education strategies. The cost of visits to GPs for minor ailments and related costs are estimated to be 25 billion ECU, but self-medication with effective input by pharmacists could cut this cost by 13 billion ECU.

NURSE PRESCRIBING AND PHARMACY

How does nurse prescribing fit into the traditional role of pharmacy?

When this question was discussed by pharmacists, a number of points were raised:

- Nurses have greater access to medical notes than pharmacists.
- There was concern that nurse prescribing legislation was ambiguous, for example could nurses prescribe products outside the 'nurse' formulary?
- Where nurses have written the prescriptions, pharmacists have acted in both an advisory manner and as a quality control measure.
- There was concern that nurse prescribing could lead to more NHS fraud than at present.
- Nurse prescribing provides a platform for intra-professional liaison.
- Pharmacists had not been sufficiently proactive within their area of expertise and thus had been overtaken by 'less pharmacologically aware' health professionals. Thus our pursuit of extended roles was slowed down and apathy was rife.

How does nurse prescribing fit into the 'new' roles of pharmacy?

The following is a summary of the points which came out of discussions about the interface between pharmacists practising new roles and nurse prescribers:

- Teamwork and communication with other health care professionals – including nurses – was seen as the key to achieving positive patient outcomes.
- Synergy would be seen in some therapeutic areas (e.g. asthma, diabetes, etc.).
- All interventions would need to be documented by all health care professionals to demonstrate accountability.
- Accreditation schemes would be needed for specialised services that should incorporate all the prescribing health care professionals. For pharmacists to be suitably accredited would be in the best interests of patients.

However, many barriers exist before we can turn the theory of pharmacist prescribing into practice. A consultant physician admits that the prescribing of a drug is a challenge and three factors must be taken into account before a drug is prescribed for a patient:

1. Correct diagnosis
2. Past medical and drug history
3. Drug choice itself.

He maintains that doctors are the experts on prescribing and pharmacists only have a role in complementing the doctor's advice. He believes that the following criteria should be adopted by all doctors to implement effective prescribing:

1. A full assessment of the patient and a correct diagnosis
2. Is the prescribing of a drug necessary?
3. Correct prescription writing
4. Ensuring patient compliance
5. Cost-effectiveness of medication prescribed
6. Having regard for medico-legal implications
7. Paying particular care to prescribing in special patient groups.

However, the pharmacy profession would consider that, with the exception of the first point, parmacists have all the necessary knowledge and skills to fulfill the above criteria.

CONCLUSION

There is a very strong case to support pharmacist prescribing and in most cases the pharmacist is seen as the health professional most suited to the prescribing of medicines. In the future, all health care professionals may be working in a multidisciplinary and synergistic manner. The GP's role could be streamlined to include only diagnosis and an overall coordination of patient care, while the pharmacist could take on the prescribing role.

There is currently an increasing degree of apathy, especially among recently qualified pharmacists, who feel that their skills and expertise are grossly under utilised at present. Furthermore, there is no incentive for pharmacists to become involved in patient centered initiatives. Although it is acknowledged that nurses will undoubtedly have a role in the prescribing of certain medications and appliances, where there is demonstrable competence, pharmacists widely feel that this should be their domain. All groups in pharmacy are hopeful that they, as the most appropriate health care professional, will be undertaking the most appropriate role that will match their skills and expertise. The pharmacist must be given prescribing rights if patient outcomes are to be achieved optimally and to entail the most cost-effective use of resources, including medicines. The YPG believes that pharmacists already possess the skills and expertise that would enable them to prescribe and hopes that the government and other health care professionals recognise this wasted resource before it is too late. If pharmacy is not allowed to progress and flourish then it will just wither away and die, affecting all the health care professionals around it as they try to compensate for the loss.

QUESTIONS FOR DISCUSSION

- Is the Medicines Act outdated with respect to the present roles of health care professionals and will it require major changes in light of the conclusions that arise from the Crown Report?

- Are the prescribing health care professionals providing the best patient care or just the best 'possible' care? And are they making the best use out of scarce resources?

- Should working in multidisciplinary settings herald new working relationships, with the specific focus being the patient?

- Is the current method of remuneration (especially for community pharmacists) fair? Considering pharmacists are paid to dispense prescriptions as opposed to their advice, spotting forgeries, contraindications, interventions, secondary health care checks, etc.

- Do we need to address the issue of standards and the accreditation of services provided by health care professionals, especially if prescribing rights are given to more than one group of health care professionals?

Further reading

Young Pharmacists Group (1996) A Sense of Purpose: putting the patient first. Submission for the Royal Pharmaceutical Society of Great Britain's Pharmacy in a New Age initiative. Birmingham: Young Pharmacists Group, July 1996. Available from the Young Pharmacists Group, P.O. Box 2641, Birmingham B1 3EB, UK. Tel: 0121 233 0708.

This is the group's template for the future direction of pharmacy as a profession and its role in healthcare.

Harding, G., Nettleton, S. & Taylor, K., eds (1994) Social Pharmacy: innovation and development, London; Pharmaceutical Press.

This book gives a concise historical perspective of pharmacy, as well as future role(s), and is written by eminent people in a pragmatic style.

Crown, J (1998) Review of Prescribing, Supply and Administration of Medicines, part 2. Review Secretariat, Room 6E64, Quarry House, Quarry Hill, Leeds LS2 7UE, UK.

This encompasses the viewpoints of all health care professionals and what roles they would like to fulfil in the future. It is the clearest reference to the potential future changes in the role as health care professionals, especially in regard to the prescribing of medicines.

Mackie, C., ed. (1998) 'Who should accredit?' Chemist and Druggist, 249: 26–29.

This gives a comprehensive guide to setting of standards for specialist services, and in particular suitable accreditation of these standards.

Royal Pharmaceutical Society of Great Britain (1997) Building the Future Strategy for 21st-Century Pharmaceutical Service. London: Royal Pharmaceutical Society of Great Britain. Available from RPSGB, 1 Lambeth High Street, London SE1 7JN, UK.

This document spells out the pharmacy profession's vision of the future of pharmacy and is a blueprint for the future of pharmacy.

ACKNOWLEDGEMENTS

The YPG Executive would like to acknowledge the granting of copyright permission by Charles Fry (Director of Publications at the Royal Pharmaceutical Society of Great Britain). Thanks too to Austin Gibbons (also at the Royal Pharmaceutical Society) for his invaluable assistance in carrying out a literature search; but most of all, a big vote of thanks go to all the delegates who attended the YPG Midlands Conference, April 1998.

REFERENCES

Agnew, T. (1998) Why we must talk to patients in the new NHS. *Pharmacy in Practice*, **May**, 180–183.

Anderson, R. (1997) Conducting a review of prescriptions for dressings. *Prescriber*, **19 March**, 83–84.

Britten, N. *et al.* (1995) Continued prescribing of inappropriate drugs in general practice. *Journal of Clinical Pharmacy and Therapeutics*, **20**, 199–205.

Britton, M. & Lurvey, P. (1991) Impact of medication profile review on prescribing in a general medicine clinic. *American Journal of Hospital Pharmacy*, **48**, 265–270.

Burnby, J.G.L. (1983) *A Study of the English Apothecary from 1660 to 1760*. Medical History Supplement No. 3. London: Wellcome Institute for the History of Medicine.

Carrin, G. (1987) Drug prescribing: a discussion of its variability and (ir)rationality. *Health Policy*, **7**, 73–94.

Christense, D.B. & Bush, P.J. (1981) Drug prescribing: patterns, problems and proposals. *Social Science and Medicine*, **15**, 243–255.

Corbett, J. (1997) Provision of prescribing advice for nursing and residential home patients. *Pharmaceutical Journal*, **259**, 422.

Cotter, S.M. (1995) Give pharmacists a leading role. *Medical Interface*, **October**, 48–50.

Culshaw, M. & Davies, S. (1998) Assessing the value of a discharge pharmacist. *Pharmacy Management*, **14(2)**, 22–23.

Department of Health (1998) *Review of Prescribing, Supply and Administration of Medicines. A report on the supply and administration of medicines under group protocols*. London: Department of Health.

Doran, K. (1997) Prescriber support – the practice pharmacist team. *Prescriber*, **5 February**, 73–74.

Eisenberg, J.M. & Williams, S.V. (1981) Cost containment and changing physicians' practice behaviour. *Journal of the American Medical Association*, **241**, 2195–2201.

Eng, H.J. & McCormick, W.C. (1990) Assessment of the Florida pharmacists self care consultant law using patient profile and prescription audit methods. *DICP*, **24(10)**, 931–935.

Farrell, J. North-Leurs, P. & Cross, M. (1997) Pharmacist prescribing in the United States. *Pharmaceutical Journal*, **259**, 187–190.

Flanagan, M.E. (1995) State prescribing authority. *American Pharmacy*, **10**, 12–18.

George, B. (1994) How nurses view ward pharmacy. *Hospital Pharmacy Practice*, **June**, 245–246.

Gilbert, L. (1997) The community pharmacist as a member of the primary health care team in South Africa – perceptions of pharmacist, doctors and nurses. *International Journal of Pharmacy Practice*, **5**, 112–200.

Harding, G., Nettleton, S. & Taylor, K. (1994) *Social Pharmacy: innovation and development*. London: Pharmaceutical Press.

Hospital Pharmacist (1997) Medicine management. *Hospital Pharmacist*, **4**, 245–259.

Mackie, C. (1998) Who should accredit? *Chemist and Druggist*, **30 May**, 26–29.

Matthews, L.G. (1967) The spicers and apothecaries of Norwich. *Pharmaceutical Journal*, **198**, 5–9.

Oakley, P. (1998) Pharmacist prescribing. *Hospital Pharmacist*, **5**, 86.

Paton, C. (1998) Are we clinically effective? *Pharmacy in Practice*, **May**, 198–202.

Pharmaceutical Journal (1997a) Editorial. *Pharmaceutical Journal*, **258**, 387–388.
Pharmaceutical Journal (1997b) Importance of pharmacists in achieving effective prescribing. *Pharmaceutical Journal*, **259**, 556–557.
Royal Pharmaceutical Society of Great Britain (1997) *Building the Future Strategy for 21st-Century Pharmaceutical Service*. London: RPSGB.
Sharp, L.K. (1985) Prussic acid, patients and professors. *Pharmaceutical Journal*, **235**, 821–822.
Smith, F.J. (1993) Community liaison: pharmacists and primary care consultations. *International Journal of Pharmacy Practice*, **2**, 85–89.
Soumarai, S.B. *et al.* (1990) Withdrawing payment for non scientific drug therapy: intended and unexpected effects of a large scale natural experiment. *Journal of the American Medical Association*, **263**, 831–839.
Soumarai, S.B. *et al.* (1991) Effects of medicaid drug-payment limits on admissions to hospitals and nursing homes. *New England Journal of Medicine*, **325**, 1072–1077.
Stimmel, G.L. (1981) The pharmacist as prescriber of drug therapy – the USC pilot project. *Drug Intelligence Clinical Pharmacy*, **15**, 665–672.
Stimmel, G.L. (1983) Political and legal aspects of pharmacist prescribing. *American Journal of Hospital Pharmacy*, **40(8)**, 1343–1344.
Trease, G.E. (1964) *Pharmacy in History*. London: Baillière, Tindall and Cox.
Wood, J. & Bell, D. (1997) Evaluating pharmacist involvements in drug therapy decisions. *Pharmaceutical Journal*, **259**, 342–345.
Wood, K.M. (1997) Influencing prescribing in primary care: a collaboration between clinical pharmacology and clinical pharmacy. *International Journal of Pharmacy Practice*, **5**, 1–5.
Wyatt, T.D. *et al.* (1992) Short lived effects of a formulary on antiinfective prescribing – the need for continuing peer review? *Family Practice*, **9**, 461–465.
Young Pharmacists Group (1996) *A Sense of Purpose: putting the patient first*. Submission for the Royal Pharmaceutical Society of Great Britain's Pharmacy in a New Age (PIANA) initiative. Birmingham: Young Pharmacists Group, July 1996.

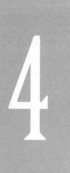

4

Nurse prescribing

The lawmakers

Sir Roger Sims   Elizabeth Gardiner

Key issues

♦ The political climate associated with nurse prescribing.

♦ The lobbying process and the campaign for nurse prescribing.

♦ Tactics used to achieve legislative change to facilitate nurse prescribing.

INTRODUCTION

The legislation allowing nurse prescribing finally reached the statute book in early 1992, just before the general election. This was 6 years after the Cumberlege Report had first recommended its introduction (DoH, 1986), and several months after the deadline set in the Crown Report. Yet it was something of a triumph for the Royal College of Nursing (RCN), and for the dedicated members of both houses of parliament who supported the measure, that it reached the statute book at all.

Despite the government's acceptance of the proposal, there was no intention to give the issue priority in terms of parliamentary time. This is perhaps unsurprising given that the Department of Health was in the process of overseeing one of the most fundamental changes to the health service since its establishment. Having successfully steered the National Health Service and Community Care Act 1990 through all its legislative stages, perhaps the reluctance of the health ministers and their civil servants to argue the case for more parliamentary time for a relatively small Bill such as nurse prescribing is understandable. Yet this was a source of great frustration for the supporters of nurse prescribing and the RCN determined to take action. If the government would not introduce a Bill, then the RCN would try to use the private member's Bill procedures to allow a backbench MP to introduce the legislation.

Private member's Bills have very little chance of success without three key ingredients: luck, dedication on behalf of the MP introducing the Bill, and a large dose of publicity to ensure that a worthy measure does not fail simply because there are too few MPs around to support it. This chapter describes the history of the legislation and the roles played by the RCN – particularly the Parliamentary office – and the backbench Conservative MPs Dudley Fishburn and (Sir) Roger Sims.

KEEPING THE ISSUE ALIVE

The Queen's Speech of November 1990, setting out the government's proposals for the forthcoming Parliamentary session, contained no reference to nurse prescribing. So the RCN determined to bring the matter to parliament's attention in other ways. Much work had been undertaken already to persuade both doctors and pharmacists of the benefits of nurse prescribing and the Crown Report had clearly set out a number of beneficial outcomes for patients. Some members of parliament, however, had yet to be convinced.

Members of parliament have more issues to deal with than time available to consider them. Bringing a new matter to their attention requires more than a few letters and a couple of parliamentary briefings, although these were certainly part of the package. Only a coordinated campaign and constant reminders from the RCN would ensure that nurse prescribing remained on the parliamentary agenda. The issue of nurse prescribing had been discussed in parliament before, for example in 1987 the report of the Commons Social Services Select Committee on primary health care recommended that the government introduce enabling legislation to permit appropriately trained nurses limited prescribing powers; 4 years later, however, the issue was not at the forefront of MPs minds. Some sceptical MPs needed to be convinced that nurse prescribing was not simply about substituting nurses for doctors, and that it would not be a costly waste of time. Above all, they wanted to know how their constituents would be affected.

The RCN's parliamentary panel

One group of MPs in particular were committed to the cause, and very well briefed on the importance of nurse prescribing. This group was the RCN's Parliamentary panel. The RCN does not sponsor MPs and peers but has a Parliamentary panel comprising about 12 members from all parties who support the RCN in parliament, and who meet on a regular basis to discuss nursing issues. Included in the RCN's panel are two of the nurses in parliament, Baroness Cox and Baroness McFarlane of Llandaff. There were, until the 1997 general election, no nurses in the House of Commons, but other panel members were chosen for their interest in health, their ability to work on a cross-party basis, and their commitment to promote the interests of nurses and nursing.

Private members ballot 1990

A private member's Bill is the device by which a backbench MP can introduce his or her own legislation, irrespective of the government's programme. The RCN sought in November 1990 to use the private member's Bill procedure to introduce a Bill on nurse prescribing. Private members wishing to sponsor a Bill enter a ballot (held at the beginning of each session of Parliament). Those coming top of the ballot have priority in the limited amount of parliamentary time allocated to backbenchers. Such is the pressure on parliamentary time that even if their proposals are relatively uncontroversial, and not opposed by the government, then only the top six in the ballot have any real chance of success.

Given the reluctance of the government to introduce legislation, the RCN drew up its own four-clause Bill, simply called Nurse Prescribing Bill. The RCN wrote to a large number of those entering the ballot, including its own panel members, suggesting that they consider the issue of nurse prescribing, should they be successful. When the result of the ballot was announced, this was followed up by another letter to the 20 selected in the ballot, enclosing the draft Bill. Unfortunately, those with most chance of success were already committed to introducing Bills on other issues. RCN panel members were not high in the list. Nevertheless, the letter writing campaign did result in many letters of support from a wide range of MPs. Number nine in the ballot was the Conservative MP for Kensington, Dudley Fishburn. Although he had little chance of being allocated parliamentary debating time, he did express his strong support for the issue, and announced his intention to introduce the RCN's Bill under the 10-minute rule procedure.

Seeking wider support

In early 1991 the RCN initiated a campaign to raise the profile of nurse prescribing – through the media and through seeking wider support. One way in which the RCN sought to convince a wider audience of the benefits of nurse prescribing was by seeking the support of leaders of patient and client groups. From a parliamentary point of view, the connection between nurse prescribing and direct benefits to constituents could be established. The British Association of United Patients, the Association of Community Health Councils of England and Wales, the Patients' Association, Shelter and the then Spastics Society were enlisted to write to the secretary of state for health, then William Waldegrave MP, calling for the speedy introduction of nurse prescribing.

DUDLEY FISHBURN MP'S BILL

Dudley Fishburn introduced his Bill on 30 January 1991 under the 10-minute rule with all party support (House of Commons, 1990), at the beginning of business in the House of Commons immediately after questions. The introduction of such a Bill is usually simply a device to have a matter aired and it is rare that it goes further. The proposer of such a Bill has 10 minutes to speak its virtues and asks the 'leave of the House' to introduce it. If the House agrees, it is then printed by the official publishers – Her Majesty's Stationery Office. While a first reading of a government Bill normally precedes a wider debate on the actual text of legislation, a 10-minute rule Bill will usually receive no more parliamentary time. However, luck and the RCN external affairs department intervened. Work was undertaken to get agreement on the consumer group's letter and it was press released on the day of the Bill's introduction to the Commons. The British Medical Association (BMA) agreed to support the RCN's Bill and the RCN press office rolled into action to ensure that the maximum publicity was given to the Bill.

Newsline, the RCN's own internal newsletter for activists and stewards, carried the story of Dudley Fishburn's Bill as the main story under the headline 'RCN Campaign Takes Off' (RCN, 1991). *Newsline* encouraged local activists to write to their local newspapers outlining the benefits of nurse prescribing, and congratulating those MPs who were prepared to support the new Bill. A special *Newsline* was also issued to community health nurses, again with the intention of seeking local publicity in relation to the Bill.

Thus, by the time of the Bill's introduction, in January 1991, nurse prescribing was on many lips and had received considerable airing in local press and radio stations, as well as some national newspaper coverage. A large number of MPs had also been prepared through letters highlighting the importance of the Bill sent from the RCN's general secretary, Christine Hancock. Among the cross-party sponsors of the Bill (that is, those MPs prepared to sign their names on the Bill being introduced) were members of the RCN's parliamentary panel from the Labour, Liberal Democrat and Scottish Nationalist parties, from Plaid Cymru, and from Conservative Party panel member Roger Sims MP.

The Bill was officially 'read a first time' (that is, spoken to by Dudley Fishburn) and, having received no objections, it was 'ordered to be read a second time upon Friday 26 April and to be printed'. However, subsequently a rescheduled date of 3 May 1991 was set, and this gave the RCN time to increase the amount of publicity for the measure, and to secure broader support from MPs.

Government opposition

To some extent, the government still needed convincing that the time was right and that the cost was manageable. A full parliamentary programme and the introduction of restrictions on prescription only medicines which GPs were allowed to prescribe suggested that the time was not right. Nevertheless, constant pressure on the government did lead to further action. In reply to a question from another RCN panel member, Emma Nicholson MP, the then minister of state, Virginia Bottomley, announced that the government would commission an independent cost–benefit analysis of the advisory group's proposals. An interim report from the cost–benefit analysis was expected to be available in the spring of 1992. 'Depending on the nature of the results, we would hope to introduce legislation as soon as a suitable opportunity arises' (Bottomley, 1991a).

MPs' opinion poll

Aware that there was a possibility of Dudley Fishburn's Bill receiving a fuller debate on its second reading, the RCN commissioned an independent opinion poll of 100 MPs from all parties (Market Access, 1991). The poll asked two questions of MPs:

1. Whether they agreed with the principle of nurse prescribing
2. Whether they believed that the government should make time available to introduce the legislation.

The results of the poll were announced in a press conference, timed to coincide with the publication of the Bill on 18 April 1991. The survey revealed overwhelming support from MPs for nurse prescribing:

- 69% of MPs supported without reservation nurse prescribing in principle
- 97% of MPs were generally supportive of the principle
- 87% of MPs believed that parliamentary time should be made available to introduce the legislation
- 93% of Conservative MPs believed that time should be made available to introduce the legislation.

Not only did the opinion poll provide extra ammunition by way of publicity for the Bill, but it clearly demonstrated support from MPs across the political spectrum. Significantly, this meant that the proposal would almost certainly become law if the government chose to introduce the legislation.

Speeding up the cost–benefit analysis

A few days after the RCN's press conference on the opinion poll, the government announced that the cost–benefit analysis was progressing well. Management consultants Touche Ross had been commissioned to undertake the work and Mrs Bottomley announced that 'the results are due by the end of August' (Bottomley, 1991b). This was encouraging news, and interpreted by some as a signal that the government might find time in their own programme to introduce a Bill in the autumn. Such optimism was somewhat dissipated by the outcome of the second reading on Dudley Fishburn's Bill.

Second reading

On Friday 3 May 1991 time was found for a second reading of the Bill (House of Commons, 1991). This time Dudley Fishburn set out once again the case for the Bill, announcing that it had the support of 'almost everyone in the National Health Service' and calling for the measure to be accepted as quickly as possible.

Virginia Bottomley replied for the government. She reiterated that 'The government are fully committed to the idea of nurse prescribing' but said that 'supporting the general idea of nurse prescribing does not mean that we can leap over some of the details that must be worked out'. The four remaining issues which needed to be tackled were identified by Mrs Bottomley as:

• The need for an authoritative cost–benefit analysis
• The establishment of the consequences for nurse education and training
• The determination of the precise type of drugs that nurses can prescribe
• The working out of detailed administrative arrangements.

While the government were clearly undertaking much of this work, and in discussion with all the relevant bodies and professions, decisions about implementation would not be taken until the results of the cost–benefit analysis were known. Mrs Bottomley concluded by saying that the government would work 'with determination and all possible urgency' to give effect to the proposals introduced by Dudley Fishburn.

The rules of the House ensure that the second reading debate on a government Bill concludes at a specified time and a conclusion is reached, but those governing private member's Bills are more complex. One effect of these is that if a member, minister or backbencher is on his or her feet speaking to the Bill when the time to end the sitting arrives, debate is adjourned and the Bill has to go to the end of the list on another of the few days allocated for such Bills, with no prospect of future progress being made. So instead of opposing the Bill, all that was necessary was for the government to ensure that a backbencher was speaking at 2.30 p.m. This is exactly what happened and the Bill was effectively dead.

Summer 1991

The RCN did not disguise its disappointment with the government's decision to block Dudley Fishburn's Bill. While accepting that there were many detailed issues yet to be determined, the RCN believed that the strength of feeling in support of the principle of the Bill could have been acknowledged. The RCN argued that an enabling piece of legislation could have progressed through Parliament and be on the statute book, ready to be implemented when the technical details were completed. Immediately letters from the RCN president, chair of council and general secretary expressing disappointment and frustration were sent to national newspapers. As Christine Hancock wrote to the editor of the *Daily Telegraph*: 'Securing almost total consensus for nurse prescribing within the NHS – from the Secretary of State down – has turned out to be the easy part. Getting a measure through Parliament with which no one disagrees, is proving to be rather more difficult.'

The RCN began another parliamentary letter writing campaign. MPs were reminded of the overwhelming support which the opinion poll had revealed, and asked to write to the government seeking an explanation of the decision to delay the introduction of nurse prescribing. This campaign served to keep up the pressure on the government, and also assisted the parliamentary officers in identifying MPs who strongly supported the proposal. This information was invaluable as the opinion poll had been anonymous, and there was another opportunity for another private members' ballot in the autumn.

In her reply to numerous MPs letters on the subject, the minister continued to express her support in principle, and to outline the obstacles and reiterate the need to await the cost–benefit analysis before announcing plans for legislation. It was particularly disappointing that the summer and autumn of 1991 passed with no publication of the Touche Ross report.

November 1991

In May 1991, at RCN Congress, the secretary of state, William Waldegrave MP, had said that nurse prescribing would go ahead unless the analysis turned up unexpected problems. At the Conservative Party Conference in October 1991 he had said that nurse prescribing would go ahead in the next financial year and that enabling legislation would be introduced in the new parliament. It was, therefore, surprising and disappointing that the Queen's Speech of November 1991 failed to include provision in the government's programme for nurse prescribing legislation. Once again the only option open to the RCN was to pursue the matter through the private member's Bill procedures.

PRIVATE MEMBERS BILL MARK II

The RCN sought to attract attention to the issue of nurse prescribing in advance of the ballot for private members' Bills in the autumn of 1991. A further letter writing campaign was initiated, based on an increasingly sophisticated database of potential supporters, which had been refined in the light of responses to letters sent out in May. RCN panel members were encouraged to enter the ballot and this time luck intervened. RCN panel member Roger Sims (Conservative MP for Chislehurst) came third in the ballot for private member's Bills and in response to press enquiries indicated that he was minded to introduce a Bill to facilitate nurse prescribing.

He was immediately invited by the minister for health to a meeting at the department, where the minister and her officials sought to divert him from this course. They were, they explained, wholly in support of the principle but the time was not yet ripe for legislation. The Touche Ross report had yet to be received and considered, time was needed for detailed work on training, formularies and protocols, various professional bodies had to be consulted ... etc., etc. The department had several small uncontroversial Bills for which there was no government time but which lent themselves to the private member's procedure – perhaps Mr Sims would like to promote one of these instead?

Roger Sims was adamant. He had publicly committed himself to nurse prescribing – which, in the light of ministerial announcements, the RCN and others had expected the government itself to introduce. His Bill was simply an 'enabling' one, giving ministers power to make regulations the details of which could be worked out after the Bill was on the statute book. He could see no reason why he should not proceed. He also pointed out that if he were to withdraw his Bill this would be bound to be ascribed to 'government pressure', putting ministers in a bad light. In any case an opposition MP a little further down the list would then pick up and introduce the Bill and the government would have difficulty in opposing it.

The minister and her officials conceded. They accepted that Roger Sims would go ahead, they promised full cooperation in facilitating the drafting and passage of the Bill, and on 28 November 1991 he issued a press release announcing his intention to use his balloted time to promote nurse prescribing. Government support for the Bill was more forthcoming than it had been the previous year. William Waldegrave, the then secretary of state for health, welcomed the Bill, saying: 'The government itself firmly intended to introduce legislation at an early opportunity, once the necessary groundwork was complete, and we are pleased that Roger Sims has now provided the necessary vehicle' (Waldegrave, 1991).

Even more importantly, the drafting of the Bill itself was placed in the hands of parliamentary counsel. The RCN's earlier 'draft' Bill was rewritten, not to change the principles or the intention of the Bill, but to make sure that it satisfied the parliamentary draftsmen that it would result in workable legislation.

To become law, any Bill has to pass through the same procedures in both

Houses of Parliament, so Roger Sims had to secure a sponsor in the House of Lords. But no sooner had he announced his intention than he was offered the support of the most obvious candidate to steer nurse prescribing through the Upper House, the producer of the original report which advocated it – Baroness Julia Cumberlege.

The newly titled Medicinal Products: Prescription by Nurses etc. Bill received its formal first reading in the Commons on 4 December 1991. This was followed by publication of the document itself bearing the names of MPs of all parties to demonstrate the breadth of support for it.

The oxygen of publicity

Although more encouraging signals were being received at last from the Department of Health, two outstanding issues meant that nothing could be left to chance. First, the Touche Ross report still had not been published. Second, Parliament had entered its last session before the general election. An election had to be held before 9 July 1992. Any Bill, whether government or backbench, which has not completed its passage through parliament before the House is dissolved for a general election falls. It has to begin all over again in the new Parliament. Once again RCN activists were enlisted, through *Newsline*, to write to their local papers explaining the benefits of the measure, to seek support from local patient groups and to write to their own MPs calling on them to support the Bill at its second reading.

When the Bill was officially printed, on 15 January, Roger Sims and the RCN called a joint press conference at the House of Commons to ensure that the maximum number of supporters – both inside and outside parliament – were aware of the Bill's existence. The RCN also prepared regional press releases for that date, identifying how many patients in each region were currently being treated by health visitors and district nurses and thus highlighting the number of potential beneficiaries of the legislation.

Behind the scenes

Having already received numerous indications of the government's 'support in principle' for nurse prescribing legislation, Roger Sims undertook to establish how far the government's support would go in practice. His position as a prominent and long-standing Conservative backbencher with some interests in health and a member of the Health Select Committee was highly advantageous to the RCN: an opposition MP might not have had the access to the minister which Roger Sims was able to secure. Prior to the press conference on 15 January, Roger Sims had a private discussion about the Touche Ross cost–benefit analysis report

(DoH, 1992) – the most significant remaining hurdle for the legislation. He was given privileged access to the report, which was now finalised. His discussions and his reading of the report strengthened the case for the Bill.

The Touche Ross report itself was finally published on 21 January 1992, between the publication of the Bill and its second reading. The Touche Ross report estimated the cost of nurse prescribing at around £15 million a year, but the benefits would be improved patient care and the ability of community nurses to use their professional skills to the full.

Announcing the publication of the report in the House of Commons, the minister of state offered Roger Sims's Bill 'the government's full support' (House of Commons, 1992). Although there was wide support for the principles of the Bill, there was some concern among professionals about how it would be put into practice, and Roger Sims received a number of representations. He and the RCN stated that their intention was that under the Bill appropriately trained health visitors and district nurses would have the right to prescribe a limited range of drugs and dressings. There were other groups of nurses, such as those working in small cottage hospitals and hospices without a 'resident' doctor, who wanted to be included, whilst the British Medical Association were anxious that the Bill should not extend to hospital nurses. Both groups were given assurances which ensured their support for the legislation.

In fact, of course, the Bill simply enabled the minister to make regulations specifying those categories of nurses who could prescribe. It was clear that practicalities dictated that, at least initially, these should be limited, and health visitors and district nurses were obvious first choices. While at the time many doctors treated the proposals with a degree of suspicion, they have since become far more supportive of, and in some cases enthusiasts for, nurse prescribing.

THE PASSAGE OF LEGISLATION

The Bill's second reading, on 31 January, was accompanied by more publicity as nurses from all over the country travelled to Westminster to show their support for the measure. Parliamentary briefing was widely circulated to encourage as many supporters in the Commons as possible to attend the House and register that support. The Bill was first business that day. Roger Sims opened the proceedings by summarising the background to the Bill and its provisions and invited the House to support it. There was no opposition to the Bill and representatives of all the main political parties expressed their commitment to nurse prescribing. Indeed several MPs urged the government to grant practice nurses the same prescribing rights which were to be given to district nurses and health visitors. Others argued that hospital nurses, as well as those in the community, should be allowed to prescribe.

The minister of state was able to respond positively to the Bill. She cautiously set out the remaining issues which had to be determined and warned that the proposed government timetable was to allow nurses to begin to prescribe in October 1993. However 'we are working to a good timetable. We shall begin work on the regulations as soon as the Bill becomes an Act. There should be no problem in preparing the regulations in accordance with that timescale' (Bottomley, 1992). She concluded by wishing the Bill 'extremely well'. After a 3-hour debate, the Bill received its second reading, without a vote.

Committee stage

In accordance with normal procedure, the Bill was then referred for consideration to a standing committee of 16 MPs from all sides of the House. This is the stage at which members can give a Bill detailed scrutiny, raise questions, and propose amendments. It may be brief or it may be protracted – indeed many a private member's Bill has foundered altogether in committee. On this occasion the lobbying done beforehand paid off. When the committee met there were no questions, no amendments, all the six clauses of the Bill were agreed together without discussion; the whole proceedings took exactly 1 minute (all duly recorded in a few lines in the Official Report (Hansard) of Standing Committee A, published by HMSO at £7.50)! Similarly, when the Bill returned to the floor of the House for third reading this was given 'on the nod'.

By 28 February the Bill received its second reading in the House of Lords, introduced as promised by Baroness Cumberlege. Once again the Bill received unanimous support from all parties. It seemed that, finally, the Bill would reach the statute book. But there was one final obstacle: the general election.

Up against the clock

All Bills pass through similar procedures in both houses of parliament. In each they require a formal first reading, a second reading (debate on the principle of the Bill) and the opportunity in committee and on report to discuss any amendments before being given a final, third reading. Any amendments then need to be agreed by the two houses before the Bill is given the royal assent and becomes an Act. Obviously, such procedures usually mean that a Bill may take a matter of months to pass through both houses.

On 11 March 1992 a general election was called for 9 April 1992. The Bill had yet to complete its passage through parliament and was in danger of being lost, along with many other worthy measures, when parliament was dissolved. However, it received its third reading in the House of Lords on 12 March, without debate.

On 16 March a Royal Commission of senior peers assembled in the House of Lords with authority to act on behalf of Her Majesty. Under the watchful eye of Roger Sims in the MPs' Gallery, its first task was to give royal assent to several Bills, including the Medicinal Products: Prescription by Nurses etc. Bill, with the traditional Norman French words 'La reine le veult' (The Queen wishes it). The Commission went on the proclaim the dissolution of parliament prior to the forthcoming general election. So the Bill had just made it, was now an Act, and nurse prescribing was on the statute book.

CONCLUSION

For an apparently uncontroversial measure, nurse prescribing became embroiled in a complex political battle. The RCN had successfully demonstrated at every possible opportunity the strength and range of support for the measure – from fellow professionals such as the BMA and the Royal College of General Practitioners, from patient and user groups, and from MPs across the political spectrum. Yet the experience of the legislative process, and the government's apparent reluctance to speed the measure, demonstrates the intensity of competing demands for government time.

It is to the credit of the many contributing officials and activists of the RCN, to the persuasive and persevering MPs Dudley Fishburn and Roger Sims, as well as Baroness Cumberlege, and to the supporters of the Bill that continuous publicity and pressure or 'lobbying' finally had a beneficial effect. Luck, of course, played its part – for example when Dudley Fishburn found time for a second reading, and when Roger Sims secured a prominent position in the private members' ballot. However, it was a well orchestrated and increasingly sophisticated campaign over a period of several years which finally culminated in the required legislative change.

It may be that the delays and setbacks are symptomatic of a wider problem which nurses face in the world of politics: that nursing issues are often sidelined in discussions about the future of the health service. There were no nurses in the House of Commons to speak directly for the profession. The RCN and others rely heavily on committed supporters, such as the parliamentary panel who, in turn, have many competing demands on their time. The subsequent delays in the implementation of nurse prescribing have further fuelled the belief that nursing issues are of secondary significance in the eyes of many politicians. Cynics may argue that the pressure of a general election creates the opportunity for nurses to be heard by a government keen to seek support wherever it can. Just as with the successful passage of the Bill prior to the 1992 election, so prior to the 1997 election the final stages of implementation of nurse prescribing were announced.

A number of incidents which led to the setting up of the Nolan enquiry and the subsequent report (House of Commons, 1995) have given the impression that 'lobbying' is a disreputable activity. Providing legislators with information and seeking to persuade them as to the strength and justice of a case is in fact an essential part of the parliamentary democratic process, but of course there are a variety of ways of doing this. The manner in which this activity has been carried out in recent years has, in some instances, reflected no credit on either the lobbyists or MPs involved, and has sadly tarnished the reputation of parliament as a whole.

The Royal College of Nursing's method of operation could be said to be a model of how lobbying can, and should, be done. The RCN 'cultivates' a handful of members from both houses of parliament and from all parties who form their panel, arranging occasional meetings and an annual working dinner with the general secretary and senior officers. The RCN provides large numbers of MPs with succinct briefs on current issues and has a high profile presence at Party Conferences. It thus ensures that, when they are needed, the RCN has at Westminster a core of activists and a wide, sympathetic and informed body of support. The story of nurse prescribing shows what this can achieve.

QUESTIONS FOR DISCUSSION

- Would the presence of nurses in the House of Commons have made any difference to the passage of this legislation?

- What distinguishes disreputable lobbying activity from pressure groups acting as an essential part of the democratic process?

- Would any other profession have to have worked so hard or so long to achieve so uncontroversial an aim?

REFERENCES

Bottomley, V. (1991a) HC Deb 4.2.91 c 53W. London: HMSO.
Bottomley, V. (1991b) HC Deb 26.4.91 c 576W. . London: HMSO.
Bottomley, V. (1992) HC Deb 31.1.92 c 1232. . London: HMSO.
Department of Health and Social Security (1986) *Neighbourhood Nursing – A Focus for Care. Report of the community nursing review.* (Cumberledge Report.) London: HMSO.
Department of Health (1989) *Report of the Advisory Group on Nurse Prescribing.* (Crown Report.) London: HMSO.
Department of Health (1992) *Nurse Prescribing Final Report: a cost benefit study by Touche Ross.* London: HMSO.
House of Commons Social Services Committee (1987) *Primary Health Care First report of the committee, 1986–87.* HC 37. London: HMSO.
House of Commons (1991) *Nurses Prescribing Bill.* (Bill 71 of 1990–91.) Introduced under the 10-minute rule by Dudley Fishburn. HC Deb 30.1.91 c 944.
House of Commons (1991) HC Deb vol 190 c 593–97. London: HMSO.
House of Commons (1992) HC Deb 21.1.92 c 174. London: HMSO.
House of Commons (1995) House of Commons Committee on Standards in Public Life. *Standards in Public Life. First report.* Cm 2850–1 London: HMSO.

Market Access (1991) Survey conducted as part of Market Access Political Opinion Panel April 1991.

Royal College of Nursing (1991) *Newsline*, **16(1)**, January.

Waldegrave, W. (1991) Department of Health press notice H91/591, 29.11.91. London: Department of Health.

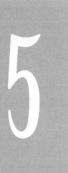

5

Nurse prescribing

A legal minefield?

Helen Caulfield

Key issues

♦ Prescribing powers for nurses are determined by the Medicines Act 1968, and subsequent legislation.

♦ The advantages and disadvantages of different sources of law are explained; these place the legislation of prescribing into context.

♦ A detailed examination of the provisions of the legislation which controls prescribing powers sets out the structure of the legislation and looks in detail at the provisions which most significantly affect nurses.

♦ Definitions in the legislation which have caused confusion in interpretation are set out in a separate section.

♦ Legal implications of protocols and the future development of nurse prescribing through protocols are examined.

♦ Government reviews of the legal situation relating to prescribing powers and protocols will affect practice for all nurses.

INTRODUCTION

The political, social and economic arguments for the development of prescribing powers for nurses need to take into account the legal aspects which can permit or prevent the supply, administration and prescription by nurses. The legal framework is set out in legislation which is not readily understood on the first time of reading, and the old clichés that lawyers always have a supply of cold towels to hand when studying Acts of parliament was never as true as when studying the legislation for prescription only medicines.

The Medicines Act 1968 is a vast piece of legislation which covers the establishment of the Medicines Agency, the manner and type of licence needed for research on medicinal products, the manufacture, import and storage of medicines, and – of particular relevance to nursing and midwifery – the manner in which medicines can be supplied and administered by health professionals such as doctors, pharmacists, nurses and midwives. A detailed study of the Statutory Instruments which accompanies the study of the primary legislation throws up some curious anomalies. For example, occupational health nurses have specific authority to supply prescription only medicines under provisions in a Statutory Instrument, (Part 3, Schedule 3, the Medicines (Products other than Veterinary Drugs) (Prescription Only) Order 1983 SI 1983 no. 1212), and anyone, including non health care professionals, can administer a medicine in an emergency (Regulation 5, the Medicines (Products other than Veterinary Drugs) (Prescription Only) Order 1983 SI 1983 no. 1212), which is a useful power for teachers, but may cause some concern for school nurses.

The introduction of prescribing powers for nurses in the Medicinal Products: Prescriptions by Nurses etc., Act 1992 provides new boundaries in prescribing for nurses. As concern grows about consistency across Europe, it is possible to trace the development of collaboration between member states of the European Union in order to safeguard consistency of practice in prescribing across member countries.

Understanding the legal framework will assist any nurse interested in developing prescribing skills to understand the core legal elements, and how these relate to the current practice in community and acute settings. An analysis of the legislation will separate out these issues to ensure that any nursing development within prescribing remains legal. The legislation which governs prescribing sets out some precise definitions and parameters of practice which must be followed by health professionals. Failure to do so may be a criminal offence. A glossary of definitions is shown at the end of the chapter, with direct reference to the legislation.

One of the main problems with the Medicines Act 1968 is that it is now 3 decades old, and it no longer fully takes into account the way in which nursing practice has developed over the last 30 years. Patient demand and the increasing use of technology require an approach from nursing which is not permitted under the Medicines Act 1968. Several sections of the Medicines Act 1968 would need to be amended to bring the provisions up to date to reflect the demand from both nurses and patients for increased prescribing powers for nurses.

SOURCES OF LAW

1. Legislation

Legislation is found in primary sources known as Acts of parliament, and secondary sources known as Orders, or Statutory Instruments. The parliamentary process requires that all primary legislation is debated in both the House of Commons and the House of Lords before coming into effect. The general route for an Act to be passed into law is that proposals for new legislation are set out in a consultation document known as a Green Paper. This outlines the area of concern and the way in which the legislation can address the issues. This is followed by a White Paper which outlines the course of action the government proposes to take in relation to the proposed new legislation. A draft of the proposed Act of parliament, known as a Bill, is then introduced in parliament, and follows a process which includes first and second readings, a committee stage and a report stage. Once this process has been finished, a vote on introducing the new Act is passed in both houses of parliament. Once the Act is passed, it is given the royal assent by the Queen and then becomes law.

Statutory Instruments are not debated in parliament, although they are approved by parliament. As a result, Statutory Instruments can become law more quickly than Acts. Once passed, Statutory Instruments have the same legislative status as the primary legislation. Failure to comply with either the statute or the Statutory Instrument will be unlawful. It may be a criminal offence and the penalties (usually a fine, or in some cases imprisonment) will be set out in the legislation.

One advantage of legislation is that it creates certainty. There is a growing body of statutes which relate to the provision and the regulation of health care which have an impact on nursing practice, and which govern an increasing part of the nurse/patient relationship. Examples include the Abortion Act 1967, the Access to Health Records Act 1990, the Medicines Act 1968, the Mental Health Act 1983 and the Children Act 1989.

There can be disadvantages in relying on legislation to determine health matters. Legislation is rigid, and generally does not allow for any flexibility in the development of nursing practice. One example of this arises from the Medicines Act 1968 which does not give powers to prescribe to registered nurses, and which has since required amending legislation in the Medicinal Products: Prescriptions by Nurses etc., Act 1992. In many ways, legislation relating to health care can only provide a snapshot of nursing practice at the time the Act was passed. In addition, if defects in the wording of the legislation are discovered at a later stage, the amending procedure needed is onerous and time-consuming.

The main advantage of secondary legislation is that it allows detailed drafting of specific matters which are too wide to be included in primary legislation. The Medicines Act 1968, for example, allows for Statutory

Instruments to be drafted to detail which medicines should be considered prescription only medicines.

2. Common law

Common law is decided by a judge in court who hears an individual case and who makes a decision on the facts of that case. The decision is known as the judgement. The judgement will create a precedent which can be used in future court hearings. This ensures that there is consistency in judgements. It is possible to appeal against a judgement. The decision of a High Court judge can be challenged in the Court of Appeal, and a further appeal may be taken to the House of Lords. A significant amount of health law has been decided in the courts. The procedure used in most of these cases is known as judicial review, where the aim of one party is to test the legality of legislation or other matters such as National Health Service circulars.

It is an increasing feature of the common law that the courts are willing to hear cases brought by individuals or by organisations who wish to challenge the decision of a public body. Where there is a conflict between the common law and legislation, the legislation always takes precedence. Interpretation of an Act of parliament takes place in court and not in parliament. Those decisions on how the Act should be interpreted then form part of common law and determine the way in which the legislation is interpreted in the future. For example, Diane Blood challenged the wording of the Human Embryology and Fertilisation Act 1990 which only allowed her to receive her dead husband's sperm with his prior written consent. The interpretation of the relevant part of the legislation was heard in the High Court and then on appeal to the Court of Appeal. The court decided that the legislation did in fact require the prior written consent. As a result of the case, calls were made to amend the legislation.

In many health care situations, an application can be made to the court for guidance on legal issues where no legislation exists. In 1993, the legal issues surrounding the withdrawal of treatment from a patient in a persistent vegetative state were discussed in court in the first case dealing with the best interests of a person with persistent vegetative state, in *Airedale NHS Trust* v. *Bland* (Airedale NHS Trust, 1993). Among the arguments raised were questions of whether it was lawful to withdraw artificial hydration and nutrition from the patient, knowing that it would lead to his death. This was the first time this situation had been raised, and no legislation existed to clarify any of the issues involved. Such cases become legal precedent so that future decisions can refer back to the judicial reasoning which took place in earlier cases.

The advantage of case law is that the courts can assess in detail the factual content of the case which is brought before it for determination. This can be particularly useful in health issues where new matters may arise which have not been considered by any other forum. The development of new technology, the pace of change in the National Health Service, the increase in the number of specialist nurses, and the increasing demand by users of the service to be informed and participate in their care are all factors which suggest that the courts will continue to be used to determine issues of importance to the health professions as a whole.

Many trusts are prepared to take cases to court for determination by a judge to establish a particular legal principle which will affect their own policy in the future and those of other trusts. Case law can provide useful precedent for health professionals in determining clinical practice. The court may lay down guidelines to be followed in all cases where similar facts arise. If nursing practice or technology alters within the near future, it would be open to another trust or individual to approach the court to ask that a reconsideration of those guidelines take place. If the court agrees, this can enable professional practice to develop. The publicity given to the case of a woman who refused intervention in labour is one example. The trust asked the court for a declaration which would allow them to provide intervention, even though the woman refused to consent. The court gave permission for the intervention and the child was delivered by caesarean section against the mother's wishes. The mother later appealed against this decision and her case was heard on appeal in the Court of Appeal which has now issued guidelines which now apply to all situations where a person refuses to consent to treatment considered to be necessary for their health (St George's Healthcare NHS Trusts, 1998).

There are significant disadvantages with relying on case law to promote certainty amongst health professionals. The courts can only deal with the cases which are referred to them. There may be many situations in which nurses are unsure about their standing legally, but are unable to seek further guidance without making an application to the court. In these situations, lawyers for nurses and trusts need to 'second guess' the reaction of the court in providing advice in a particular situation, and this does not provide certainty in advance of the hearing. Another disadvantage of relying on case law is that completely novel issues may be presented to the court where the judges do not feel that they have the experience or expertise to make important decisions. In such cases there is a danger that health professionals believe that the judge is the best qualified person to make these decisions. Very often the reality is that the clinical staff themselves have the expertise, professional standing and experience to guide a path through the difficulties.

3. Codes of conduct and codes of practice

The UKCC is the statutory regulatory body of the nursing, midwifery and health visiting professions and was set up by an Act of parliament in

1979. The legislation which governs the UKCC has been amended since then and the current Act setting out its functions was passed in 1997 (Nurses, Midwives and Health Visitors Act, 1997). The regulatory body is charged with acting as parliament's representative in regulating the nursing professions. The UKCC Code of Conduct (UKCC, 1992a) sets out the extent of the professional duty required of a nurse, midwife or health visitor. It is a requirement of the statutory regulatory body that the professions adhere to the Code of Conduct, and failure to do so may lead to a nurse, midwife or health visitor being made the subject of a complaint to the regulatory body and where appropriate, being removed from the register.

The regulatory body determines the professional duty of nurses and midwives. In some cases this may be more extensive than their legal duty. If a nurse appears in court for any reason, he or she may be found liable in negligence, or guilty of a criminal offence. While the courts have power to order a nurse to pay compensation, or to impose a criminal sentence, they do not have the power to order that the nurse be prohibited from working as a nurse. There is, for example, no legal duty for a nurse 'to safeguard and promote the interests of individual patients and clients', but there is a professional duty to do so under Paragraph 1 of the Code of Conduct. The regulatory body alone holds the power to determine whether or not the nurse has behaved in a professional manner, sufficient for him or her to remain on the register.

Codes of practice differ from codes of conduct in that they are produced by groups of professional organisations which give guidance to those professions on the extent to which practice should be followed. One example is the code of practice for use by health professionals under the Mental Health Act 1983. Another code of practice has been developed as required under section 25 of the Human Fertilisation and Embryology Act 1990. Codes of practice are a form of law in which the rules are not legally binding. These codes of practice are different from codes of conduct established by the regulatory body for health professionals, such as the UKCC and the GMC. It is likely that the courts would place enormous significance on any code of practice where a health care case was referred to the court for determination. The advantage of this is clear; the court would be able to assess immediately the view of the profession on a particular aspect, and to be much clearer about determining the extent of professional practice in relation to a particular health issue. A further advantage of a code of practice is that it is easy to amend to keep it in line with current philosophical and practice issues.

The disadvantages of a code of practice appear to be minimal. Although a code of practice does not have the same weight in law as a statute or a court judgement, it is difficult to see why it could not take on a quasi legal form and be used as a standard bearer for practice in a particular field.

4. Department of Health directives

The Secretary of State for Health is given power under sections 13–17 of the National Health Service Act 1977 to issue directions which, because they arise from a statutory basis, must be obeyed. Further guidance from the NHS Executive on how trusts and health authorities should discharge their functions may be contained in directives or in executive letters, guidance and circulars. The matters contained in these directives are usually of an internal nature and do not affect the rights of patients. They do not have a statutory impact and a voluntary compliance is intended. These directives are capable of legal challenge. In one case, the High Court held that a health authority had a duty to give serious consideration to the contents of an executive letter when discharging its functions, and that failure to do so was unlawful. The judge ordered the health authority to implement a policy which took into account the policy expressed in the executive letter within 14 days of the judgement (*R* v. *North Derbyshire Health Authority ex parte Fisher*, 1997).

5. European law

A further source of legislation comes from Europe which requires member states to implement community law through their own Acts of parliament. European legislation (also known as European Directives) includes a variety of issues. In health matters, the European Directive on the manual handling of loads in 1990 and that on the protection of pregnant workers rights are now part of UK law. Matters relating to the standardisation of medicines and controls for the safe use and development of new pharmaceutical products are also European issues.

PRESCRIBING: THE LEGISLATION

The law which governs prescribing is found in the following legislation:

1. Medicines Act 1968
2. Medicinal Products: Prescription by Nurses etc., Act 1992
3. Medicines (Products other than Veterinary Drugs) (Prescription Only) Order 1983 SI 1212

1. Medicines Act 1968

The primary legislation is the Medicines Act 1968. The Medicines Act covers a vast range of powers and duties in relation to the manner in which medicines can be described as prescription only medicines, and sets out the basis on which they can be imported, manufactured, stored, sold, supplied and administered. The Act is divided into eight main parts with separate provisions for each aspect of the safe control of medicines. Most importantly for nurses, the Act sets out the groups of professionals who can prescribe, and the manner in which prescription only medicines can be supplied and administered. It is this aspect of the Act which will be described in detail and discussed, although a short description of the eight main parts of the Act is set out below:

Part 1 establishes the Medicines Commission, the body which advises the licensing authority on the safety and quality of medicines and on the granting of licences allowed under the legislation.

Part 2 sets out the provisions for the procedures to be adopted when a licence is granted to manufacturers and suppliers of medicines. Under this section it is unlawful to manufacture or assemble medicinal products without a licence. It is also unlawful to sell, supply, or to procure the sale, supply or manufacture of medicinal products without a licence.

Part 3 deals with situations where a sale, supply or administration of a medicine is made without a licence. The general rule is that it is a criminal offence to sell or supply any prescription only medicine unless it is in certain specified circumstances.

Part 4 covers pharmacies, their registration and qualification.

Part 5 covers the packaging, labelling and identification of medicinal products. For example, section 66 gives power to the appropriate ministers to draw up regulations to deal with the accommodation, storage, safe-keeping, disposal, record keeping, sanitation, use of apparatus and disposal of refuse from premises of medicinal products.

Part 6 covers the advertisement and sales promotion of medicinal products.

Part 7 covers the provisions for publications such as the British Pharmacopoeia which provide information on substances and articles used in the practice of medicine, surgery, dentistry and midwifery. Part 7 does not cover nursing practice. These publications include the names of substances and articles and can be updated and published as the British Pharmacopoeia, the British National Formulary, as well as other lists of names and compendiums prepared.

Part 8 covers miscellaneous provisions.

2. Medicinal Products: Prescription by Nurses etc., Act 1992

This Act is very short. It amends the Medicines Act 1968 to include registered nurses, midwives and health visitors as appropriate practitioners in section 58 'who are of such a description and comply with such conditions as may be specified in the order'.

3. The Medicines (Products other than Veterinary Drugs) (Prescription Only) Order 1983 Statutory Instrument 1212

The Medicines Act 1968 allowed for the introduction of Statutory Instruments to provide in more detail the naming of prescription only medicines. There have been over 17 other Statutory Instruments since then which largely deal with the adding or deletion of certain drugs from the various schedules. The most significant Statutory Instrument relating to prescribing was introduced in 1983. This contains many definitions relating to the prescribing of prescription only medicines and it must be read in conjunction with the Medicines Act 1968, and the Medicinal Products: Prescription by Nurses etc. Act 1992.

SPECIFIC PROVISIONS OF THE LEGISLATION
The legal requirements for a prescription

Regulation 12 of the 1983 Statutory Instrument specifies the conditions which need to be in place before a prescription is lawful. The prescription must be in writing and signed by the practitioner giving it. The prescription must have the name of the practitioner giving the prescription and state whether the practitioner is a doctor or dentist. The prescription must contain the date on which it was written; and where the patient is under 12 years of age the prescription must show the patient's date of birth. The prescription is valid for 6 months. The prescription may include a repeat prescription, in which case the prescription only medicine can be dispensed once more within 6 months. After that time, a new prescription is needed.

The purpose of the requirements is to ensure that prescription only medicines are only provided by way of written prescription. The same Statutory Instrument took into account the practical issue arising in a hospital situation where it may place excessive demands on doctors there to write out every prescription needed on each occasion for each patient. Regulation 10 of the 1983 Statutory Instrument removes the need for a prescription to be in writing for the supply of prescription only medicine in a hospital where that medicine is supplied 'in accordance with the written directions of a doctor'. The contrast between a prescription in writing and written directions is significant. This allows doctors in hospital settings the authority to enter prescribing directions onto a computer by code, for example, where there were written directions in place that authorised this to happen.

Section 9 of the Medicines Act 1968 deals with the types of licence which need to be granted before a person can supply or sell a prescription only medicine. Licences are granted by the Medicines Agency. Under this section doctors and dentists are allowed to import for administration or to supply or sell a particular product without a licence where this is to a particular patient of his or hers (section 9(1)(a)). Nurses have no such legal authority. Registered nurses and midwives are allowed to assemble a product without a licence (section 11(1)), but registered nurses or midwives cannot import prescription only medicines in order to sell, supply or administer to patients unless they have a licence. Any development in the powers to prescribe for nurses may need to include an amendment to section 9 to avoid the prospect of a registered nurse having to apply for a licence to import for the purpose of supplying or administering a prescription only medicine where a medical colleague is exempt from doing so.

Clinical trials of prescription only medicines

The Medicines Act 1968 contains provisions relating to clinical trials. For example, under section 31, it is forbidden to sell or supply a medicine for a clinical trial without a licence unless the clinical trial is carried out by a doctor or dentist. This section would also need to be amended to bring some aspects of nursing practice relating to research into the effects of prescription only medicines so that nurses involved in clinical trials could be allowed to obtain prescription only medicines without a licence.

Premises on which prescription only medicines can be supplied or administered

Section 52 of the Medicines Act 1968 prohibits the sale or supply of prescription only medicines unless the person is a pharmacist, or the sale or supply takes place in a pharmacy. This part of the legislation was subject to analysis by the High Court in 1997. A GP practice had applied for outline consent to dispense medicines to patients living in its practice area, but more than 1 mile away from a pharmacy. The local family health services authority (FHSA) granted the application which was then opposed by the pharmacist who subsequently sought a judicial review of the decision. The pharmacist argued that the arrangements for dispensing would contravene the Medicines Act as the FHSA were granting unlawful authority for persons other than a doctor to and who may not be qualified, to do the dispensing. The High Court held that section 52 (c) of the Medicines Act 1968 allowed for another person, in this case a doctor, the authority to act on behalf of the pharmacist. The High Court found that a doctor had 'a particular personal responsibility' in a locality in which he or his practice would remain, and this responsibility could not be avoided, (*R* v. *FHSA Appeals Authority*, 1997).

Section 53 prohibits the sale or supply of prescription only medicines at premises other than a pharmacy unless:

[the] place at which the medicinal product is sold, offered, exposed or supplied ... must be premises of which the person carrying on the business ... is the occupier and which he is able to close so as to exclude the public ... and the prescription only medicine has been assembled for sale elsewhere. The business ... must be carried on in accordance with such conditions as may be prescribed for the purposes of this section.

This means that the conditions in which prescription only medicines can be stored or kept for supply are controlled by the legislation. The restrictions in sections 52 and 53 which control the type of premises on which prescription only medicines can be sold or supplied are softened by the provisions of section 55 which do not apply to the sale or supply of a medicine by doctors or dentists to their patients, or to persons under their care (section 55 (1)(a)). This section means that doctors or dentists can supply a prescription only medicine to patients anywhere. This section, for example, allows doctors to supply prescription only medicines to patients in their own homes. Because this section specifies doctors and dentists only, it would need to be amended with any extension to the powers for prescribing to nurses in order to allow them to prescribe and supply prescription only medicines away from a clinic.

The provisions in sections 52 and 53 do not apply to the sale or supply of a medicine where this takes place 'in the course of the business of a hospital or health centre'. The legislation has included the additional provision that where the sale or supply is to be administered in the hospital, the health centre or elsewhere this must be done 'in accordance with the directions of a doctor or dentist' (section 55 (1)(b)).

The consequences of sections 52–55 of the Medicines Act 1968 are that prescription only medicines can be supplied to a patient in any location by a doctor. Where nurses want to supply prescription only medicines, they can do so only if they are normally based in a hospital or a health centre, and they have 'directions' to do so from a doctor. These directions can be written or oral. This section would cover, for example, all community nurses visiting and supplying prescription only medicines to patients at home.

Supply and administration by registered nurses and midwives

There are important provisions in section 55 which give specific powers to some registered nurses and to midwives. Section 55(2)(a) allows registered nurses to sell or supply a prescription only medicine in the course of their professional practice where a Statutory Instrument has specified which prescription only medicines can be sold or supplied. This section does not, however, give registered nurses the power to administer prescription only medicines in the course of their professional practice. The arrangements are more extensive for midwives who can be given authority to sell, supply or administer prescription only medicines under local arrangements made by a health authority or a health board under section 55 (2)(b).

Section 55 is the provision in the primary legislation which gives legal authority for registered nurses and midwives to sell or supply prescription only medicines. This power is activated once any Statutory Instrument is passed which specifies the prescription only medicines which can be supplied. There is no requirement that the registered nurse or midwife needs to have specific prescribing rights. This power has already been activated in the Medicines (Products other than Veterinary Drugs) (Prescription Only) Order 1983 Statutory Instrument 1212 Schedule 3, which gives authority to both occupational health nurses, and to midwives to sell or supply prescription only medicines.

Section 57 gives authority to the Secretary of State for Health to introduce a Statutory Instrument which provides that section 55 (1)(b) or (2) shall cease to have effect, or shall have effect subject to such exceptions or modifications as may be specified in the Statutory Instrument. For example, a new Statutory Instrument could expand the definition in section 55 of 'the business of a hospital or health centre' to include the business of a trust or of a primary care group, and this would allow for the sale, supply or administration of prescription only medicines to take place outside a clinic. This would cover for example, the provision which would allow nurses to supply or administer prescription only medicines to the homeless from a variety of settings.

SECTION 58, PRESCRIBING POWERS FOR NURSES?

Section 58 is a key part of the legislation and is the section of the Medicines Act 1968 which has caused the greatest confusion in relation to nurses being able to supply and administer prescription only medicines under protocols (see Box 5.1).

There are two separate powers in section 58 in relation to providing prescription only medicines. These two powers are 'supply' and 'administration'. The use of language in this section is critical to the understanding of the way in which nurses can be involved in the supply and administration of medicines. It is therefore important that nurses have an understanding of the definitions used in this section.

Appropriate practitioner

The provisions of section 58 mean that only doctors, dentists, and veterinary surgeons have the legal authority to prescribe. This is because they

Box 5.1 Section 58 Medicines Act 1968

58(1) The appropriate Ministers may by order specify descriptions or classes of medicinal products for the purposes of this section; and, in relation to any description or class so specified, the order shall state which of the following, that is to say–

(a) doctors,

(b) dentists, and

(c) veterinary surgeons and veterinary practitioners, are to be appropriate practitioners for the purposes of this section.

58(2) Subject to the following provisions of this section–

(a) no person shall sell by retail, or supply in circumstances corresponding to retail sale, a medicinal product of a description, or falling within a class, specified in an order under this section except in accordance with a prescription given by an appropriate practitioner; and

(b) no person shall administer (otherwise than to himself) any such medicinal product unless he is an appropriate practitioner or a person acting in accordance with the directions of an appropriate practitioner.

58(3) Subsection (2)(a) of this section shall not apply–

(a) to the sale or supply of a medicinal product to a patient of his by a doctor or dentist who is an appropriate practitioner, or

(b) to the sale or supply of a medicinal product, for administration to an animal or herd under his care, by a veterinary surgeon or veterinary practitioner who is an appropriate practitioner.

are the only professionals to be described as 'appropriate practitioners'. As an 'appropriate practitioner' they have authority to provide a prescription. Section 58 is the key provision of the Medicines Act 1968 which limits the power to prescribe to doctors, dentists and vets.

It is this section which is amended by the Medicinal Products: Prescription by Nurses etc., Act 1992. This Act amends section 58(1)(a) by adding nurses as an additional group of professionals with power to prescribe. This power to prescribe for nurses, however, is subject to the introduction of further Statutory Instruments which specify the qualifications those nurses are to have, and the extent to which they are to be able to prescribe. The introduction of pilot sites for nurse prescribing has been by way of Statutory Instrument which was triggered by the amendment to section 58(1)(a). Those nurses who worked in the demonstration sites were given specific powers to prescribe from a limited formulary.

Supply

Section 58 is clear in the use of its language that there are no provisions which allow a nurse to supply a prescription only medicine unless the nurse has the prescription from the doctor or dentist. There are some exemptions to this in regulation 10 of the 1983 Statutory Instrument. These exemptions cover hospitals and allow for the possibility that a nurse can supply a prescription only medicine where the sale or supply is 'in the course of the business of a hospital' and the prescription only medicine is sold or supplied in accordance with the written directions of a doctor or dentist, even when the directions do not comply with the legal requirements of a prescription. This provision allows doctors, for example, to write on a patient's chart or in a patient's notes the prescription to be supplied by the nurse, without following the requirements for the prescription under regulation 12 which specify the conditions for the prescription to be lawful.

Directions

Much of the speculation surrounding the development and use of protocols, whether they are for an individual or for a group, appears to arise from the use of the facility in section 58 which allows an appropriate practitioner to give 'directions' to another person to administer prescription only medicines. There is no definition in the legislation which describes the extent or the meaning of 'directions'. This is an unfortunate omission in the drafting of the legislation. Because there is no definition of directions, nurses and doctors have interpreted this phrase as the legal authority through which they can develop clinical practice in prescribing based on protocols.

It is important to understand that the use of the facility of 'directions' applies only to the administration of medicine. It does not apply to the supply of medicine. Where an appropriate practitioner wishes to develop a protocol which will allow nurses to be involved in the prescribing process, this can only be lawful when the process relates to the administration of medicines. It is lawful to use the protocol where an administration is indicated. It is not lawful to use a protocol where a supply is indicated.

There is no provision that directions need be in writing or relate to a specific patient. It appears lawful, for example, for a practice nurse to administer 'flu vaccines to a category of patients on the verbal directions of a doctor without the need for a specific prescription.

Because there is no definition of 'directions' in the legislation, the law is unclear here, and it is appropriate that nursing practice follows a proper course of action that written directions in the form of a protocol would allow for clear and adequate understanding between the doctor and nurse in such cases. Directions contained in a protocol should be specific enough to ensure that the administration is clinically proper. Nurses would be advised to require a written protocol rather than oral directions to avoid any misunderstanding.

Administration

Section 58(2)(a) of the 1968 Act applies to the administration of prescription only medicines. 'Administer' is defined by the Medicines (Products other than Veterinary Drugs) (Prescription Only) Order 1983 SI 1983 1212 as 'parenteral administration covering administration by breach of skin or the mucus membrane'. This has the odd effect that administration by injection falls within section 58(2)(b), but administration to the body does not. Parenteral administration would cover all injections, but provides a curious anomaly which suggests that polio vaccines and dressings are not included in the definition of the Medicines Act 1968, and therefore fall outside the provisions of the legislation. Application of prescription only medicine dressings does not fall within the section, neither does the placing of a prescription only medicine on a patient's tongue. As a result, the legislation does not cover these situations and on this analysis, nurses do not need a prescription or a protocol in order to give a lawful polio vaccine.

The 1983 Statutory Instrument Schedule 3 is divided into three parts. Each part of Schedule 3 lists those persons who are exempted from following the provisions of section 58. This schedule names the group of persons exempted, the names of the prescription only medicines which the group can sell, supply or administer, and the conditions attached to the group.

Part 1 describes those groups who can sell or supply prescription only medicines. Midwives are one group who are exempt from the provisions of section 58 for the sale or supply of prescription only medicines containing various substances (for example chloral hydrate, and in the case of ergometrine maleate only when contained in a medicinal product which is not for parenteral administration). The conditions are that the sale or supply shall only be in the course of their professional practice.

Part 2 describes those groups who can supply. One of these groups covers: 'persons requiring prescription only medicines for the purpose of enabling them, in the course of any business carried on by them, to comply with any requirements made by or in pursuance of any enactment with respect to the medical treatment of their employees.' This group can supply prescription only medicines specified in the relevant enactment.

'Persons operating an occupational health scheme' are allowed to supply prescription only medicines which have been sold or supplied to the occupational health scheme in response to an order signed by a doctor or a registered nurse. The conditions are that if the supply is made by the nurse, he or she must be acting in accordance with the written instructions of a doctor as to the circumstances in which the prescription only medicine is to be used.

Part 3 describes the groups who can administer prescription only medicines. One such group are registered midwives, who can administer from a list of prescription only medicines including, for example, lignocaine. The conditions are that the administration shall be only in the course of their professional practice and, in the case of three specified prescription only medicines, shall only be while attending a woman in childbirth.

Another group are 'persons operating an occupational health scheme'. They are allowed to administer prescription only medicines for parenteral administration in response to an order in writing signed by a doctor or a registered nurse. If the individual administering the prescription only medicine is not a doctor or acting in accordance with the directions of a doctor, he or she must be a registered nurse acting in accordance with the written instructions of a doctor as to the circumstances in which the prescription only medicine is to be used in the course of the occupational health scheme.

A further group are persons who work in osteopathy, naturopathy, acupuncture, or 'other similar field', except chiropody. They are allowed to administer prescription only medicine for parenteral use only. The conditions are that 'the person administering the prescription only medicine shall have been requested by or on behalf of the person to whom it is administered and in that person's presence to use his own judgement as to the treatment required.'

Emergency requirement for prescription only medicines

Regulation 5 of the 1983 Statutory Instrument lessens the strict effect of section 58(2)(b) of the Medicines Act 1968, and allows named prescription only medicines to be administered, apparently by anyone, without the directions of a doctor where the situation is an emergency for the purpose of saving a life. This means that parents or teachers who need to administer adrenalin for the purpose of an emergency, perhaps where a child has suffered anaphylactic shock, are covered for such an action which under the legislation is lawful.

Regulation 6 of the 1983 Statutory Instrument lessens the strict effect of section 58(2)(a) of the Medicines Act 1968, and allows the emergency supply of a prescription only medicine by a pharmacist where the request to supply has come from a doctor who is unable to issue a prescription immediately but who undertakes to do so within 72 hours. The pharmacist must supply the prescription only medicine in accordance with the directions of the doctor and make a record in the register. Pharmacists are also allowed to supply a prescription only medicine themselves where there is an immediate need for a prescription only medicine, it is impractical for the patient or the pharmacist to obtain a prescription, the patient has already had the prescription only medicine under prescription, and the dose is appropriate. Pharmacists can provide a supply for 5 days or a full cycle of an oral contraceptive drug. A pharmacist cannot supply the morning after pill unless the woman can show that she has already had it before.

Miscellaneous provisions

Section 58 gives power to the appropriate ministers to specify in a Statutory Instrument the descriptions or classes of medicinal products which can be supplied or administered by an appropriate practitioner (i.e. doctors, dentists, vets and now nurses). Before making such an order, the appropriate ministers shall consult the appropriate committee (section 58 (6)). The order may also allow for specified exemptions (section 58 (4)(a)), and these exemptions may be subject to conditions or limitations specified in the order (section 58 (5)).

The Pharmaceutical Society has a duty to enforce the provisions of section 58 in England and Wales concurrently with the minister (section 108(6)) except where the activity takes place in a hospital or 'so much of any premises as is used by a practitioner for carrying on his practice' (section 108(9)). It is interesting that none of the professional bodies are included in this monitoring. This implies that nurses with prescribing powers need to be monitored by the Pharmaceutical Society and this may indicate the Pharmaceutical Society would need to be involved in consultation about the training courses and development of practice for nurses with prescribing powers.

Before making any regulations or orders under the Act, the minister shall consult with 'such organisations as appear to them to be representative of interests likely to be substantially affected by the regulations or order.' (section 129(6)). The ministers must consult with a committee or the Medicines Commission with respect to the proposal they intend to make by the regulations or order and shall take the advice into account before proceeding with the proposals (section 129(7)).

PROTOCOLS: LEGAL IMPLICATIONS

For several years now, certainly prior to the passing of legislation enabling limited prescribing by nurses, it has been common practice for nurses to supply prescription only medicines under protocol arrangements. This practice is particularly prevalent in family planning clinics and with practice nurses.

Essentially, a protocol in this context is a written directive from a doctor, authorising nurses to give patients prescription only medicine from a predetermined list. The nurses have to acknowledge their competence and accept professional responsibility in this regard. For example, a patient attending a GP practice for travel immunisation could be seen by the nurse alone and the nurse could decide which vaccines would be required from the agreed list, administering them to the patient as appropriate. Similarly, a patient could be seen by a nurse in a family planning clinic or an asthma clinic, and the nurse could supply an oral contraceptive or an inhaler from an agreed list of products.

So far it has been assumed that the use of such a protocol is a convenient utilisation of section 58 of the Medicines Act 1968, which is believed to permit doctors to delegate responsibility to others, including nurses, for the decision as to what drugs should be given to patients in specified circumstances. The UKCC standards for the administration of medicines (UKCC, 1992b) also acknowledges this facility.

The government's review of the legal standing of protocols has been examined in depth in a review headed by June Crown in 1997. The interim report, published in March 1998, reported on the practical and legal implications of group protocols. The report found that:

Advice to the Department of Health is that group protocols may not meet the requirements in sections 55(1)(b) and 58(2)(b) of the Medicines Act 1968 for the supply and administration of medicines 'in accordance with the directions of a doctor', and that in order to meet the requirement of current legislation, protocols should leave the minimum of discretion to the health professional involved. Protocols which specify the patient by name (patient specific protocols) are more likely to be within the law than those which apply to groups of patients.

The interim report recommended that the law should be clarified to ensure that the health professionals who supply or administer medicines under approved group protocols are acting within the law.

Nurses have used the protocol facility to circumvent the fact that they are not legally allowed to prescribe. In general practice, nurses are providing patients with a wide range of prescription only medicine ranging from bronchodilators to analgesia and antibiotics, in addition to the administration of vaccines. Increasingly, family planning nurses have been seeking to develop the use of protocols in order to facilitate them using their own professional and expert knowledge to make decisions about the supply of oral contraception without necessarily involving a doctor in every patient consultation.

When authority for the provision of prescription only medicine by doctors is delegated to another, a nurse for example, then the authority for such a delegation must be considered in the context of both supply and administration of such medicine.

Section 58(2)(a) of the Medicines Act 1968 is clear that nurses cannot supply prescription only medicine unless a prescription is completed by an 'appropriate practitioner', such as a doctor. The 1983 Statutory Instrument sets out the criteria for the prescription itself which must, amongst other things, be in ink and contain the name and address of the patient (and age if under 12 years). The prescription must be in existence at the time the prescription only medicine is supplied. Therefore a nurse who seeks to supply a prescription only medicine to a patient under a protocol arrangement without a prescription would be acting unlawfully. Supply means handing over prescription only medicines which are in a 'disposable or alienable form', so a nurse who provides a bronchodilator to a patient is involved in a supply. This is unlawful without a prescription.

Nurses working in hospitals do not fall within these strict limits. The 1983 Statutory Instrument allows the supply of prescription only medicine 'in accordance with written directions of a doctor', and there are no rules as to how these written directions are made up. This would imply that the use of protocols in a hospital setting for the supply of prescription only medicines is lawful. The Medicines Act 1968 defines hospital as including a clinic, nursing home and similar institutions but does not extend to GP surgeries or family planning clinics outside the NHS.

Section 58(2)(b) of the Medicines Act 1968 deals with administration. Administration is defined in the 1983 Statutory Instrument as piercing the skin or mucus membrane. Administration by a nurse is lawful by way of protocol because the administration can take place under the directions of an appropriate practitioner. It is not therefore necessary for a prescription to exist or to be completed by a doctor before the administration takes place. As such, we have the unusual position that a nurse giving a travel or 'flu vaccine, or a family planning nurse administering a depot contraceptive agent would be engaged in an act of administration, and could work from a protocol without needing a doctor's prescription. If the Medicinal Products: Prescription by Nurses etc. Act 1992 were fully implemented this particular problem would be immediately overcome as nurses could prescribe items in their own right without having to resort to protocols.

One issue that has been raised in the discussion about the lawful use of protocols is whether administration of a prescription only medicine also involves a supply. A nurse who administers by injection a measles vaccine, for example, is clearly involved in the administration of a prescription only medicine, but does it also involve supplying the vaccine to the patient? It would appear that the legislation intended that the two activities are distinct since the supply provisions of section 58(l)(a) involve receiving a prescription only medicine in a disposable form such as tablets or pills. Giving an injection does not involve this since the patient cannot receive the supply in an identifiable disposable form.

The government review of the use of group protocols should enable clearer practice in nursing to develop. This will benefit patients and will allow the opportunities for greater collaboration between those nurses without prescribing powers to develop their practice in a manner which is consistent with the requirements in the legislation.

CONCLUSION

The future of nurse prescribing will depend upon the demand made by professionals and the public for the extension of prescribing powers. In order for this to be legal, it is appropriate that the legislation is drafted in terms which allow development in a manner that is safe and effective, and which contains sufficient flexibility to ensure that future practice is not rigidly bound by statute.

The Medicines Act 1968 sets out the criminal liability where the provisions in relation to the supply and administration of prescription medicines are not followed. A detailed examination of the provisions of section 58 of the Act has produced the surprising conclusion that protocols are not a legal form of allowing responsibility to pass from a doctor to a nurse in the supply of any prescription only medicine. This is in spite of a flourishing and diverse range of protocols which are appearing in family planning clinics throughout the country.

The provisions for the supply of vaccines by use of protocol is lawful, although the directions which are required to be given by a doctor are not defined. It therefore remains the responsibility for individual nurses to assess the patient and act according to professional practice and guidance issued to nurses involved in these areas of work.

Any nurse who fails to comply with the provisions of the Medicines Act 1968 commits a criminal offence and can be prosecuted accordingly. However, any ambiguity in construction would be resolved in favour of the nurse. No evidence exists that a nurse has been prosecuted to date for supplying prescription only medicine in accordance with a protocol and it would therefore appear unlikely that this will happen before further guidance is issued by the Department of Health in relation to this matter.

The government review into the legal issues surrounding the use of patient specific protocols and group protocols is likely to lead to further legislation which will reduce the confusion in practice for nurses.

QUESTIONS FOR DISCUSSION

- The legislation distinguishes between community services and acute services in the requirements for certain aspects of prescribing. Do you think that such differences can be justified?

- Do you believe that the distinction between supply and administration is appropriate for today's nursing practice?
- What do you consider to be the best source of law for the classification of the law relating to prescribing?

GLOSSARY

Administer: means administration whether orally, by injection or by introduction into the body in any other way, or by external application, whether by direct contact with the body or not, section 130(9) Medicines Act 1968. This definition is amended in the Statutory Instrument (see below for *Parenteral administration*).

Business: includes a professional practice and includes any activity carried on by a body of persons whether corporate or unincorporate, section 132 Medicines Act 1968.

Certified midwife: means a midwife certified under the Midwives Act 1951, as amended, section 11(2) Medicines Act 1968.

Directions: has no definition.

Group protocol: has a suggested meaning of a specific written instruction for the supply or administration of named medicines in an identified clinical situation, Crown review, Interim Report, March 1998.

Health prescription: means a prescription issued by a doctor or dentist under the NHS Act 1977 and appropriate NHS Acts for Scotland and Northern Ireland, regulation 1 Statutory Instrument 1983, 1212.

Hospital: includes a clinic, nursing home or similar institution, section 132 Medicines Act 1968.

Medicinal product: means any substance or article for medicinal use on a human or animal by administration or as an ingredient in the preparation of a substance for administration, section 130(1) Medicines Act 1968. This definition is amended in regulation 1, Statutory Instrument 1983, 1212 to exclude any medicinal product for use by a vet.

Medical prescription: has the same meaning as in Article 1(2) of the Council Directive 92/96 EEC.

Occupational health scheme: means a scheme in which a person, in the course of a business carried on by him, provides facilities for his employees for the treatment or prevention of disease, regulation 1, Statutory Instrument 1983, 1212.

Parenteral administration: means the administration by breach of the skin or mucous membrane, regulation 1, Statutory Instrument 1983, 1212.

Prescription only medicine: means a medicinal product specified in Article 3, regulation 1, Statutory Instrument 1983, 1212.

Practitioner: means a doctor, dentist, or vet, section 132 Medicines Act 1968.

Prescribed: means prescribed under regulations, section 132 Medicines Act 1968.

Registered nurse: is a nurse registered under the Nurses Act 1957 as amended, section 11(2) Medicines Act 1968.

Repeatable prescription: means a prescription which contains a direction that it may be dispensed more than once, regulation 1, Statutory Instrument 1983, 1212.

Supply: means supply in circumstances corresponding to retail sale, section 131 Medicines Act 1968.

Supplying anything in circumstances corresponding to retail sale: means supply without a sale, for a purpose which is not to do with administration or supply, section 131(4) Medicines Act 1968.

Writing: means any form of notation, whether by hand or by printing, typewriting or any similar process, and *Written* has a similar meaning, section 132 Medicines Act 1968.

REFERENCES

Airedale NHS Trust (1993) *Airedale NHS Trust* v. *Bland* [1993] 1 All ER 821.
St George's Healthcare NHS Trust (1998) *St George's Healthcare NHS Trust* v. *S* (no 2) *Times*.
Medicinal Products: Prescriptions by Nurses etc., Act (1992) London: HMSO.
Medicines Act (1968) London: HMSO.
Medicines (Products other than Veterinary Drugs) (Prescription Only) Order (1983) SI 1983 no. 1212. London: HMSO.
Nurses, Midwives and Health Visitors Act (1997) London: Stationery Office.
R v. *FHSA Appeals Authority*, 10 October 1997, QBD.
R v. *North Derbyshire Health Authority ex parte Fisher*, 1997.
United Kingdom Central Council for Nursing, Midwifery and Health Visiting (1992a) *Code of Professional Conduct*. London: UKCC.
United Kingdom Central Council for Nursing, Midwifery and Health Visiting (1992b) *Standards for the Administration of Medicines. A report on the supply and adminstration of medicines under group protocols*. London: UKCC.

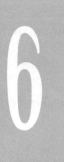

6 Nurse prescribing
Education, education, education

Maggie Banning

Key issues

♦ Critique of current educational preparation for nurse prescribing.

♦ The reality of the extent to which nurses need to be prepared as prescribers.

♦ Suggestions for an ideal educational pathway for nurse prescribers.

INTRODUCTION

One of the fundamental prerequisites for the further expansion of pre-scribing rights to nurses is the provision of a comprehensive educational programme. This chapter looks at existing provision for nurse prescribing education and suggests an appropriate model for nurse prescribers of the future.

EDUCATION FOR THE NURSE PRESCRIBING PILOTS

For the nurse prescribing pilot project, the English National Board for Nursing, Midwifery and Health Visiting (ENB) developed a short course in nurse prescribing. The ENB course comprised a taught course and an open learning pack. The taught element of the course was carried out in institutions of higher education that offered either district nurse or health visitor training. The open learning pack was developed by the working party in liaison with consultants and learning materials design experts. Students enrolled on the course received the open learning pack 2 months prior to commencing the taught programme. Students were then expected to complete a self-assessment questionnaire that addressed their learning needs before beginning the open learning pack.

The open learning pack aimed to:

1. Increase education and training of nurses beyond that of the taught element of the course
2. Provide equivalent theoretical underpinning for all nurses on the course
3. Increase flexibility within the working environment.

These aims would be achieved by completion of the course and students would feel that they had:

- Improved confidence
- Enhanced professional knowledge
- Developed the ability to relate nurse prescribing to their specific nursing practice
- Identified individual learning needs
- Improved analytical skills
- Continuous peer support
- Enhanced skills to meet the needs of nurse prescribing
- Reviewed current ideas.

The open learning pack was divided into sections, these included getting to grips with nurse prescribing, accountability, and prescribing safely and effectively.

The open learning pack

Core content

This introductory section provided a description of the recommendations on nurse prescribing following the initial community nursing review (DHSS, 1986), the Crown Report (DoH, 1989) and the development of the Nurse Prescribers' Formulary (NPF) found in the British National Formulary (BNF). An excerpt from the Crown Report (DoH, 1989) was provided with questions for nurses to consider regarding their feelings about nurse prescribing and the impact that this might have on patient care and existing workloads. In this section students were asked to prioritise their own training requirements and educational deficits with respect to wound healing and tissue viability, use of various forms of compression bandages, adverse drug reactions, general practitioner referral and new products. This was followed by a review of the UKCC codes of conduct, influences on nurse prescribing in terms of professional liability, and the rights of nurses to exercise their own accountability in relation to safe and effective prescribing. This section was underpinned by student current knowledge of physiology, pharmacology and therapeutics, pathology and disease progression. Practical prescribing problems were reviewed with regard to specific preparation found in the NPF used to treat common ailments. Students were expected to read the BNF and develop an understanding of current formulation, routes of administration, dose, therapeutic range for safe management, indications for use, adverse effects and mode of action of specific agents.

However, one has to question how students could be expected to sufficiently investigate these variables from the BNF, which is only a guide for the prescribing of drugs and does not provide sufficient detail to permit the individual to discriminate between specific drugs. Any choice of drug has to be supported with an existing knowledge of the pathophysiological condition that is being treated and mode of action of the chosen drug. Furthermore, it is unclear how students were expected to conceptualise when to give specific drugs without first addressing the underpinning pathophysiological theory of the conditions they were attempting to treat. In addition to knowing how drugs act, one must also know why the various forms of treatment differ in terms of their respective suitability for an individual patient.

Consideration should also have been given to the amount of time that had elapsed since these nurses had completed their initial nurse training and subsequent courses. Even though the theoretical components of nurse training are now taught at diploma level, the inclusion of pathophysiology and pharmacology in nurse training has not always been addressed as well as it should be. Academic levels of educational provision within colleges of nursing do tend to vary. Moreover, the emphasis on scientific components within any one course will depend on available resources and experience; this means that comprehension of existing scientific knowledge may be extremely weak.

In the final part of this section, students were expected to critique a research paper prepared by a drug company and answer methodologically focused questions that assessed ability to assimilate information from a research paper. The core textbooks offered (Ogier, 1989) might provide students with sufficient knowledge, but little consideration seems to have been given to the experience and skills necessary to critique a rationalistic paper using an experimental design. There is also little evidence of teaching of research methods within the course content. It was unfortunate that nurses were expected to critique a research paper with very little basic knowledge of the research process, particularly as the inclusion of research based learning is a fairly new concept in nurse education: it is unlikely that nurses who qualified in the 1970s and before will have studied any form of research methods.

Reference material offered for this section of the course was limited. The content focused on reports, UKCC codes of conduct (UKCC, 1989, 1992a, 1992b), a textbook of pharmacology beneficial only as an introductory text, one research textbook and two journal articles. Further reading included the community nursing review (DHSS, 1986), the Crown Report (DoH, 1989), the UKCC code of conduct on standards for administration of medicines (UKCC, 1992c) and clinical supervision and mentorship

(Butterworth and Faugier, 1992). For specific reading material students were expected to provide their own sources. This must have posed multiple problems for students undertaking this course as it is likely that most were in full time employment, with very little support and probably limited access to library facilities. Furthermore, many students may not have studied pathophysiology and pharmacology to the depth required for prescribing and this would raise problems when attempting to understand the pharmacodynamic (mode of action) principles of specific therapeutic agents.

The final sections of this pack focused on ethical issues related to nurse prescribing, working as part of team and measuring clinical effectiveness. Students were expected to complete a self-assessment questionnaire to assess their individual learning needs prior to commencing the learning pack. In addition they were expected to maintain between 10 and 15 hours of independent study. The taught course comprised 15 hours of tuition addressing the issues described in the open learning pack. Prescribing safely and effectively and evaluating effectiveness were assigned only 5 and 2 hours respectively. These issues are obviously pertinent to nurse prescribing, particularly as this is a new role that raises numerous accountability issues. Clearly the deficit in time allocated to these areas in the course, and the lack of pharmacology and therapeutics demonstrate that nurses who undertook this course were inadequately prepared for this initiative. Support for students appeared to also be limited.

It is difficult to see how prospective students following the ENB approved course could be expected to take on the new responsibility of prescribing without adequate support, supervision and guidance on the academic content and on how to handle challenges met. Moreover, it would have been difficult for students not only to decipher the level at which to study, but also to appreciate the association between pathophysiology and pharmacology. Students would have required some guidance on specific areas to study and appropriate journals to review with respect to pathophysiological conditions and their respective treatments. Often such journals are not available within the nursing literature; this raises problems of access and sometimes of comprehension.

Training for nurse prescribing educators

The ENB provided guidelines for tutors to facilitate the planning of this educational course. Guidelines did not include the actual syllabus for the course, but did provide a video from the Southern Derbyshire Community Health Service. As the academic level of the course and its assessment were not addressed in the course documentation, it is unclear what quality assurance procedures were involved in the selection of educational institutions and course leaders.

Selection and assessment of students

Practitioner profiles and telephone interviews aided the selection of candidates and helped in gaining knowledge of the participating audience. The self-assessment questionnaire was used as an indicator of student competency and ability to complete the course. The selection of appropriate course assessment strategies was deemed the responsibility of course leaders from individual colleges. Several forms of assessment were thought applicable for the assessment of the learning outcomes for the course; short answer questions, case study analysis, continual peer assessment (if available) and reflective casebook or diary. The course documentation does not state how these assessments were graded and whether external examiners were involved in the assessment. The lack of clarity on the selection of students and on assessment also raises the following issues:

- How were students supported during the course?
- What measures were undertaken if a student failed the course assessment?
- What was the expected pass rate for the course?
- How was the course evaluated?
- Was external lecturer/examiner support involved?

In view of these considerations and the course literature, this educational course did not appear to provide sufficient educational learning material and support for students to effectively prepare them to undertake this new role. Student centered learning is not an appropriate teaching strategy for subjects such as pharmacology and therapeutics when the majority of material is being viewed for the first time and when students require a foundation in physiology, biochemistry and chemistry to help understand basic principles.

RCN NURSE PRACTITIONER IN PRIMARY CARE PROGRAMME

Nurse prescribing content

The RCN BSc in health studies nurse practitioner programme aims to provide students with an overview of the tenets of sociology, health education and promotion related to primary health care. This degree utilises a modular scheme based on a fourfold curriculum incorporating its higher ordering principles (Beattie, 1987). It aims to provide students with the basic principles of sociology, biology, research, education, health assessment, interpersonal psychology, pharmacology, health promotion and nursing. Applied pharmacology is a compulsory module for students wishing to undertake the RCN programme for nurse practitioners in primary health care.

Generally, this degree programme is attractive to nurses who work predominantly in the community, working as practice nurses within a general practitioner surgery, as district nurses or health visitors, or as nurses within accident and emergency departments. Although nurses may possess abundant experience of these these specific areas of nursing, often their fundamental knowledge of science is limited; this may be a reflection of the inadequate scientific education in state registration training and post registration courses. This presents a problem when attempting to teach pharmacology as the deficiencies in comprehension of normal physiology, pathology and biochemistry are not addressed within the current degree programme.

Prior to studying pharmacology, students study the basic principles of life sciences in a 12-week module taught at diploma level. Due to time constraints, the limited quantity of science that can be discussed is insufficient as a prerequisite for the applied pharmacology module. This module aims to provide students with an understanding of the principles of pharmacology with specific application to clinical practice. By building on existing scientific knowledge, one hopes to achieve an appreciation of pharmacology and its relationship to nurse prescribing. It is important for students to understand the theory underpinning how drugs work before addressing specific examples of therapies and their role in the management of specific diseases. This module is also only 12 weeks in duration and therefore is insufficient to meet the needs of the nurse prescriber who may wish to prescribe drug therapy. In the time allocated, one can only provide an overview of the principles of pharmacology – pharmacokinetics, or what the body does to a drug, and pharmacodynamics, or what the drug does to the body – and provide some analysis of systemic pharmacology with application to clinical practice. Only a limited number of pathophysiological conditions can be addressed in sufficient detail for comprehensive understanding.

Pharmacokinetic principles

Pharmacokinetics can be described as the mathematical assessment of how the body deals with drugs and their effects on specific variables. These can be organised into four main divisions, namely drug absorption, drug distribution, drug metabolism and drug excretion (see Box 6.1).

Nurses who administer drugs to patients need to have an appreciation of what happens to a drug following its absorption. This requires a good comprehension of the basic principles of normal physiology, chemistry and factors influencing drug absorption. Nurses administer drugs in several forms by numerous routes. Successful drug absorption is dependent on the formulation of the drug, its ability to be absorbed by the plasma membrane of the epidermis, lungs, or the gastrointestinal tract. Nurses also need to

Box 6.1 Pharmacological phases for drug effectiveness

Pharmaceutical phase   Drug administration
          Disintegration of dosage form into solution
Pharmacokinetic phase   Drug ready for absorption
          Distribution, metabolism and excretion
Pharmacodynamic phase   Drug available for action
          Metabolites available for action and drug related effect

appreciate how age and mechanical or physiological factors might influence drug absorption.

The age of the patient is important, particularly in neonates due to the immaturity of the epidermis and erratic gastric absorption. In contrast, in the elderly patient, drug absorption may be influenced by age-dependent changes in gastric pH, blood flow to the stomach, gastric ulceration, and polypharmacy or the administration of multiple drug therapies concurrently (Calloway, Foley and Lagerbloom, 1965). In order to minimise problems with absorption of prescribed drugs, nurse prescribers require a sufficient knowledge of the patient's medical history, and of the characteristics of the drug and influencing factors.

It is essential for the nurse prescriber to be aware of the need for routine monitoring to ensure that serum levels remain within the therapeutic index or therapeutic level required for safe and effective management, particularly when new therapies are commenced (Reynolds and Aronson, 1993).

Perhaps one of the most important pharmacokinetic parameters is that of drug metabolism or biotransformation, as this allows drugs to become water soluble to permit their elimination via the kidney or the bile (Pacifici *et al.*, 1988; LaBella, 1991). The efficiency by which the body undertakes this process is dependent on the organ systems involved. A working knowledge of this aspect of pharmacology is essential to the nurse prescriber for the following reasons:

• Most drugs undergo some form of biotransformation to reduce their toxicity which renders the drug more water soluble and enhances excretion.
• Drug metabolism is a rate dependent response that can be overruled by numerous chemicals such as those consumed in the diet or produced during digestion of food, alcohol or cigarette smoking.
• Extremes of age can have a negative influence on drug metabolism.
• Pathophysiological changes can alter the ability to metabolise drugs; this is particularly prevalent in hepatic disorders.
• Enterohepatic recycling can prolong the half-life of drugs that are usually excreted by the faecal route.

- Genetics and pregnancy can adversely influence the ability of the individual to metabolise drugs.
- Polypharmacy can contribute to the development of drug interactions.
- Increasing quantities of drugs increase the tendency for adverse drug reactions to develop.

As the majority of patients will administer more than one medication on a daily basis, it is crucial that the nurse prescriber has a sufficient understanding of the phases of metabolism and of its importance to health. Drug elimination is dependent on the ability to biotransform drugs into metabolites that are chemically less harmful and provides the basis for assessing serum levels of drugs prior to administration of the next dose and assessment of toxicity.

A knowledge of drug metabolism will enhance the nurse prescriber's understanding of the effects of age on the ability to eliminate drugs (Schmucker *et al.*, 1990; Rowland, 1993) and of the importance of the recognition of adverse drug effects and drug interactions (Vestal *et al.*, 1979). Furthermore, it will enable the nurse to understand the importance of ensuring that drug levels are within therapeutic limits and the need to educate the patient with regard to the administration of drug therapy, hence promoting drug compliance (Urquhart, 1994).

Drug excretion aims to reduce the toxicity of chemicals and prevent the build up of seriously high serum levels that can be detrimental to the patient's health (Zauderer, 1996). Drugs are eliminated via sweat and saliva, by exhalation, rectally or via the kidney. The chemistry of the drug will determine the predominant route of elimination. With regard to nursing knowledge, it is imperative that the nurse prescriber understands the processes involved in the excretion of drugs and parameters such as age that can influence it (Meyer, 1989; Meyer and Hirsch, 1990; Kee, 1992). These are listed below:

- Normal physiology and anatomy of the nephron and biliary and gastrointestinal tract
- Physiological parameters involved in the maintenance of glomerular filtration and renal dynamics
- Influence of drugs on renal dynamics, acidity and alkalinity of drug excretion
- Influence of cardiac pathologies and age on glomerular filtration
- Relationship of pharmacokinetic parameters to drug elimination
- Effect of hepatic and gastrointestinal pathologies on faecal elimination of drugs.

Limitations of the module do not permit discussion of variables that influence those pharmacokinetic parameters which are pertinent to nurse prescribing: for example the effects of nutrition, alcohol and cigarette smoking and the nutritional status of the patient (Bailey *et al.*, 1989, 1991; Shyu *et al.*, 1991; Soons *et al.*, 1991; Vestal *et al.*, 1979), or the effects of the development of tolerance to drug therapy, the propensity for displacement reactions, and how pathophysiological change can influence the efficacy of drug therapy (Watson *et al.*, 1987).

Systemic pharmacology

To understand the principles of drug action pertinent to the treatment of specific conditions, nurses are expected to study the potential targets for drug action and indications for use of a specific therapy (John and Stevenson, 1995; Schwartz, 1991). The importance of the recognition and reporting of adverse drug reactions in accordance with UKCC guidance (1996) is also examined. The treatment of pathological conditions relevant to community based nursing is discussed within the current module. Treatments include the pharmacological and non-pharmacological management of asthma, hypertension and depression, and the use of anti-microbial chemotherapy in the treatment of infections. The choice of pathological conditions discussed reflects the types of conditions common to community based nursing.

Lack of time in the module prevents any review of pathophysiological conditions pertaining to multiple body systems; this results in large deficits in knowledge that could only be filled by a course designed to better meet the needs of prospective nurse prescriber students.

THE FUTURE

In future, nurse prescribers may be allowed to prescribe extensively from the British National Formulary. This will require these individuals to possess an extensive understanding of science based subjects underpinned by the ability to physically examine patients from both normal and pathophysiological perspective in order to support the clinical decision being proposed. For nurse prescribers to succeed in this respect, they will need to operate at a level comparable to that of the general practitioner. This requires a sound foundation knowledge in anatomy, basic and systemic pathology, biochemistry, cell biology, cardiology, endocrinology, haematology, immunology, physiology, microbiology, neurology and virology supported by a broad understanding of clinical pharmacology and therapeutics.

To achieve this, the nurse prescriber will need to undertake extensive postgraduate training that provides not only the scientific basis to underpin decisions made but also provides extended training in the clinical assessment of patients. This will give the nurse the competencies necessary to problem solve and maintain evidence based practice. From a scientific perspective, nurse prescribers will need to understand how the body functions normally and what constitute normal physiological parameters in terms of its assessment. Once competency has been achieved in this assessment, then nurses may study pathophysiology and disease management, and develop skills in problem solving.

You may ask why such a strong scientific background is essential to the role of the nurse prescriber when nurses are already registered and may have developed expertise in the management of patients suffering from a variety of conditions. One must remember that nurse training does not prepare nurses to prescribe drugs or to assess patients clinically and make undifferentiated diagnoses. The scientific basis of nurse education has often been either poorly taught, or omitted, hence nurses have not been developed scientifically. How often does one meet nurses who can tell you how to undertake specific procedures but cannot provide a scientific basis for what they are doing?

The current nurse practitioner course also operates in a similar manner: the scientific basis of this programme is extremely weak. The basic principles are taught at diploma level which is commensurate with current first level education Diploma in Nursing courses. It does not prepare nurses to take on this new role as generalists, since the omission of an appropriate scientific foundation cannot be met within a 12-week module in pharmacology. The problem of inadequate educational preparation may contribute to the dilemma recognised by official nursing bodies when attempting to validate the nurse practitioner qualification. This new role for nurses requires specific educational preparation that can only be achieved through a training and development programme that is clinically based and is rigorous. The reasons for this are multiple.

Firstly, nurse prescribers require an explicit knowledge of the condition they are attempting to treat, if they are to assess patients clinically, make undifferentiated diagnoses and prescribe the appropriate form of either pharmacological or non-pharmacological treatment. To achieve this the nurse prescriber will not only require an appreciable understanding of normal physiology, biochemistry and cell biology in order to assess the patient with regard to normal reference ranges of physiological parameters, but also be able to differentiate between a multitude of possible diagnoses.

Asthma

Once an in-depth knowledge of these aspects of the human body is achieved, then and only then will the nurse prescriber possess the foundation with which to study altered diseased states. For example to understand the altered disease state that occurs when a patient presents with a chronic inflammatory condition such as asthma, it is imperative that the nurse prescriber:

- Understands the difference on examination of a normal lung and those of a patient suffering from airflow limitation
- Is able to interpret lung function tests such as spirometry and peak expiratory flow rate and their relationship to respiratory physiology.

One can also measure the oxygen saturation as an estimate of tissue perfusion and hypoxia. Used in conjunction with the patient's history and presenting symptoms, these estimates will allow the examiner to judge the severity of the condition for the individual patient. The correct diagnoses of the condition can only be made by understanding how the respiratory physiology is altered by immunological stimulants and triggers, how this response manifests itself pathophysiologically in the development of the pathognomic or pathologically relevant signs and symptoms of asthma. The nurse prescriber should also understand the mechanisms behind the biochemical responses that induce asthmatic attacks in children and in adults (Jones and Bowen, 1994; Kolnaar *et al.*, 1994; Luyt *et al.*, 1994).

An understanding of the relationship between occupational pollutants, chemicals, drugs, sensitisers, microorganisms, cigarette smoke and genetic elements in the induction of pathognomic changes characteristic of asthma is important to its prevention (Patten and Holt, 1992; McKenzie, 1994). By understanding the biochemistry of the immune response, nurse prescribers should be able to relate the role of chemical mediators to the severity of the presenting symptoms. A knowledge of pharmacology and therapeutics will then allow the nurse prescriber to assess the suitability of current drug therapy or therapies to treat the condition, supported by a good comprehension of the physiological parameters measured and the examination of the individual patient.

We need to ask what pharmacological knowledge the nurse practitioner would require to prescribe drugs to treat an asthmatic patient. If one commences with the route that the drug is to be administered, respiratory therapies are usually inhaled in the form of a fine powder of <2 μm in diameter. Such a small size is essential to achieve absorption across the alveolar plasma membrane. One has to understand what plasma membranes are and how drugs are absorbed across them in order to explain to patients how their drugs work. Knowledge of the characteristics for drug absorption are important here. For example, the occupation of the patient can influence the lung environment, and this may often be related to the development of allergic lung conditions. One can then enquire how this may influence drug absorption.

Additional influences on drug absorption might include the type of inhaler or inhaler technique. Numerous inhalers are available; the ability of individual patients to use a specific inhaler will depend on their dexterity, age, severity of the disease, type of drug used in the treatment and social circumstances. Inhaler devices generally deliver drugs at speeds of up to 60 miles per hour, however, this varies with type of device and inhaler technique (Rickenbach and Julious, 1994). Invariably one will find that roughly 10% of the drug will be swallowed, with the greater percentage absorbed directly into the lungs. Spacer devices are commonly used to avoid systemic absorption and increase drug delivery to the lungs (O'Callaghan and Barry, 1997).

If a patient has a poor inhaler technique and continually swallows a large percentage of the prescribed drug, it will be ineffective as it will not reach the target site within the lungs. So the potential benefits of the drug will appear negligible and the patient will complain that the drug is useless, when really the drug may have been excreted on first passage through the liver (Back and Rogers, 1987; Tam, 1993). It is important to understand this concept and how it can influence therapeutic efficacy and to educate patients accordingly (Reinke and Hoffman, 1992).

In the case of inhaled steroids, Flixotide undergoes total first pass metabolism and is therefore excreted via the bile (Allen and Hanbury, 1993). In contrast, budesonide and beclomethasone have lower rates of first pass metabolism and therefore can be re-absorbed systemically which augments the development of systemic adverse effects – which may in turn reduce patient compliance with respect to taking medication and controlling symptoms (Ninan and Russell, 1992).

To differentiate between the variety of drugs available to treat a specific condition, the nurse prescriber needs to be able to compare how drugs work and the benefit to the individual patient at this stage in the disease process. Often, guidelines will be available which provide a recommended sequence of drug administration for a given condition. In the case of asthma, guidelines are produced by the British Thoracic Society.

Knowing how drugs act can also help to establish potential adverse effects that may become problematic with increasing administration. For example, salbutamol is the first line of therapy for patients with asthma (see Box 6.2).

If nurse prescribers are to undertake extensive prescribing of drugs they must understand the pharmacological actions of the drugs they are

---

Box 6.2 Pharmacological action of salbutamol

Pharmaceutical phase. Drug administered by inhaler
Pharmacokinetic phase. Drug absorbed across alveolar plasma membrane, distributed to heart and liver, metabolised by catechol-O-methyltransferases and excreted in bile and urine
Pharmacodynamic phase. Activates β2-receptors mimics action of isoprenalin and noradrenalin to bronchodilate bronchiolar smooth muscle

prescribing. This can only be achieved by possessing an extensive knowledge of drugs and their potential side-effects. Such knowledge and expertise will only be provided by the in-depth study of multiple organ systems, in addition to extensive experience of treating conditions being investigated. This is pertinent to all nurses, but is essential for nurses aiming to prescribe drugs independently.

Chronopharmacology investigates the influence of circadian rhythms on chronokinetics and chronodynamics (TPS Drug Information Centre, 1992). The scientific evidence of this is established from chronopathological parameters whereby the symptoms of the respective disease may be influenced by the 24-hour rhythm or monthly cycles. Drugs that influence circadian rhythms are those that possess a narrow therapeutic index such as theophylline (Colli *et al.*, 1988). The timing of administration of a drug has been shown to benefit the patient's control of the organ-based disease. In asthmatic patients, the use of morning doses of prednisolone minimises reductions in bone density and suppression of the hypothalmo–pituitary–adrenal axis. Theophylline administered as an evening dose helps to suppress the physiological triggers that contribute to nocturnal asthmatic conditions (high serum histamine, increased reactivity to acetylcholine, poor airway patency causing a drop in the FEV or forced expiratory volume), with little adverse influence during the daytime.

Knowledge of the complexity of asthma can be used to educate patients to monitor their condition, maintain compliance with respect to drug therapy, and understand the signs of a deteriorating condition (for example how infections may alter airway patency and have a negative effect on their condition). The nurse prescriber can be used as a health educator specifically for the elderly and for children and their families. Asthma can be a debilitating and frightening disease that can have a direct effect on the equilibrium of the family unit. Support can be given through effective communication and education of patients and their families; the nurse prescriber, if trained and educated appropriately, can offer this.

Infections

Nurse prescribers will be expected to examine patients who present with a multitude of infections. To be able to differentiate between the numerous forms of microorganisms, the nurse prescriber should have studied the behavioural characteristics of microorganisms. This means examining the morphological, biochemical and growth characteristics of bacteria, viruses, fungi and parasites, how the body responds to infection, and the role of drug therapy in the treatment of a specific infection. This is particularly important as nurse prescribers often provide health education advice on international travel, administer vaccinations and examine patients with suspected infections.

By reviewing the pertinent aspects of each form of microorganism and how they initiate an immune response and develop infection, the nurse prescriber will then understand the need to culture microorganisms and for sensitivity testing before prescribing the appropriate drug therapy. Many infections will be viral in origin and therefore will not respond to anti-microbial therapy. By possessing this information, the nurse prescriber will be able to differentiate between viruses, bacteria, fungi, protozoa and helminths and correlate the history of the infection to the symptoms and the microorganism most likely to be responsible for that particular infection. This ability to correlate the history, source of infection and treatment most sensitive to the microorganism responsible will reduce the incidence of bacterial resistance to antibiotics and hopefully speed up the recovery rate for the individual patient.

Education of the patient is also an important parameter in the treatment of infections with antimicrobial chemotherapy. Patient compliance with respect to administering drug therapy is a continual problem (Evans and Spelman, 1983; Beardon *et al.*, 1993). Reduced compliance arises from a lack of belief that the therapy will be beneficial, or a lack of knowledge that there is a requirement to complete the regime once commenced, especially when the individual feels better (Cargill, 1992). Partial compliers exist who administer their medication on appointment days only or when they feel the need. The financial cost of this form of behavior is huge (Madden, 1995). Often, antibiotics interact with dairy produce, reducing drug absorp-tion and limiting therapeutic efficacy (Neuvonen, Kivisto and Lehto, 1991). If patients feel no benefit from administering medication they will not complete the antibiotic regime. This is an important aspect of patient education.

An additional difficulty pertinent to administering antibiotics is the potential for adverse reactions and drug interactions. Penicillin and also vaccines can initiate immunological reactions, causing histamine release leading to life-threatening situations such as acute bronchospasm, uncon-sciousness and syncope. Nurse prescribers need to be aware of the propensity for these reactions to occur and review patient history of allergies to such preparations before prescribing them.

Nurse prescribers can be extremely influential in advising patients about how long a treatment should be sustained, the timing of the therapy and any potential side-effects; they can also dispel any misconceptions that patients may have regarding treatment, discuss issues related to feelings patients may have regarding drug therapy and administration, issues of denial and the need for additional interventions, and arrange a suitable follow-up appointment.

By providing nurse prescribers with an understanding of microbiology, the inflammatory response and the use of chemotherapy in the treatment of microorganisms, patients will be given safe and reliable management options. These will be based on a concrete body of knowledge and current research rather than experiential learning, thus emphasising how evidence based practice can be used and maintained. Perhaps in this way existing antibiotics will remain selectively bacteriocidal or bacteriostatic in the new millenium.

Cardiac patients

In a similar manner, to examine and treat cardiac patients nurse prescribers require an in-depth knowledge of normal cardiac anatomy and conduction of the heart, cardiac biochemistry and analysis of electrocardiograph rhythms. This background will provide the nurse prescriber with the understanding of cardiology that is necessary to advise and treat cardiac patients safely.

Additional study is required in the various organ based specialties such as neurology, dermatology, endocrinology, gastroenterology, paediatrics, psychiatry, opthalmics, urology and obstetrics and gynaecology. The importance of a broad understanding of clinical pharmacology and thera-peutics is essential in future for extensive nurse prescribing and can only be achieved through the completion of appropriate courses that specifically aim to train suitably qualified nurses to become nurse prescribers. This level of knowledge and its application is what is required for extensive nurse prescribing. This raises the following immediate problems:

- Should students undertake this training as a taught degree supported by health assessment and clinical decision making skills?
- What time factors are involved in the duration of this course?
- How does one assess the suitability of candidates? Are prior knowledge and skills essential for admission to such a course of study?
- At what academic level should this course be assessed?
- How should this course be taught and assessed?
- Should this course be based in an academic institution or in the clinical environment or both?
- Is this form of preparation for nurse prescribers sufficient for only the community based environment or will it also be suitable for secondary care settings?
- What preparation will lecturers require to teach this type of course?
- Should funding be made available?

THE SUGGESTED COURSE

For this course to gain recognition by nursing and medical professionals, it is essential that it be taught at postgraduate level with accreditation by appropriate facilities. Secondly, to be provided with an educational award, theory must be supported by relevant clinical experience of health assessment and decision making skills; the only way to develop these skills is to learn them as an important aspect of a health assessment course.

To allow nurses to access this type of course, the duration for completion needs to be flexible but contained within an appropriate time-frame that is manageable and provides ample time for learning to become established. A time-scale of around 4 years on a full-time basis or 8 years on a part-time basis is probably necessary to provide the depth and breadth of theory to permit the nurse to develop appropriately. This would need to be approved by the educational establishment awarding the qualification.

Entry criteria for such a course will always be a debatable issue. However, it should be realised that not everyone can become an advanced practitioner. Necessary skills will include the ability to conceptualise theory, to differentiate the possible pathophysiological conditions and to make the correct decisions for an individual patient based on knowledge of the condition itself, and of pharmacology, health assessment and the influence of socioeconomic variables. Due to the changing face of health care, an increasing number of patients are being nursed within the community; nurses will need to appreciate how sociological, psychological and economical factors can influence patient care in this health care setting. It is imperative therefore that nurses possess a first degree that provides a foundation in primary health care with the inclusion of the basic principles of interpersonal psychology and research. Nurses will be expected to be effective communicators. This skill is essential to the provision of patient education through discussion of diagnosis, management using non-pharmacological and pharmacological therapy and to ensure patient compliance. It is likely that a BSc in health studies would be the expected entry criteria.

If this form of course were available it would need to be taught at post-graduate level. There are numerous reasons for this. The most compelling is that nurse prescriber is currently thought of as a generalist who is trained to bachelors level. However, if advancements in the delivery of care and nurse prescribing are to succeed, nurses need to be equipped with the knowledge, skills and approval to initiate this care. This can only develop from jointly accredited clinically based courses taught at postgraduate level. Commensurate with the concept of advanced practice, the nurse prescriber in this instance would be functioning at an advanced level and would have the approval and authority to do so.

As with any good academic course, a variety of teaching methods are essential to help facilitate learning. De Vries *et al.* (1995) found that the incorporation of experiential learning within medical training assisted medical students in their understanding of pharmacological theory. The use of didactic exposition, problem solving through case history analysis, clinical examination and assessment of pharmacological therapy are skills that will enhance the development of students to a level that may be consistent with that of the general practitioner.

To attain joint accreditation this course should be developed and taught within an academic department with all physical assessment skills undertaken by clinical attachment to the necessary hospitals. Nurses require both academic theory and clinical input to support and facilitate the form of learning required for this type of course. Assessment can therefore only occur within the clinical environment, and so the inclusion of clinical placements is essential to the learning outcomes of the course. Only in this way can continuous evaluation of physical examination skills, competence in determining the diagnoses and assessment of potential treatments be undertaken.

Patient care is becoming more community orientated so it is essential that nursing developments be focused in this direction. However, the advanced nurse prescriber role could also be an important development within secondary care settings such as accident and emergency or acute care. The core general theory and clinical assessment skills could easily be utilised within the triage setting in these departments or in acute ward settings.

Lecturers should be trained to PhD level in the specialty they teach. The possession of a postgraduate teaching qualification would also be desirable, with experience of teaching at both undergraduate and postgraduate standard. Evidence of nursing/medical training pertinent to the specialty being taught would be essential to maintain standards and to link theory to clinical practice. This would ensure that graduate standard teaching was produced which was of a quality commensurate with university standards. Academic staff would be encouraged to undertake research to encourage its application in teaching and evidence based practice.

Funding in the form of grants, bursaries or fellowships could be made available from a variety of sources to support graduate nurses for the duration of the course. The long term usefulness of this course to local trusts, general practitioners and educational establishments should be made apparent to funding bodies. The benefits of such developments in nursing should be immediately apparent to general practitioners as they change their functional role from generalist to one that is more specialist, involving carrying out minor surgery or running specialist clinics.

A model for learning

If this form of education were available it would provide a means by which the nurse prescriber might develop expert knowledge and skills through continuous theoretical and clinical assessment. The nurse prescriber would be developing along a continuum from novice to expert (Benner, 1984). This could be achieved through a curricular approach utilising four predominant concepts: liberal humanism, progressivism, instrumentalism and reconstructionism, as outlined by Beattie (1987) (see Box 6.3).

> **Box 6.3** Nurse practitioner educational content based on Beattie's fourfold curriculum (Beattie, 1987)
>
> **Liberal humanism**
> - Applied and organ based sciences
> - Pharmacology
>
> **Progressivism**
> - Experiential learning
> - Clinical experience
>
> Advanced practitioner
>
> **Reconstructionism**
> - Communication
> - Nursing leadership
>
> **Instrumentalism**
> - Clinical assessment and prescribing

Typical framework for such a course

This programme of study would provide the student with the basic principles of applied scientific knowledge. It would commence with a foundation course in human anatomy and physiology, biochemistry, cell biology, haematology, microbiology, immunology, basic pathology and virology. This would be followed by a foundation course in clinical pharmacology and therapeutics in which students would learn the basic principles of pharmacokinetics, pharmacodynamics, the importance of pharmacovigilance, therapeutic drug monitoring and pharmacoeconomics. Theoretical input would be assessed by examination and clinical skills by successful completion of a full physical examination with interpretation of biochemical and physiological parameters by reference range. Generally, this would normally take 2 years to complete on a full-time basis.

Following successful completion of the foundation course, students would be required to study organ based specialty modules focusing on basic cardiology, neurology, endocrinology, gastroenterology, respiratory medicine, nephrology, paediatrics, psychiatry, dermatology and other sub-specialties (e.g. oncology, public health medicine) with application to clinical pharmacology and therapeutics. Continuous assessment of clinical decision-making skills would be undertaken and involve the interpretation of clinical data providing an accurate diagnoses and treatment profile.

Outline for a model of clinical excellence for nurse prescribers (Box 6.4)

During the first 2 years of the course students would be expected to attend lectures, carry out practical experiments, and attend clinical sessions to learn physical assessment skills and interpretation of biochemical and physiological reference parameters. The teaching and assessment of the foundation course could be undertaken with medical students.

Box 6.4 Example of a progression map for MSc clinical pharmacology and therapeutics for nurses

Section
Foundation.
Year
1 and 2.
Theory
Applied sciences and pharmacology.
Clinical assessment
Physical assessment and biochemical reference ranges, interpret ECG, blood picture, blood gases and lung function tests.
Theory assessment
Perform a total body physical assessment. Foundation examinations in human anatomy and physiology, biochemistry, cell biology, haematology, microbiology, immunology, basic pathology and virology. Problem solving exercises in, pharmacokinetics.
Section
Specialties.
Year
3 and 4.
Theory
Pathophysiological conditions pertinent to the following areas: cardiology, dermatology, neurology, endocrinology, gastroenterology, respiratory medicine, nephrology, paediatrics, psychiatry, and sub-specialties.
Clinical
Students would prepare seminars based on clinical cases examined from each organ based specialty. Discussion would focus on clinical and biochemical assessment, diagnosis, pharmacological and non-pharmacological management and follow-up. Presentations would provide research based clinical evidence to support clinical decisions relevant to practice. At the end of the clinical attachment, students would present seminars in the form of a portfolio of cases for summative assessment.
Pharmacology
Students would present a drug diary that contained summaries of up to 70 commonly used drugs. Each summary should provide research based evidence in support of indications for use supported by pharmacodynamic and pharmacokinetic considerations, contraindications, and potential adverse effects and established drug interactions.

Box 6.4 *contd*

Examination

Written examination, clinical assessment skills, and decision-making processes, problem solving and portfolio assessment would be undertaken to assess students at the end of each clinical specialty.

Theoretical and clinical assessment

Perform a total body physical assessment of a patient with pathophysiological condition pertinent to organ based specialty. Interpret physiological and biochemical parameters pertinent to the condition being examined.

Example: cardiology

Theory

ECG analysis, in depth cardiac anatomy, physiology and biochemistry. Examination of the pathophysiology of ischaemia and reperfusion arrhythmias, myocardial infarction, cardiomegaly, cardiac failure, hypertension.

Clinical assessment

Over a 6-month period, present case studies of atrial and ventricular arrhythmias, hypercholesterolaemia, cardiac failure, myocardial infarction, hypertension, and mitral stenosis and left ventricular failure. Discussion would focus on clinical and biochemical assessment, diagnosis, pharmacological and non-pharmacological management and follow-up. Presentations would provide research based clinical evidence to support clinical decisions relevant to practice. At the end of the clinical attachment, students would present seminars in the form of a portfolio of cases for summative assessment.

Pharmacology

Drug diary of summaries of the research based evidence in support of indications for use of β-blockers, cardiac glycosides, diuretics, ACE inhibitors, Ca^{2+} channel blockers, amiodarone (type III antiarrhythmic), alpha antagonists, vasodilator preparations and anti-cholestrolemic agents. Evidence would be supported by pharmacodynamic and pharmacokinetic considerations, contraindications, and potential adverse effects and established drug interactions.

Theoretical assessment

Undertake a physical assessment of a patient with a pathophysiological condition pertinent to cardiology. Interpret physiological and biochemical parameters pertinent to the condition being examined, and treatment.

Following completion of the foundation course in applied sciences as assessed by examination, students would attend specific organ based specialty clinics for a period of 4–6 months. The placements would provide students with the opportunity to review clinical expertise through formal and summative assessment of patients attending outpatient clinics in organ based specialties.

These clinical sessions would complement lectures provided for each organ based specialty and would involve a full physical assessment of patients in both community and hospital based environments. Students would be assessed by the clinician/nurse lecturer for competence in general physical assessment, diagnostic skills and clinical management decision making. In each specialty students would be expected to maintain a portfolio of patients they had examined and assessed with regard to the proposed diagnosis and its potential management. This would be assessed for accuracy and proficiency of clinical assessment, diagnosis and treatment by the clinician/lecturer specific for that particular clinical specialty.

Students would be expected to maintain a drug diary of summaries of 70 commonly used drugs. Each summary should provide research based evidence describing the indications for use supported by pharmacodynamic and pharmacokinetic considerations, contraindications, potential adverse effects and established drug interactions, in addition to patient specific issues that might be an issue of importance.

Students would prepare seminars based on clinical cases examined from each organ based specialty. Discussion would focus on clinical and biochemical assessment, diagnosis, pharmacological and non-pharmacological management and follow-up. Presentations would provide research based clinical evidence to support clinical decisions relevant to practice. At the end of the clinical attachment, students would present seminars in the form of a portfolio of cases for summative assessment.

Examination, clinical assessment skills, and decision-making processes, problem solving and portfolio assessment would be used to assess students at the end of each clinical specialty. Pass marks would be assessed at 50% in theoretical examination and 70% in clinical presentation, assessment skills, diagnosis and management. Such a high pass mark is essential to maintain rigorous academic standards, since qualified nurse prescribers would be given the authority to manage and treat patients independently. In view of this, any student failing an examination within the foundation programme would be allowed only one retake per annum. Students requiring to resit three or more examinations in any section of the course would be removed from the programme. Obviously not all graduate nurses could become nurse prescribers.

On successful completion of the course, students would be monitored for 1 year with respect to assessment and clinical decision-making skills, appropriateness and effectiveness of prescribing prior to attaining a certification of competence. Students would then be provided with an advanced practice nursing qualification. This would permit nurse prescribers to prescribe drugs independently from the BNF under the jurisdiction of a suitably qualified practitioner. Registration would be reviewed every 5 years. For nurse prescribers to be maintained on the existing register they would need to successfully complete an assessment of competence. This would form the basis for insurance and legal requirements.

Following one successful period of registration (normally 5 years experience), advanced nurse prescribers should be permitted to practise independently and set up autonomous practices. Moreover, nurse prescribers should be allowed to register to study for fellowships/specialist practice qualifications in sub-specialties such as paediatric respiratory care, dermatology or opthalmics. This would allow nurse prescribers to differentiate knowledge, expertise and undertake research while functioning as a generalist practitioner with specialist knowledge in a particular field of health care.

CONCLUSION

The concept of advanced nursing practice focuses on the initiation of extensive prescribing rights that may become an issue for nurses in the future. Such an initiative is not without its drawbacks, the most obvious being the educational requirements and clinical decision-making skills needed to make this initiative worthwhile for nursing and safe and effective for patients. This chapter aimed to alert the reader to some of the potential problems of such an initiative, but also to outline its merits.

QUESTIONS FOR DISCUSSION

- If nurse prescribers are to prescribe extensively from the BNF, what level of knowledge of science, clinical pharmacology and therapeutics is required?
- Should nurses completing this form of training be provided with a recordable nursing qualification that denotes advanced skills offered by the UKCC and/or an MSc in nursing and clinical pharmacology and therapeutics?
- What postgraduate assessment would be required to maintain nurse prescribers on this part of the register?
- Would nurse prescribers be recognised as working at an advanced level?

Further reading

Becker, K.L., Zaiken, H., Wilcox, P.M., Kirk, B., Levitt, M.K. & Pasternak, N.S. (1989) 'A nurse prescriber job description.' Nursing Management, 20: 42–44.

This reference is included to assist the nurse practitioner comprehend nursing issues pertinent to prescribing medication, particularly as this is an extended role and hence a constantly developing one.

Holmes, S. (1991) 'Clinical leadership: a role for the advanced practitioner.' Journal of Advanced Health Nursing Care, 1: 3–20.

This reference examines how nurses working at an advanced level need to consider the complexity of the nature of their role external to prescribing of medication.

Manley, K. (1996) 'Advanced practice is not about medicalising nursing roles.' Nursing in Critical Care, 1: 1–2.

This paper reviews the relationship with nursing and the implications for the advanced role.

Mundinger, M.O. (1994) 'Advanced-practice nursing - good medicine for physicians?' New England Journal of Medicine, 330: 211-214.

Examines the issues of advanced nursing practice and the relationship with medicine.

REFERENCES

Allen & Hanbury, (1993). Flixotide. [Product monograph.] Middlesex: Allen & Hanbury.
Back, D.J. & Rogers, S.M. (1987) First-pass metabolism by gastrointestinal mucosa. *Alimentary Pharmacology and Therapeutics*, **1**, 339–357.
Bailey, D.G., Spence, J.D., Bayliff, C.D., Arnold, J.M.O. (1989) Ethanol enhances the haemodynamic effects of felodipine, *Clinical Investigations Medicine*, **12**, 357–362.
Bailey, D.G., Spence, J.D., Munoz, C. & Arnold, J.M.O. (1991) Interaction of citric juices with felodipine and nifedipine. *Lancet*, **337**, 268–269.
Beardon, P.H.G., McGilchrist, M.M. & McKendrick, A.D. (1993) Primary noncompliance with prescribed medication in primary care. *British Medical Journal*, **307**, 846–848.
Beattie, A. (1987) Making a curriculum work. In *The Curriculum in Nursing Education*, ed. Allan, P. & Jolley, M. London: Croom Helm.
Benner, P. (1984) *From Novice to Expert: excellence and power in clinical nursing*. California: Addison-Wesley.
Butterworth, T. & Faugier, J. (1992) *Clinical Supervision and Mentorship in Nursing*. London: Chapman & Hall.
Calloway, N.O., Foley, C.F. & Lagerbloom, P. (1965) Uncertainties in geriatric data II: organ size. *Journal of the American Geriatrics Society*, **13**, 20–28.
Cargill, J.M. (1992) Medication compliance in elderly people influencing variables and interventions *Journal of Advanced Nursing*, **17**, 422–426.
Colli, A., Buccino, G., Cocciolo, M., Parravicini, R. & Scaltrini, G. (1988) Disposition of a flow-limited drug (lidocaine) and a metabolite capacity-limited (theophyllines) in liver cirrhosis. *Clinical Pharmacology and Therapeutics*, **44**, 642–649.
De Vries, T.P.G.M., Henning, R.H. *et al.* (1995) Impact of a short course in pharmacotherapy for undergraduate medical students: an international randomised controlled study. *Lancet*, **346**, 1454–1457.

Department of Health (1989) *Report of the Advisory Group on Nurse Prescribing.* (Crown Report.) London: Department of Health.

Department of Health and Social Security (1986). *Neighbourhood Nursing – A Focus for Care.* (Cumberlege Report.) London: HMSO.

Evans L & Spelman M (1983) The problems of non-compliance with drug therapy. *Drugs,* **25,** 63–76.

John, A. & Stevenson, T. (1995) A basic guide to the principles of drug therapy. *British Journal of Nursing,* **4,** 1194–1198.

Jones, A. & Bowen, M. (1994) Screening for childhood asthma using an exercise test. *British Journal of General Practice,* **44,** 127–131.

Kee, C.C. (1992) Age-related changes in the renal system: causes, consequences, and nursing implications. *Geriatric Nursing,* **13(2),** 80–83.

Kolnaar, B.G.M., Van Lier, A., Van Den Bosch, W.J.H.M. *et al.* (1994) Asthma in adolescents and young adults: relationship with early childhood respiratory morbidity. *British Jounral of General Practice,* **44,** 73–78.

LaBella, F.S. (1991) Cytochrome P450 enzymes: ubiquitous 'receptors' for drugs. *Canadian Journal of Physiology and Pharmacology,* **69,** 1129–1132.

Luyt, D.K., Burton, P., Brooke, A.M. & Simpson, H. (1994) Wheeze in preschool children and its relation with doctor diagnosed asthma. *Archives of Disease in Childhood,* **71,** 24–30.

McKenzie, S. (1994) Cough – but is it asthma? *Archives of Disease in Childhood,* **70,** 1–2.

Madden, V. (1995) The economic and clinical costs of noncompliance. *Prescriber,* **19 April 1995,** 64–65.

Meyer, B.R. (1989) Renal functioning in aging. *Journal of the American Geriatrics Society,* **37,** 791–800.

Meyer, B.R. & Hirsch, B.E. (1990) Renal function and the care of the elderly. *Comprehensive Therapeutics,* **16(9),** 30–37.

Neuvonen, P.J., Kivisto, K.T. & Lehto, P. (1991) Interference of dairy products with the absorption of ciprofloxacin. *Clinical Pharmacology and Therapeutics,* **50,** 498–502.

Ninan, T.K. & Russell, G. (1992). Asthma, inhaled corticosteroid treatment, and growth. *Archives of Disease in Childhood,* **67,** 703–705.

O'Callaghan, C. & Barry, P. (1997) Spacer devices in the treatment of asthma. *British Medical Journal,* **314,** 1061–1062.

Ogier, M. (1989) *Reading Research.* London: Scutari Press.

Pacifici, G.M., Franchi, M., Bencini, C., Repetti, F. & Di Lascio, N. (1988) Tissue distribution of drug metabolising enzymes in humans. *Xenobiotica,* **18,** 849–856.

Patten, B.C. & Holt, J.A. (1992) When your patient is allergic. *American Journal of Nursing,* **September,** 58–61.

Reinke, L.F. & Hoffman, L.A. (1992) Breathing space: how to teach asthma co-management. *American Journal Nursing,* **October,** 40–47.

Reynolds DJM & Aronson JK (1993) Making the most of plasma drug concentration measurements. *British Medical Journal,* **306(48),** 31.

Rickenbach, M.A. & Julious, S.A. (1994) Assessing fullness of asthma patients' aerosol inhalers. *British Journal of General Practice,* **44,** 317–318.

Rowland, M.(1993) Variability and the individual. *Pharmaceutical Journal,* **251,** 408–410.

Schumucker, D.L., Woodhouse, K.W., Wang, R.K., Wynne, H. & James, O.F. (1990) Effects of age and gender on in vitro properties of human liver microsomal monooxygenases. *Clinical Pharmacology and Therapeutics,* **48,** 365–374.

Schwartz, D.W. (1991) Basic principles of pharmacologic action. *Nursing Clinics of North America,* **26,** 245–262.

Shyu, W., Knupp, C.A., Pittman, K.A., Dunkle, L. & Barbhaiya, R.H. (1991) Food-induced reduction in bioavailability of didansoine. *Clinical Pharmacology and Therapeutics,* **50,** 503–507.

Soons, P.A., Vogels, B.A.T.M., Roosemalen, M., Schoemaker, H.C. & Uchida, E. (1991) Grapefruit juice and cimetidine inhibit stereoselective metabolism of nitrendipine in humans. *Clinical Pharmacology and Therapeutics,* **50,** 394–404.

Tam, Y.K. (1993) Individual variation in first-pass metabolism. *Clinical Pharmacokinetics,* **25(4),** 300–328.

TPS Drug Information Centre (1992) The right time? Chronopharmacology – a new science. *Nursing RSA Verpleging,* **7,** 23–25.

United Kingdom Central Council for Nursing, Midwifery and Health Visiting (1989) *Exercising Accountability*. London: UKCC.

United Kingdom Central Council for Nursing, Midwifery and Health Visiting (1992a). *Code of Professional Conduct*. London: UKCC.

United Kingdom Central Council for Nursing, Midwifery and Health Visiting (1992b). *Scope of Professional Practice*. London: UKCC.

United Kingdom Central Council for Nursing, Midwifery and Health Visiting (1992c) *Standards for the Administration of Medicines*. London: UKCC.

United Kingdom Central Council for Nursing, Midwifery and Health Visiting (1996) *Guidelines for Professional Practice*. London: UKCC.

Urquhart, J.(1994) Role of patient compliance in clinical pharmacokinetics. *Clinical Pharmacokinetics*, **27(3)**, 202–215.

Vestal, R.E., Wood, A.J.J., Branch, R.A., Shand, D.G. & Wilkinson, G.R. (1979) Effects of age and cigarette smoking on the disposition of propranolol in man. *Clinical Pharmacology and Therapeutics*, **26**, 8–15.

Watson, R.C.P, Bastain, W., Larkin, K.A., Hayes, J.R. & McAinsh, J.A. (1987). A comparative pharmacokinetic study of conventional propranolol and a long acting preparation of propranolol in patients with cirrhosis and normal controls. *British Journal of Clinical Pharmacology*, **24**, 527–535.

Young-Jin, S. & Shannon, M. (1992) Pharmacokinetics of drugs in overdose. *Clinical Pharmacokinetics*, **23**, 93–105.

Zauderer, B. (1996) Age-related changes in renal function. *Critical Care Nursing Quarterly*, **19(2)**, 34–40.

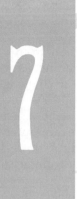

Nurse prescribing

Essential practice or political point

Eileen Shepherd   Anne Marie Rafferty
Veronica James

Key issues

♦ Nurse prescribing challenges the conventional boundaries of nursing practice and its jurisdiction.

♦ The socio-legal context in which prescribing practice develops acts as a brake as well as an enabling force for change.

♦ Public protection and inter-professional professional rivalry balance the forces for and against change.

INTRODUCTION

Arrangements for the supply of medicines to patients are constructed around a division of labour which includes three key health care professionals: doctors prescribe, pharmacists dispense, while nurses administer medication (UKCC, 1992a). From October 1994 a limited number of nurses in Britain in eight demonstration sites were able, for the first time, to prescribe from a range of products defined in the Nurse Prescribers' Formulary, a new addendum to the British National Formulary.

It could be argued that the move to nurse prescribing, a change in the traditional hierarchy of health care labour, has major implications for the relationships between the professions which control the supply of medicines to patients. The earlier processes surrounding the implementation of nurse prescribing have been lengthy and complex (Poulton, 1994; Carlisle, 1990). The Treasury presented the main stumbling block to the proposed change on cost grounds (Poulton, 1994), although it has been argued that changes in practice enhanced the need for such change (RCN, 1995). Nevertheless it was the economic implications of setting up and maintaining a system of nurse prescribing that prevailed over opposition from other health care professionals. This economic dominance is intriguing, as giving authority to nurses to prescribe could be perceived as a challenge to medical hegemony within the division of health care labour. However, it also begs the question as to whether nurse prescribing represents a genuine advance in the status of nursing practice or can more accurately be characterised as an act of tacit delegation by the medical profession, leaving nurse prescribing open to challenge from the countervailing influence of the pharmacist (RPS/RCN, 1995).

Drawing on nurse prescribing as an example of the expansion of nurses' roles, this chapter explores the regulation of nursing, taking special account of nursing's boundaries, as they are mediated by law and education, with doctors and pharmacists. An examination in the first section of the introduction of nurse prescribing is followed in the second by consideration of the factors which delineate professional boundaries. A closer examination of regulation in nursing and medicine as it applies to prescribing is considered in the third section. The final section discusses the issues involved in renegotiating boundaries, in which key implications of nurse prescribing are identified.

INTRODUCTION OF NURSE PRESCRIBING

The reform process: a history of nurse prescribing

The 1986 Cumberlege Report on neighbourhood nursing (DHSS, 1986) highlighted publicly, for the first time, the issue of nurse prescribing. The report expressed the concerns of community nurses about the complex procedures that surrounded the prescribing process. The report recommended that the then Department of Health and Social Security (DHSS) should agree a limited list of medicines which could be prescribed by nurses as part of a nursing care programme. It also advised that guidelines be issued to enable nurses to control drug dosages in certain, defined circumstances. These recommendations were interpreted as an integral part of a much wider scheme which aimed to establish a more effective and responsive neighbourhood nursing service.

The recommendations of the Cumberlege committee were endorsed and developed in 1989 in the Crown Report on nurse prescribing (DoH, 1989). The Crown Report was compiled by a committee of nurses, doctors and pharmacists who concluded that only district nurses and health visitors, who were seen to have clear responsibility for care and management, should be granted prescribing rights. Community psychiatric nurses (CPNs) and specialist nurses were excluded from this category because of their dual role in acute and community units. However, CPNs were seen to be appropriately placed to alter the dosages and timings of drugs, while other specialist nurses might prescribe specific items for a named group of patients (DoH, 1989).

COSTS AND BENEFITS OF NURSE PRESCRIBING

The Crown Report concluded that its recommendations should be implemented without a pilot study. The decision to establish a number of demonstration sites was a response to concerns voiced by the Treasury as to the potential costs of a nationwide nurse prescribing scheme (Poulton, 1994). The chosen sites were subject to economic and qualitative evaluation of the effects of nurse prescribing prior to any further decision on the expansion of the scheme.

In 1994, the cost of drugs supplied to National Health Service patients accounted for 10% of total NHS expenditure – a drug bill which, since 1980, has risen dramatically from £1 billion to £3.3 billion. Despite national cost containment measures such as the 'limited list', generic prescribing initiatives, and the introduction of indicative prescribing schemes for general practitioners (GPs), expenditure on drugs continues to grow (Maynard and Bloor, 1993).

With the publication of the Cumberlege Report came concerns that nurse prescribing could result in an increase in drug costs and bureaucracy (Devlin, 1986). Contradicting this, it has been argued that as the basis of the proposed prescribing scheme is substitutive in nature, with nurses prescribing only what doctors would have prescribed, it will be a zero cost development (Devlin, 1986; NHS Executive, 1994). Against this background, the need to identify the costs and benefits of nurse prescribing led the Department of Health to instigate the country's only economically led evaluation of the changes advocated by the proponent's of nurse prescribing (DoH/Touche Ross, 1991).

The resulting Department of Health/Touche Ross cost–benefit analysis of nurse prescribing suggested that community nurses already made effective use of resources, thereby limiting opportunities for savings through more effective prescribing. Furthermore, the report also notes that the potential for increased prescribing of over-the-counter (OTC) medicines could have the effect of shifting cost from the patient onto prescribing budgets. This has obvious implications for government policy, which has consistently aimed to transfer the cost of prescribing from the NHS to the citizen and is reflected in ongoing deregulation of prescription only medicines (POM) to pharmacy (P) status (Booth, 1994).

A different view is offered by the authors of the Crown Report (DoH, 1989). They claimed that the increased efficiency of nurse prescribing will save 2.84 million hours per annum for patients, carers, GPs and nurses. However, such a saving is predicted by the Department of Health/Touche Ross cost–benefit analysis to have little effect on global costs as the time saved translates into as little as 1 hour per district nurse per week. Meanwhile, the cost of implementing a full nurse prescribing scheme was estimated at £7.06 million for systems and training in 1991. In addition, training costs will absorb 389 000 hours of nurses' time at a nominal cost of £3.8 million. Annual costs of £15 million are predicted for additional items and for data collection. District nurses included in the study suggest that they currently initiate an average of 5.9 prescriptions per week, of which half would be eligible for signature by a prescribing nurse trained under the new regulations. For health visitors the comparable figure was 2.6 prescriptions initiated per week.

While American studies on nurse prescribing abound, it has been suggested that such evidence and experience is incompatible with British plans in view of variation in formulary content and profound differences in arrangements for primary health care provision that exist between the two countries (DoH/Touche Ross, 1991). Despite the difficulty of transatlantic translation, evidence from the USA does suggest that where the medical monopoly of prescribing has been broken by nurse prescribers, such deregulation has resulted in savings on administrative overheads and the elimination of unnecessary communication (Moran and Wood, 1993). Although information on American nurse prescribing is limited to small-scale studies, some findings have suggested that nurse practitioners in the USA prescribe less than physicians (Mahoney, 1992; Safriet, 1992). Limitations of these studies are that they do not control for severity of illness, or the caseload of the practitioner (Mahoney, 1992). Furthermore, it is clear that nurses are more likely to prescribe OTC drugs (Hadley, 1989). This is particularly significant for the British demonstration sites where the Nurse Prescribers' Formulary does not include any prescription only medicines and so nurses are able to prescribe only medicines and other products which are already currently available over the counter and by GP prescription.

LEGISLATION AND EDUCATION

The Medicinal Products: Prescription by Nurses Etc. Act 1992 (DoH, 1992) amended the Medicines Act 1968 (DoH, 1968) to allow nurses (and anyone else deemed appropriate by the Secretary of State) to prescribe from a defined list of medicines. This measure helped overcome the hiatus caused by nurses assessing the need for and identifying the appropriate product, but having to go through the legal formality of waiting for a doctor to sign the prescription. An amendment to the NHS Act 1977 was also made to enable pharmacists to dispense prescriptions signed by a nurse.

The secondary legislation clarifying changes in prescribing law, and the final content of the Nurse Prescribers' Formulary were agreed in September 1994 prior to the commencement of the eight demonstration projects in England, set up in compliance with Crown Report recommendations

(UKCC, 1994). This legislation provides the framework within which an appropriately qualified community nurse (district nurse, health visitor, practice nurse) can prescribe a defined number of medicines. This framework is firmly fixed and can be changed only by further secondary legislation (J. Morris, UKCC, personal communication). Responsibility for the registration and education of prescribing nurses has been delegated by the Secretary of State to the UKCC, with the ENB being designated to design a training package and requiring the nurse to register with the UKCC before being allowed to prescribe (Pharmaceutical Journal, 1994a). The training package consists of 10–20 hours of open learning and 15 hours of formal college education. The content of the course covers:

- Pharmacology and therapeutics
- Effective prescribing
- Understanding the roles of other professionals
- The legal framework
- Maintaining high standards of accountability and professional responsibility
- Understanding the economics of prescribing (Brew, 1994).

The course is followed by an assessment, but further education is the responsibility of nurses and their employers (NHS Executive, 1994; Brew, 1994).

CHANGING PROFESSIONAL BOUNDARIES

The processes identified here as leading to legislative changes in prescribing illustrate some of the sociopolitical and economic factors through which the state plays a key role in shaping professional boundaries. As the government has sought to reduce public dependency and public spending on National Health Service provision (Appleby, 1992), so a politically and economically led health policy has facilitated a change in the professional boundaries of prescribing, dispensing and administering drugs. The precise mechanisms through which professional boundaries are defined can be further explored using the example of prescribing.

Qualified doctors of medicine have been granted a virtual monopoly over the prescription of prescription only medicines and controlled drugs by the Medicines Act 1968 which effectively prevents rival providers from entering the market-place. Moran and Wood (1993) suggest that the regulations which govern the exchange of goods and services, including pharmaceuticals, can be separated into four distinct areas:

1. The control of market entry and exit: identifying the kinds of individuals who can carry out the intervention and the conditions they have to fulfill.

2. The regulation of competitive practice: defining the conditions under which the market will operate.

3. The regulation of market structure: identifying through which institutions and organisations the service can be provided.

4. Market organisation and remuneration: methods and scales of charging.

Thus it is that government controlled and delegated regulatory processes determine who will benefit from the operation of the market. At one end of a continuum, the state has a direct role as a regulator – for example passing primary legislation which defines statutory obligations, such as health and safety requirements, with which all organisations must comply. Further along the continuum is a form of independent self-regulation. This is characterised by free markets in which professionals and occupations dominate the market entry and competition via systems of elaborate control (Moran and Wood, 1993). Between these two positions is the most common form of regulation in the UK – state sanctioned self-regulation. For example, the General Medical Council (GMC) carries out the detailed tasks of regulating medicine, under the supervision of the state, as the UKCC carries out the same delegated function for nursing, midwifery and health visiting within constraints laid down by the Secretary of State and the European Commission.

The advantage of this arrangement is that it protects the state from the financial and administrative burden of direct regulation, but to achieve this issues of delegation of power and attendant accountability have to be clearly defined (Moran and Wood, 1993). In the case of prescribing, the monopoly of the medical profession has been maintained by professional control over diagnostic and curative processes through functions delegated by the state to the GMC.

Professionalisation

Any changes brought about by introducing and expanding nurse prescribing occur both within the context of the state and market mechanisms described, and are also subject to the professional control and regulation from the disciplines involved – medicine, nursing and pharmacy. This ability to regulate and define practice is, arguably, a core characteristic of a mature profession (Montgomery, 1992; Freidson, 1970). It is accepted that medicine is a profession whereas nursing has struggled throughout the 20th century to achieve such status (Witz, 1992; Davies, 1995). Freidson (1986) has suggested that doctors are the key professionals from whom the legitimacy of other professionals is derived, and that the superordinate position of doctors is possible because of the subordination of other occupations such as nursing, whose members undertake delegated activities.

While a number of attempts have been made to characterise the constituents of a profession, they tend to ignore the role of power and privilege that enables professional bodies to manipulate and control their clients and markets and the microdynamics associated with the social processes through which professions are shaped (Turner, 1987; Hugman, 1991; Johnson, 1972). Professionalisation has been said to develop strategies to ensure a monopoly in three important dimensions (Freidson, 1986):

1. They possess a unique body of knowledge that is underpinned by formal education and systematic entry requirements.
2. They maintain and cultivate an extensive clientele which is exclusive of other professions or occupations. This may require legislative and state support in promoting a monopoly.
3. They maintain certain privileges at work in terms of their skills and clients.

While there are clear parallels between these dimensions and the key features that differentiate forms of regulation, Abbott (1988) argues that this configuration of professional components ignores the core motivation of professions – inter-professional competition. His claim is that it is the history of jurisdictional disputes, that is competing claims over legitimate areas of expertise, that encapsulates the real history of professions, and that these disputes can be examined, initially, only through case studies. In his view, while medicine has full jurisdiction over health matters, the subordination of nursing is the result of an uneasy public and legal settlement, but one which leaves nursing absolutely necessary to the good practice of medicine (Hunt, 1994). Approaching this issue from the route of gender analysis, Davies (1995) argues that autonomy for some professional groups is only ever possible through 'adjunct' work of others: 'Autonomy therefore turns out to require considerable work by others and without this work it cannot be sustained' (Davies, 1995, p. 60). This has implications for the negotiating power of nursing, and presents an opening through which nurse prescribing becomes possible in inter-professional terms. However, such a move becomes intelligible not only in terms of the professionalising projects of nursing and medicine, but in relation to that of pharmacy, too (Cotter, Barber and McKee, 1994). Evidence is beginning to emerge that pharmacists are not going to react passively to prescribing initiatives by nurses. Indeed nurses may find themselves on the receiving end of critical scrutiny as pharmacists sharpen their 'gaze' on prescribing practice under the pressure of and for professionalisation (Pharmaceutical Journal, 1996a).

Extending the boundaries

Prescribing is the only area in which the law defines the nature of the work carried out by health care professionals. Such criteria are determined by statutory bodies, and the limits to practice are established in accordance with the role of the occupation and its associated educational requirements. At the periphery of these boundaries there is freedom to develop skills which cross the line of demarcation between occupational and professional groups (Wainwright, 1994; Dimond, 1994).

Throughout their history, nurses have come to absorb many tasks previously the preserve of doctors; for instance, they now administer drugs, measure blood pressure and catheterise patients. Doctors have delegated, over time, a range of duties which have now become established as the defining features of nursing work. Such acts of delegation have been a one-way process and have reinforced the dominant position of medicine within the division of labour. The acceptance of such tasks by nurses has, however, been accompanied by an emphasis on the need for formal training and proof of competence (Dimond, 1994). This process was reflected in the use of the now obsolete certification practice involved in the 'extended role' defined by Zarnow as 'carrying out some function in a protracted context' to fill perceived gaps in the health care system (Zarnow, 1977). The legislation which defined the extended role served to emphasise delegation, training and competence, but restricted nurses' abilities to act in a flexible and knowledgeable way. The principles which underpinned such a role appeared to confirm that registration marked the end of a nurse's development.

In 1992, extended role legislation was abandoned in favour of the UKCC's *Scope of Professional Practice* (UKCC, 1992b), which emphasised the notion of role expansion. McGuire (1980) suggests that role expansion occurs when nurses take on responsibility for a role where training is a prerequisite and where nurses' skills are drawn upon. Expansion enables the nurse to introduce new components or practices into health care. The notion of expansion has proved attractive to those seeking to rationalise medical tasks in an attempt to contain costs in the secondary care setting. The potential that role expansion offers to policy makers is reflected in the comments of Caines (1980), who welcomed *The Scope of Professional Practice* as a move by nurses to be more responsive to fluctuations in professional boundaries: 'Nurses are multi-skilled and we accept this. All we are talking about is the shifting of boundaries and the sorts of responsibilities that allow nurses to become more flexible' (Caines, 1980, p. 7).

It has been suggested that the technicalisation of nursing in secondary care will continue to be regarded in terms of extended roles, with proof of competence underpinning acceptance of delegated tasks (Dimond, 1994). Since the expansion of the nurse's role is an important consideration for nurses seeking professional status (Wainwright, 1994; McGuire, 1980; Pickersgill, 1993), prescribing by community nurses can be claimed as an example of increased occupational control over the context of their work (Hunt, 1994). Nevertheless, the possibility of an alternative reading of the evidence in which prescribing by community nurses can be considered in terms of acceptance of delegated authority cannot be discounted.

Together, the expanded role, coupled with the concept of the 'named nurse' (DoH, 1992), nurse prescribing and increasing numbers of master's level courses in nursing practice, creates a synergy that might facilitate the development of advanced nurse practitioner roles. However, additional responsibility without commensurate autonomy in decision making may merely expand the role by absorbing delegated technical tasks (McGuire, 1980). This is clearly significant in the case of nurse prescribing where the sites chosen for nurse prescribing are ones in which there is clear budgetary control by the GPs. The prescribing could therefore be interpreted as a form of role extension, with little increase in autonomy, nurses being under the direct delegation and financial control of the provider practice.

REGULATION OF NURSING PRACTICE

The Nurses, Midwives and Health Visitors Act 1979 was heralded by commentators as an opportunity for nursing to function as an independent discipline. The Act led directly to the formation of the UKCC, which had a remit to:

- Provide guidance on professional standards and conduct
- Determine rules of registration and maintain a single professional register
- Protect the public from unsafe members of the profession.

The UKCC worked with the four National Boards (England, Northern Ireland, Scotland, Wales) responsible for nurse education across the UK. The constitution and function of the UKCC and the national boards was clarified and streamlined by the Nurses, Midwives and Health Visitors Act 1991, which aimed to make the UKCC directly accountable to the profession. This was reflected in the composition of its membership, two-thirds of whom were elected and one-third appointed by the secretary of state (Montgomery, 1992). The power vested in the UKCC by the state to self-regulate can be interpreted as a step forward in the professionalisation of nursing. However, despite the clear definitions of nursing competencies which appear in the Nurses Acts, no explicit reference is made to nurses' power or authority to make decisions. It has been suggested that while the Acts place an emphasis on the responsibilities of nurses, this has not been accompanied by a net increase in discretionary freedom (Wainwright, 1994).

The predominantly female character of nursing and its historical link to domestic and vocational work supports the definition of nursing as a quasi-professional occupation (Freidson, 1986). Florence Nightingale did much to define the moral nature of nurses' work, and also defined the location of nursing in a role subordinate to medicine (Holton, 1984). Yet nurses were deeply divided over the issue of registration (Dingwall, Rafferty and Webster, 1988; Abel-Smith, 1960). Historically, nursing, like medicine, had difficulty developing a recognised system of entry and practice. More recently, in the increasingly international world of nursing and health care, nursing showed its collective lobbying power by influencing the content of the European Community Directives regulating nurse education on the 'Nurse Responsible for General Care' (Russell, 1993; Keyzer, 1994), while medicine has yet to achieve such a Directive. Yet while there is shared recognition of training for 'general care', precise definitions of the role of the nurse are elusive, and professional fragmentation is illustrated by the failure to reach agreement on training requirements for specialist nursing roles (Russell, 1993).

REGULATION, NURSING AND MEDICAL POWER
Nursing and medical power

Like all professionals, individual nurses are subject to organisational and professional controls which, particularly in nursing, restrict their ability to act autonomously (Davies, 1983). Collective challenge to these controls is not an easy option for nurses who, in addition to their history of medical subordination, lack the support of an overarching professional body to equal the strength of the British Medical Association (BMA).

As nurses are challenging their subordinate role in the division of labour, medical hegemony is said to be in decline (Montgomery, 1992). The delegation of traditional medical skills to paramedical staff may reflect ongoing encroachment into medical territory (Alaszewski, 1979; Armstrong, 1976), but more importantly, economic constraint and the introduction of general management systems are said to pose a similar threat to medical dominance (Montgomery, 1992). In particular, medicine's ability to negotiate directly with government as a monopoly player (Moran et al., 1993) was challenged by the advent of the internal market. Furthermore, the increasing demands of a knowledgeable and informed public have led to a demystification of medical practice (Montgomery, 1992). Yet the state has not directly challenged the dominance of medicine or the notion of clinical freedom (Eaton and Webb, 1979), although, arguably, there have been many indirect challenges.

The origins of modern medical power can be traced to the Medical Act 1858, which united the then competing occupations of apothecaries, physicians and surgeons into one body. This unique event allowed medicine to define its own boundaries and to guard against encroachment by the incorporation of competing factions into the unitary body of the General Medical Council, albeit with some difficulty (Eaton and Webb,

1979). Like the UKCC, the GMC is responsible for disciplining those who transgress its rules (Moran *et al.*, 1993).

Yet medicine's expansion into specialist areas has required formal and informal delegation to occupations (or professions) 'allied' to medicine (PAMs). This could imply an opening of boundaries, but it can also be argued that medicine retains control over other occupations by delegating tasks, while withholding the authority to control them (Freidson, 1986). Davies (1995) identifies gender differences in professional autonomy as a dominant factor through which medicine shapes the status of nursing work, leaving nursing to challenge the dominant 'impartial rationality' of medicine, and arguing that 'the real and painful irony . . . is that there is no clear professional practice role at all'. It is thus in these contradictory contexts of state reorganisation of health care, traditional medical dominance and nursing's drive for professionalisation that development of nurse prescribing needs to be considered.

Nurse prescribing: boundary encroachment?

The forces driving the expansion of the role of community nurses have been attributed to greater emphasis on primary health care and increased demands for health care, particularly among older age groups. In addition, despite rises in the number of practising GPs from 29 336 in 1980 to 33 839 in 1991, there is a perceived shortfall in workforce numbers. Moreover, GPs now undertake more rigorous diagnostic examinations and minor surgical procedures as part of the shift in focus towards primary care (DHSS, 1986), and the development of GP fundholding schemes has created new pressures across broad areas of general practice. Such changes in the GP's role have been associated with an increase in delegation to community practice nurses. Yet Stilwell and others (1988) suggest that there is still potential for practice nurses to play a more autonomous part in patient care (Bowling, 1981; Greenfield et al, 1987). This is of particular relevance in rural communities where reductions in secondary care facilities have led to increasing pressure on GP services. In the USA, similar problems have stimulated a growth in nurse practitioners with prescribing authority prevailing in those rural areas which are considered to be under served by medical practitioners (Safriet, 1992; Bowling, 1981; Mahoney, 1992).

The limitation of prescribing rights to district nurses and health visitors in Britain has important implications for the development of the nurse practitioner role (Rickford, 1993). The use of agreed treatment protocols and standing orders is helping to alleviate the problems of GP workload management, and enabling nurses to provide a responsive service to patients (Mayor, 1994). Yet these solutions present a compromise to the nurse practitioner who still requires the signature of a GP on prescriptions.

The granting of prescribing rights to community nurses should herald a new stage in nurses' professional development. Yet some community nurses anticipate that only a small improvement in their job satisfaction will result, while others fear an increase in responsibility. Certainly nursing and medical perceptions of the degree of nursing involved in prescribing already differ, with GPs ascribing more input from nurses than nurses do themselves (RCN, 1995). The majority of nurses, however, see prescribing as a legitimisation of the status quo rather than an advancement in professional status (DoH/Touche Ross, 1991). This is reinforced by a general acknowledgement that nurses routinely circumvent existing legislation governing drug administration (DoH, 1989; Stilwell, 1988). For example, community nurses often currently obtain medicines using pre-signed prescriptions (DoH, 1989; DoH/Touche Ross, 1991).

Potentially then, the granting of prescribing rights offers community nurses the opportunity to develop their nursing practice in a flexible and adaptable way that will ultimately benefit their patients. Yet the limitations of the Nurse Prescribers' Formulary and the uncertainty which surrounds the future development of nurse prescribing suggest that the realisation of such benefits may be short-lived. Further, while it has been argued that the development of nurse prescribing will increase nurses' control of patient care at the expense of medical hegemony, informal nurse prescribing is known to occur currently with the sanction of GPs (Stilwell, 1988) and without fear of boundary encroachment (Eaton and Webb, 1979).

In practice, the subordination of community nurses to medical staff is played out in the doctor–nurse game (Stein, 1967). This 'game' has, in the past, proved to be mutually beneficial in confirming the authority of doctors and shielding nurses from responsibility for their decisions (Mackay, 1993). Community nurses exert some influence over GPs' prescribing activity and in doing so, Stein suggests, the 'rules' of the doctor–nurse game are changed so that nurses no longer adopt a subservient role but are acting as stubborn rebels (Stein, 1990). Yet despite this influence nurses have failed to take control of treatment and have left the core of physicians' prescribing activity largely intact (Eaton and Webb, 1979). This is reinforced by studies of hospital nurses and their compliance with doctors' orders for medication. Such studies illustrate that nurses will follow doctors' instructions, even when they may directly endanger patients (Hofling et al., 1966; Milgram, 1974).

The functioning of nurse prescribing removes the power of delegation from the doctor for those medicines that are included in the Nurse Prescribers' Formulary. The signature of a nurse prescriber is then sufficient to initiate a course of treatment, albeit with readily available medicines and products. While it could be argued that this legislative change has forced medicine to relinquish some of its control to nurses keen to expand into medical territory, an alternative interpretation is that delegation of the responsibility through the state is politically expedient in the light of the expanding workload of GPs. The latter is commensurate with the acceptance of nurse prescribing by the Royal College of General Practitioners, and its subsequent calls for the extension of prescribing rights to practice nurses without district nurse or health visitor status (Royal College of General Practitioners, personal communication).

Legal responsibilities

Although community nurses will have responsibility for their prescribing practice, it has been suggested that the GP, who bears final responsibility for the patient, will retain ultimate control over treatment options. The Crown Report recommended that in the event of a dispute between a prescribing nurse and community pharmacist, the GP would have the final say (DoH, 1989). This raises the question as to the legal responsibilities surrounding nurse prescribing, and fails to address the position of the nurse who prescribes for a patient who is not registered with a GP. Guidance for nurse prescribers from the National Health Service Executive suggests that when a nurse prescribes as part of his or her nursing duties with the employer's consent, the employer is held vicariously liable for the nurse's action. For practice nurses with prescribing rights, this liability will fall upon the GP practice. For district nurses and health visitors, local trusts and commissioning agencies will bear similar responsibility. However, the guidelines suggest that nurses should obtain additional professional indemnity through their professional organisations (NHS Executive, 1994). The guidance does not address the issue of dispute between the professionals which will have to be played out in the practical arena of the demonstration sites. Comments from professional bodies seem to support the view that nurses will be considered liable for their actions, and therefore will be professionally responsible (Medical Defence Union; Medical Protection Society, personal communications).

Existing case law appears to reinforce the position of the community nurse as subordinate to the GP. Although there has been some legal recognition of the work of nurses and midwives, the dominance of medicine remains, despite the multidisciplinary nature of modern health care. While doctors are not responsible for nursing negligence, it has been shown that nurses can be protected from medical liability by relying on a doctor's instructions (Montgomery, 1992). However, increased litigation involving nurses suggests that this balance may change, and that it is likely that nurse prescribers will be subjects of legal action (Medical Defence Union, personal communication, 1994).

Education of nurses: self-limiting boundaries?

Hadley (1989), in her study of nurses and prescriptive authority in the USA, distinguishes between two types of nurse prescribers: those with substitutive jurisdiction who can prescribe without the supervision of a physician, and those with complementary jurisdiction, who work with a supervising physician. In market terms, substitutive prescribing can create competition between doctors and nurses, whereas complementary pre-scribing is a joint venture that is symbiotic in nature. The development of substitutive prescribing in the UK could potentially increase the flexibility of nurses' work, but it requires the elimination of established boundaries and a collaborative approach between nurses and doctors. In addition, Hadley notes that in order to prescribe competently nurses need to develop an adequate knowledge of drug therapy and pharmacology as well as the ability to diagnose. In the UK there is a recognised educational deficit among nurses relating to their knowledge of therapeutics and practical prescribing (Andrews, 1992). It has been suggested that nurses require extensive preparatory education before gaining prescribing rights (Fennell, 1991), which casts doubts upon the limited content and duration of the pilot education scheme described earlier. This contrasts markedly with arrangements in some states in the USA where nurse practitioners, clinical nurse specialists and midwives must hold a master's degree and complete 30 hours of pharmacology learning (Andrews, 1994). In the UK, district nurses and health visitors' knowledge of drugs and their effects have been questioned in a small-scale study (Andrews, 1992). In 1993, While and Rees (1993) revealed that health visitors and district nurses had a poor knowledge of pharmacology, therapeutics and the practical aspects of prescribing. These results have been reinforced by an exploratory study of clinical decision making which questioned the relationship between research based knowledge and clinical practice. The authors, Luker and Kenrick (1992), suggest that nurses are able to function as highly skilled practitioners, but are unable to articulate the source of their knowledge. Furthermore, the work of Pirie (1987) suggests that nurses are not aware of their weaknesses in relation to mathematics. The need for basic mathematical reasoning in the prescribing process suggests that this should be included in the education of nurse prescribers (Hopkins, 1990).

In view of the limits of the Nurse Prescribers' Formulary, which covers a restricted number of OTC medicines, appliances, reagents, wound management and related products, the significance of the diagnostic and pharmaceutical skills referred to can be perceived to be overplayed. Indeed the absence of any prescription only medicines from the formulary and the ongoing discussions as to their eventual inclusion (Friend, 1994) suggests that the whole scheme is characterised by legal constraints and professional boundaries rather that patient need.

Pharmacists

It is worth noting that while pharmacists have a central role in the provision of prescribed medicines, many of the issues affecting nurses' professional development in this area are being played out simultaneously at the boundary between pharmacy and medicine and at another level, pharmacy and nursing (Freidson, 1986; Eaton and Webb, 1989; Pharmaceutical Journal, 1994b). Pharmacists' search for professionalisation is focused principally on expanding their influence over the supply and use of drugs, and thereby extracting themselves from a subordinate relationship with medicine. In the primary care setting, community pharmacists are actively seeking a wider remit in the provision of drug treatment which goes far beyond their current monopoly over the supply of prescription only medicines. Consequently the development of nurse prescribing has led to calls for similar prescribing rights to be extended to pharmacists. Drawing upon initiatives and case studies from the USA, pharmacists in the UK seem set to make a bid to extend their influence over prescribing protocols in the UK. A more radical model, that of the pharmacy 'surgery', mimics medicine in its organisational format but could develop into a source of competitive rather than complementary services if medicine attempted to claw back territory lost in the labour substitution process (Pharmaceutical Journal, 1994b). Pharmacist involvement in the running of anticoagulation therapy and asthma clinics, for example, was already underway, and a similar reticence to make overt currently covert practices was expressed by some pharmacists, uncertain about where such practices would be located in relation to the law (Pharmaceutical Journal, 1996b).

Prescribing policies

Australia shines out as an example of positive and proactive prescribing policymaking. In 1991 two committees were formed to advise the government on how to implement a policy on the quality use of medicines: the Pharmaceutical Health and Rational Use of Medicines (PHARM) Working Party and the Australian Pharmaceutical Advisory Council (APAC) (CDHSH, 1994). Nurses have been particularly active in PHARM and their role transformed from one of passive to active participation (Hodge, 1995). PHARM established a task force which organised a conference on nurses and the quality use of medicines (DHSH, 1995). It could be argued that a similar research and policy initiative aimed at regularising nurse prescribing and clarifying the blurred legal boundary between nurses and doctors should be undertaken in this country. The quality criteria devised by PHARM could be usefully applied to evaluate the impact of legislative change and identify areas requiring further research. Comparative research in this sphere is urgently needed.

RENEGOTIATING BOUNDARIES: SOME CONCLUSIONS

The boundaries between the health care professions can be interpreted as being economically inefficient by granting some professionals exclusive rights to perform specific functions and preventing the efficient substitution of labour (Hadley, 1989). Labour substitution produces fears of fragmentation which threatens the dominant professional status of medicine through a process of rationalisation (Turner, 1987; Hunt, 1994). The shift in the balance of power and control initiated by nurse prescribing should result in an overall redistribution of authority over a defined number of medicines. However, it is possible to view this change as a 'renegotiation of order', whereby those who are subordinate can influence the activity of their superiors (RCN, 1995; Pharmaceutical Journal, 1994b). This moves away from the conflictual model of delegation and encroachment and concentrates on the two social groups and their interactions. In this way, the opportunity for nurses to prescribe does not necessarily mean that medicine has relinquished any rights relating to the use of medicines. Rather, as Mesler suggests, the distinction between boundary encroachment and task delegation is in reality blurred by social interactions between occupational groups which serve to 'define, establish, maintain, and renew the tasks they perform and the relationships between them' (Mesler, 1991, pp. 310–331). Such interactions can be mutually beneficial to those groups involved in renegotiation and may improve the outcome for patients. By interacting with physicians at a local and national level, nurses are negotiating their professional boundaries. This is clearly reflected in the consultation which has surrounded the development of legislation to enable nurse prescribing and the subsequent establishment of protocols and procedures to support its practice.

The extent to which nurse prescribing represents a genuine advance in nursing practice remains open to conjecture. While it can be predicted that nurse prescribers will be able to provide more effective and timely care for a small group of patients, the broader professional significance of such a development is far from easy to determine. The ambiguity surrounding the achievement of a nurse prescriber's formulary is founded upon the overwhelmingly political nature of the move towards nurse prescribing and, more importantly, on the interests of policy makers in fashioning the future. In essence, it appears that any further development of nurse prescribing will depend not on the needs of patients or the ambitions of nurses but on the economic success of the current demonstration sites and the prevailing priorities of care planners. Furthermore, the extension of substitutive prescribing will require further substantial negotiation with the medical and pharmaceutical professions, in whose interests it remains to control the sale and use of medicines, although subject to increasing government interest in drug expenditure. The continuing discussion which surrounds the inclusion of prescription only medicines in the nursing formulary could be construed as evidence of the tensions that may be generated were such an extension in nurse authority to become a reality. In particular, the role of the pharmacist and calls to assume a 'gatekeeping role' in health care may need to be taken into account in the event that pharmacists begin to take this role seriously and pursue it with vigour (Pharmaceutical Journal, 1996c).

The outcome of nurse prescribing is likely to depend on the mutual interaction and countervailing influences that nursing, pharmacy and medicine exert upon each other. The role of the professional organisations in pushing the frontiers of practice may well be pivotal. The Royal College of Nursing has demonstrated a strong commitment to campaign on behalf of nurse prescribing, and the Royal Pharmaceutical Society has followed suit in adopting an active and assertive role in promoting prescribing roles for its constituency (RPS/RCN, 1995). But all of this has to be viewed within the context of recent attempts to reconstruct the very nature of professionalism and to break down the boundaries that have hitherto separated professions into ostensibly distinct social and intellectual spheres. It will be interesting to observe the extent to which the managerial agenda for multi-skilling can infiltrate the particulars of professional practice and indeed the points at which proposals for role expansion, originating from professionals themselves, converge with those of the new managerialism (Hurst, 1995). Prescribing authority may well provide a focal point for such study. There is, therefore, considerable scope for further research into the effects of nurse prescribing on the role boundaries which separate and define medicine, pharmacy and nursing in the health care division of labour, and in particular, whether nurse prescribing can generate a renegotiation of such boundaries or will merely reinforce existing patterns of task delegation within existing relationships (Hurst, 1995). Furthermore, the interests of policy makers in maintaining a stake in the regulation of nurse prescribing provide an additional context in which the debate needs to be understood.

QUESTIONS FOR DISCUSSION

- Arguments in favour of nurse prescribing can be made on grounds of economy and efficiency, but to what extent does the delegated authority consequent upon prescribing practice represent a substantive shift in the power relations between medicine and nursing?

- Will pharmacy play more than a mediating role in balancing inter-professional tensions between doctors and nurses by seizing the substitutive initiative?

- Is residual regulatory rivalry between pharmacy, nursing and medicine likely to intensify or diminish with a quality use of medicines policy in the future?

ACKNOWLEDGEMENTS

The authors would like to thank *Nursing Times Research* and Macmillan Magazines for permission to reprint material first published in *Nursing Times Research*, 1(6): 465–478 and the Trent Institute for Health Services Research of University of Nottingham for funding the review upon which this chapter is based.

REFERENCES

Abbott, A. (1988) *The System of Professions: an essay in the expert division of labour*. London: University of Chicago Press.
Abel–Smith, G. (1960) *A History of the Nursing Profession*. London: Heinemann.
Alaszewski, A. (1979) Doctors and paramedical workers – the changing pattern of interprofessional relations. Quoted in Eaton, G. & Webb, B. Boundary encroachment: Pharmacists in the clinical setting. *Sociology Of Health and Illness*, 1, 69–89.
Andrews, P. (1994) Nurse prescribing. In *Expanding the Role of the Nurse: the scope of professional practice*, ed. Hunt, G. & Wainwright, P. Oxford: Blackwell.
Andrews, S. (1992) Prescription for success. *Health Direct*, **March 12**.
Appleby, J. (1992) *Financing Health Care in the 1990s*. Buckingham: Open University.
Armstrong, D. (1976) The decline of medical hegemony. A review of government reports during the NHS. *Social Science and Medicine*, **10**, 157–163.
Booth, B. (1994) *Over the Counter Formulary*. London: Macmillan.
Bowling, A. (1981) *Delegation In General Practice: a study of doctors and nurses*. London: Tavistock Publications.
Brew, M. (1994) Teaching nurses to prescribe. *Nursing Times*, **90(21)**, 32–34.
Caines, E. (1980) Multiskilling now accepted by nurses. *Nursing Standard*, **8(20)**, 7.
Carlise, D. (1990) Nurse prescribing: Just what the doctor ordered. *Nursing Times*, **86(29)**, 26–29.
Commonwealth Department of Human Services and Health (in conjunction with the Australian Pharmaceutical Health and Rational Use of Medicines (PHARM) Committee) (1994) A Policy on the Quality Use of Medicines, p.13. Canberra: Commonwealth Department of Human Services and Health/Australian Pharmaceutical Health and Rational Use of Medicines Committee.
Cotter, S., Barber, N. & McKee, M. (1994) Professionalisation of hospital pharmacy: the role of the clinical pharmacy. *Journal of Social and Administrative Pharmacy*, **11(2)**, 57–66.
Davies, C. (1995) *Gender and the Professional Predicament in Nursing*. Buckingham: Open University.
Davies, C. (1983) Professionals in bureaucracies: conflict thesis revisited. In *Readings in the Sociology of Nursing*, ed. Dingwall, R. & Macintosh, J. Edinburgh: Churchill Livingstone.
Department of Health (1992) *Medicinal Products: Prescription by Nurses Act*. London: HMSO.
Department of Health (1989) *Report of the Advisory Group on Nurse Prescribing*. (Crown Report.) London: HMSO.
Department of Health (1968) *The Medicines Act*. London: HMSO.
Department of Health (1992) *The Patient's Charter*. London: Department of Health.
Department of Health and Social Security (1986) *Neighbourhood Nursing – A Focus For Care*. (Cumberlege Report.) London: Department of Health and Social Security.
Department of Health/Touche Ross (1991) *Nurse Prescribing: final report. A cost benefit study*. London: Department of Health.
Department of Human Services and Health, Australian Nurses' Federation and Royal College of Nursing, Australian Pharmaceutical Health and Rational Use of Medicines (PHARM) Committee (1995) *Nurses and the Quality Use of Medicines*. Nurses and Medications: examining roles and partnerships, pp. 10, 20, 24 (Conference report.) November 1994. Canberra: Department of Human Services and Health.
Devlin, R. (1986) Power of the prescription pad. *Community Outlook*, **16, July**, 31–32.
Dimond, B. (1994) Legal aspects of role expansion. In *Expanding the Role of the Nurse: the scope of professional practice*, ed. Hunt, G. & Wainwright, P. Oxford: Blackwell.
Dingwall, R., Rafferty, A.M. & Webster, C.(1988) *An Introduction to the Social History of Nursing*. London: Routledge.

Eaton, G. & Webb, B. (1979) Boundary encroachment: pharmacists in the clinical setting. *Sociology of Health and Illness*, **1**, 69–89.

Fennell, K. (1991) Prescriptive authority for nurse-midwives. *Nursing Clinics of North America*, **26(2)**, 511–516.

Freidson, E. (1970) *Profession of Medicine*. New York: Harper & Row.

Freidson, E. (1986) *Professional Powers: a study of the institutionalisation of formal knowledge*. London: University of Chicago Press.

Friend, B. (1994) Prescribing pioneers. *Nursing Times*, **90(39)**, 20.

Greenfield, S., Stilwell, B. & Drury, M. (1987) Practice nurses: social and occupational characteristics. *Journal of the Royal College of General Practitioners*, **37, August**, 341–345.

Hadley, H.E. (1989) Nurses and prescriptive authority: a legal and economic analysis. *American Journal of Law and Medicine*, **15(2&3)**, 245–299.

Hodge, M.M. (1995) *Improving the Use of Medicines: involving all stakeholders in the policy, education, research and practice process*. Seminar at Centre for Policy in Nursing Research, London School of Hygiene & Tropical Medicine, 12 March. (Copy details from: Anne Marie Rafferty, Centre for Policy in Nursing Research, London School of Hygiene & Tropical Medicine, Keppel St., London WC1 E 7HT)

Hofling, C.K., Brotzmann, E. Dalrymple, S. *et al.* (1966) An experimental study in nurse–physician relationships. *Journal of Nervous and Mental Disease*, **143**, 171–180.

Holton, S. (1984) Feminine authority in social order: Florence Nightingale's conception of nursing and health care. *Social Analysis*, **15**, 59–72.

Hopkins, A. (1990) Modifying drug dosage and timing. *Nursing Standard*, **5(13/14)**, 26–28.

Hugman, R. (1991) *Power in the Caring Professions*. London: Macmillan.

Hunt G. (1994) New professionals? New ethics? In *Expanding the Role of the Nurse: the scope of professional practice*, ed. Hunt, G. & Wainwright, R. Oxford: Blackwell.

Hurst, K. (1995) *Progress with Patient-Focused Care in the United Kingdom*. Leeds: NHS Executive.

Johnson, T.J. (1972) *Professions and Power*. London: Macmillan.

Keyzer, D. (1994) European aspects of the nursing role. In *Expanding the Role of the Nurse: the scope of professional practice*, ed. Hunt, G. & Wainwright, R. Oxford: Blackwell.

Luker, A. & Kenrick, M. (1992) An exploratory study of the sources of influence on the clinical decisions of community nurses. *Journal of Advanced Nursing*, **17**, 457–466.

Mackay, L. (1993) *Conflicts in Care. Medicine and nursing*. London: Chapman & Hall.

Mahoney, D.F. (1992) A comparative analysis of nurse practitioners with and without prescriptive authority. *Journal of the American Academy of Nurse Practitioners*, **4(2)**, 71–76.

Mahoney, D.F. (1992) Nurse practitioners as prescribers: past research trends and future study needs. *Nurse Practitioner*, **17(1)**, 44–51.

Maynard, A. & Bloor, K. (1993) Cost-effective prescribing of pharmaceuticals: the search for the holy grail? In *Purchasing and Providing Cost-Effective Health Care*, ed. Maynard, A. & Drummond, F. Edinburgh: Churchill Livingstone.

Mayor, S. (1994) Good practice. *Nursing Times*, **90(35)**, 24–25.

McGuire, J.M. (1980) *The Expanded Role of the Nurse*. London: King's Fund College.

Mesler, M.A. (1991) Boundary encroachment and task delegation: clinical pharmacists on the medical team. *Sociology of Health and Illness*, **13(3)**, 310–331.

Milgram, S. (1974) *Obedience To Authority. An experimental view*. New York: Harper & Row.

Montgomery, M. (1992) Doctors' handmaidens. In *Law, Health, and Medical Regulation*, ed. : Wheeler, S. & McVeigh, S. Hampshire: Dartmouth Publishing.

Moran, M. & Wood, B. (1993) *States, Regulation and the Medical Profession*. Buckingham: Open University Press.

NHS Executive (1994) *Nurse Prescribing Guidance*. London: HMSO.

Pharmaceutical Journal (1994a) Nurse prescribing. *Pharmaceutical Journal*, **253**, 435.

Pharmaceutical Journal (1994b) Prescribing role for pharmacists within general medical practice. *Pharmaceutical Journal*, **253**, 453.

Pharmaceutical Journal (1996a) Study finds nurses hesitate to report medication errors. *Pharmaceutical Journal*, **257**, 401.

Pharmaceutical Journal (1996b) The conference: the pharmacist as a prescriber. *Pharmaceutical Journal*, **257**, 412–416.

Pharmaceutical Journal (1996c) Pharmacy – the new gatekeeper to health care. *Pharmaceutical Journal*, **257**, 417–418.

Pickersgill, A. (1993) A new deal for nurses too? *Nursing Standard*, **7(35)**, 21–22.

Pirie, S. (1987) *Nurses and Mathematics*. London: Royal College of Nursing.

Poulton, B. (1994) Nurse prescribing: broadening the scope of nursing practice. *International Nursing Review*, **41(3)**, 81–84.

Rickford, F. (1993) Still held back. *Nursing Times*, **89(46)**, 21.

Royal College of Nursing (1995) *Whose Prescription? A survey to examine the influence of the practice nurse on GP prescribing patterns*. London: Royal College of Nursing.

Royal Pharmaceutical Society/Royal College of Nursing (1995) Nurse prescribing and patient care. *Pharmaceutical Journal*, **254**, 163.

Russell, S. (1993) The EC: an overview. Nursing: the European dimension, ed Quinn, S. & Russell, S. Harrow: Scutari.

Safriet, B. (1992) Health care dollars and regulatory sense: the role of advanced practice nursing. *Yale Journal on Regulation*, **9**, 440–465.

Stein, L. (1967) The doctor–nurse game. *Archives of General Psychiatry*, **16**, 699–703.

Stein, L. (1990) The doctor–nurse game re-visited. *New England Journal of Medicine*, **322**, 546–549.

Stilwell, B. (1988) Should nurses prescribe? *Nursing Times*, **94(12)**, 21–23.

Turner, B. (1987) *Medical Power and Social Knowledge*. London: Sage.

United Kingdom Central Council for Nursing, Midwifery and Health Visiting (1992a) *Standards for Administration of Medicines*. London: UKCC.

United Kingdom Central Council for Nursing, Midwifery and Health Visiting (1992b) *The Scope of Professional Practice*. London: UKCC.

United Kingdom Central Council for Nursing, Midwifery and Health Visiting (1994) *Nurse Prescribing*. London: UKCC.

Wainwright, P. (1994) Professionalism and the concept of role extension. In *Expanding the Role of the Nurse: the scope of professional practice*, ed. Hunt, G. & Wainwright, P. Oxford: Blackwell.

While, A.E. & Rees, K.L. (1993) The knowledge of health visitors and district nurses regarding products in the proposed formulary for nurse prescription. *Journal of Advanced Nursing*, **18**, 1573–1577.

Witz, A. (1992) *Professions and Patriarchy*. London: Routledge.

Zarnow, R.A. (1977) The curriculum model for expanded roles. *Nursing Outlook*, **25(1)**, 43–44.

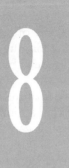

Nurse prescribing

A useful attribute?

Fiona Winstanley

Key issues

♦ Historical background to nurse prescribing.

♦ How nurse prescribing works in practice.

♦ The Nurses' Formulary – how useful is it?

♦ Accountability and professional issues surrounding nurse prescribing.

♦ Collaborative working and relationships with other professionals.

♦ Does nurse prescribing benefit patient care? Does it improve working practices? Case histories to illustrate.

INTRODUCTION

How does nurse prescribing work in reality? This chapter will explore the effect of nurse prescribing on patient care and community nursing practice. It will be viewed from the perspective of one of the district nurses involved in one of the initial prescribing demonstration sites in Ipswich, Suffolk, who has been prescribing since 1994.

HISTORICAL BACKGROUND TO NURSE PRESCRIBING

Baroness Cumberledge announced the government's intention to introduce eight demonstration sites for nurse prescribing on 21 November 1993. The pilot had been long awaited. Since 1986, when nurse prescribing was first advocated in the report *Neighbourhood Nursing – A Focus For Care* (DHSS, 1986), and subsequently endorsed by the Crown Report in 1989

(DoH, 1989), there had been delays and obstacles put in the way of taking the concept forward. One of the major hurdles, that of changing the legislation to enable nurses to legally prescribe, was overcome by the introduction of a private member's Bill by Roger Sims MP which received royal assent in March 1992 (DoH, 1994). This paved the way for nurses to be legally able to prescribe, in defined circumstances, from a nursing formulary of items that were to be used as part of a nursing care programme.

However, the government continued to delay the initiative because of fears that the NHS drugs budget would increase as a result of nurse prescribing. A cost–benefit analysis had been commissioned by the Department of Health in 1992, and had been carried out by Touche Ross, the management consultants. Their findings predicted that although nurses' time could be saved by their being allowed to prescribe, there was a danger that costs could escalate overall. Touche Ross estimated that nurses would save between 36 and 48 minutes per week, but it was felt that these benefits could be lost if nurses were expected to take on extra procedures to do with prescribing (e.g. extra paperwork). They were also concerned with the possible extra cost implications of training, which they estimated could be in the region of £107 million over 10 years, and the fact that the budgetary arrangements for reimbursement of nurse prescriptions had not been established. It had been estimated that the financial benefit of nurses being able to prescribe could be in the region of £47.5 million (Tattam, 1992). Although it was acknowledged that the costs involved were very small in relation to the overall spending on the GP drugs budget, this was nevertheless a politically sensitive time in relation to these issues. The findings were enough to fuel Treasury fears and caused delay in implementation until 1994.

THE PILOT PROJECT

Applications to take part in the pilot as one of the demonstration sites were invited, and the response was enormous. There were specific criteria for the selection of the sites (see Box 8.1). Applications had to be made and signed jointly by the practice, the community provider trust and the local family health services authority (FHSA). As one practice was to be selected from each regional health authority, the application had also to be endorsed at a regional level. The sites were to be selected to give as wide a range of comparison as possible between fundholding surgeries in terms of population size, location and demography.

The applications included letters of intent from the nurses eligible to take part in the pilot as prescribers, to endorse and back the application. An extract from the district nursing application from Ipswich illustrates why they applied to take part in the demonstration:

Box 8.1 Criteria for the selection sites for the pilot project
(Morris, 1994)

The demonstration sites had to have:

♦ A well established GP fundholding practice

♦ A well established primary health care team

♦ A contract for community health services with a single provider

♦ Practice computing systems that were able to link patient and prescribing data

♦ An adequacy of management information

♦ A willingness to participate in data collection and evaluation prior to, during and after implementation

♦ A willingness to provide representation on an implementation group

♦ A willingness to modify the existing contract, if necessary

Community nurses are very aware of the potential benefits of nurse prescribing. They feel that it will provide a much more efficient system that will benefit patients and health professionals alike and will generate considerable cost savings in terms of time and mileage. District nurses spend an unacceptable amount of time in running around chasing prescriptions, and patients do experience delays in starting treatments waiting for prescription items to be issued.

In our practice the doctors and nurses collaborate closely in caring for our patients and deciding on treatments. Our lines of communication are generally good.

The nurses are aware of the implications of costs involved in prescribing and to assist in this have drawn up their own basic dressing formulary. This identifies the most inexpensive brands of commonly used items. The district nurses currently enter their patients' prescriptions into the practice computer, which saves time and also helps the practice staff. They are hoping to have a terminal in their office which will further increase efficiency and ease congestion in the reception area.

Because the district nurses are based in the practice they have ease of access to patients' records and prescribing information which will be necessary in order to avoid duplication or omissions in prescribing.

We feel that nurse prescribing is a constructive step forward in primary health care would welcome the opportunity to be involved in its inception.

(Winstanley, 1992)

Prior to starting the pilot

The demonstration sites were announced in April 1994 and the pilot was scheduled to start in October 1994. This left a comparatively short time to set in place all the necessary arrangements. The private member's Bill had made legislative provision for nurse prescribing but final arrangements had to be made for the primary legislation to come into force. The Medicines Act 1968, the NHS Act 1990 and the Pharmaceutical Services Regulation 1977 had to be amended to enable nurses to be legally able to prescribe. This was in place by 3 October 1994.

The Nurse prescribers' formulary had been put together following recommendations to the Department of Health in July 1991 from the UKCC and the national boards. However, the legislation to enable nurses to prescribe prescription only medicines (POMS) was not set in place until January 1995, which resulted in a delay for nurses accessing that part of the formulary.

Evaluation of the pilot sites

Proper evaluation of the pilot was essential and analyses were to be made qualitatively by the University of Liverpool, and quantatively by the University of York.

Prescriptions generated by nurses had to be closely monitored during the pilot. This involved setting in place a comprehensive tracking system which would enable the Prescription Pricing Authority in Newcastle to identify and analyse the costs and prescribing patterns of the nurses involved during the pilot.

The qualitative evaluation of the demonstration sites was to involve the collection of data from the sites based mainly on semi-structured interviews with a sample of patients, nurses, GPs, practice staff, pharmacists and community provider and FHSA personnel. Initial baseline data in the form of interviews and patient diaries had to be collected prior to the beginning of the pilot. A number of patients from each pilot practice were given diaries to fill in over the period of a month, in which they recorded details of all prescriptions issued during that time and all unprescribed over-the-counter (OTC) items they had purchased themselves from chemists. These diaries were completed in June 1994 and June 1995 (i.e. prior to the pilot to give pre-prescribing data and in the final stages of the pilot to enable comparison between the two). The semi-structured interviews were held at regular intervals throughout the trial period.

Training

Training for nurses took the form of an English National Board (ENB) approved open learning pack (10–20 hours of study) and a 2 day (15 hours) training course for the taught component, followed by an examination leading to a recordable qualification. The open learning pack had been devised by the ENB in 1992 in the expectation that nurse prescribing was to be implemented in October 1993, so was more or less ready for use when the pilot was announced. Courses were run by Manchester University in the north of England, and North-East Surrey College of Technology in the south, to enable ease of access for nurses.

Several courses were held during September 1994; these underpinned the open learning pack which had been issued to nurses, and which they had been working through during the summer. Areas covered in the course included the principles and process of nurse prescribing, the Nurse Prescribers' Formulary and the relevant pharmacology, accountability, safety and ethical issues. The economics and mechanics of prescribing and prescribing in a team context were also considered. The objectives of the educational programme were to prepare nurses who could:

- Prescribe effectively from the Nurse Prescribers' Formulary
- Understand the respective roles of other professionals in relation to nurse prescribing
- Understand the legal framework for nurse prescribing
- Understand and maintain high standards of accountability and professional responsibility
- Understand the economics of nurse prescribing (Brew, 1994).

The examination, which was validated by the ENB, took place at the end of the 2-day course. It was in the form of a written paper designed to assess the nurse's competence to prescribe safely and effectively. The resulting qualification was then recorded on the UKCC's register as 'Nurse Prescriber'.

The courses, as they brought nurses from several areas together, were also an opportunity to network with other demonstration sites and share common interests and concerns. There was also the chance to establish links with the researchers, who joined the courses for some of the time to explain and discuss the approaches to the evaluation of the project.

The pilot begins

The pilot actually started on 4 October 1994. The amended legislation allowed for registered nurses with either a district nurse or health visitor qualification to prescribe if they were employed by a DHA, an NHS trust or a fundholding practice, providing they had completed the necessary educational preparation approved by a national board to the UKCC's standards (UKCC, 1994). This enabled the inclusion in the pilot scheme of practice nurses who held a district nurse or health visitor qualification, and enabled an evaluation to be made of the benefits of nurse prescribing in a practice nurse setting.

During the pilot, prescribing nurses could only issue prescriptions for patients registered with the demonstration site practice. They could not sign them for patients on behalf of other nurses who were not prescribers unless they were part of the pilot practice team. With the wider implementation of nurse prescribing this will, hopefully, be reviewed.

Initial reactions to prescribing

There were very mixed feelings amongst the prescribing nurses about being part of the demonstration. All the nurses had been involved in the initial application process and were excited to be part of such an important project, but the responsibility was felt quite keenly by many of the nurses. With such a small pilot, involving only eight sites and only about 58 nurses, we felt that the sucess or failure of the demonstration rested very heavily on our shoulders. It was only after our applications had been accepted that the rigorous nature of the proposed evaluation became apparent. We also rapidly became aware that the success of the pilot was not a foregone conclusion by any means. It became apparent that there was a great deal of scepticism and opposition from many quarters, not least the Treasury, who were extremely nervous about the escalating drug budget and were going to be very hard to convince of the benefits of nurse prescribing, and also of the fact that nurse prescribing was in reality substitute prescribing and not new prescribing.

The actual prescribing, although initially rather daunting, very soon became an integral part of nursing practice. Its value was immediately apparent, particularly in terms of meeting patients' needs and in time savings for everyone.

The Crown Report of 1989 had envisaged that nurse prescribing would result in:

- A significant improvement in the quality of patient care
- A more responsive service to patients
- Improved nurse/patient relationships
- Better use of nurses' training and skills
- Savings in terms of time and mileage, and more appropriate prescribing for nursing care needs
- Clarification in professional responsibilities leading to a strengthening of professional partnerships in primary health care teams
- GPs having to spend less time on prescribing with fewer consultations with patients under continuing care (DoH, 1989).

The aim of the demonstration sites was to test nurse prescribing to see if it would work in practice, to find out how much it would cost, and to establish just how beneficial it would really be.

Writing prescriptions

The first prescription the author wrote was, appropriately, for a retired nurse, who appreciated not only the professional significance of the prescription, but also the fact that she did not have to organise for the prescription to be collected from the practice in the usual 2 days' time by a carer or a relative, and was able to have the prescription items there for use the next day.

Identification of nurse generated prescriptions

The prescriptions had to be hand-written, using generic names on forms FP10 (CN) or FP10 (PN), and in accordance with the nurse's terms of service and legal requirements. Prescribing nurses had been issued with coloured prescription pads to aid identification. GP attached community nurses such as district nurses and health visitors were given green prescriptions, and practice nurses were issued with lilac forms. Each prescribing nurse had a stamp which printed details of her name, employer's details and UKCC pin number on each prescription form. The practice identification number was also recorded, together with the practice telephone number. This would enable tracking and monitoring of all nurse generated prescriptions and give pharmacists the means to confirm identification of prescribing nurses if necessary and to contact nurses with prescription queries if needed. Initially there were a few queries from pharmacists unfamiliar with the concept of nurse prescriptions but on the whole the actual process of prescribing took off with little difficulty.

Security arrangements

The need to ensure the security of prescriptions was emphasised repeatedly. This was due to the general rise in thefts and losses of prescription forms over recent years. Prescribing nurses have responsibility for the safeguarding of their prescription pads and have to notify both the police and the local FHSA in the event of loss or theft. The FHSA then informs the local pharmacists and decides on any necessary action to limit potential misuse of the forms. The pads should be kept out of view, and locked away whenever possible. On no account should any prescription be pre-signed.

Relationships with pharmacists

One of the generally agreed benefits of the pilot – and this was confirmed by the evaluation report (Luker, 1997) – was improved working relationships between nurses and pharmacists. Prior to the pilot, pharmacists had been perceived to have a somewhat peripheral role in community health care. Over the year communication between prescribing nurses and pharmacists increased, either as a direct result of nurse generated prescriptions, or through monthly scheduled meetings with local pharmacists to discuss progress, iron out teething problems, and share relevant information such as over-the-counter (OTC) products, advisory roles and problems concerned with compliance and delivery of medicines.

Through working more closely together locally, we came up with some solutions that have benefited patient care and increased compliance with medication regimes. The local pharmacist, for example, as part of his established delivery system, will also now undertake to fill and deliver weekly multiple dose 'dosette' boxes, on prescriptions from the practice, for patients that the district nurse or the GP have identified as having problems with obtaining and/or taking medication. This system has greatly benefited patients living alone, with no family to fill their dosette box, who have difficulty mentally or physically managing their medication. Patients have two alternating dosette boxes which the pharmacy uses to fill, deliver and collect on a weekly basis. The pharmacist holds the prescription and dispenses from it and liaises with the practice when necessary for new prescriptions etc. A newly filled box is left with the patient when the empty one is collected, on the same day each week so that the patient knows when to expect the delivery, and continuity of care is achieved. During the week the nurse can monitor that the patient is taking the medication as prescribed; compliance has been generally improved, especially with elderly mentally frail patients.

Protocols

Relationships between other members of the primary health care team were also noticeably improved as a direct result of the involvement in the pilot scheme, an advantage also highlighted by the evaluation (Luker, 1997). Although the team considered the possibility of conflict between nurses and GPs in the areas of clinical autonomy, there was also the opportunity to use the pilot to look at ways participating surgeries improved working practices. Practice teams had often agreed and established ground rules and clarified roles and responsibilities between different members of the primary health care team, which led to better collaborative working practices and improved communication. There were several areas which were in need of clarification in our own area, due to the changing nature of primary health care provision and the expansion of nursing roles to meet the more complex needs of patients in the community. The pilot served as a catalyst to tackle these issues and draw up local protocols to agree best practice and shared patient care.

Protocols were first discussed in the 1970s, but have only become widely used since the introduction of the GP contract in 1990, when GPs increasingly delegated health promotion activities and chronic disease management to practice nurses (Ogilvie, 1995). Their value lies in enabling a team approach to identifying and agreeing the standard management of either certain categories of patients (group protocols) or individual patients (patient-specific protocols). It is essentially about the way care is shared between team members, or the way decisions are reached about diagnosis and treatment (DoH, 1989).

The practice had, in the preceding year, drawn up protocols for joint working between practice nurses and GPs, but had not had a similar approach with the attached community nurses. The demonstration sites were all advised to draw up locally agreed protocols to clarify responsibilities in clinical areas in which nurses were likely to prescribe. Guidelines for the production of both group and patient-specific protocols were defined by the Crown Report (DoH, 1989) and these were used by the practice.

Working groups, consisting of community nurses, GPs, practice nurses and managers, met to discuss and agree protocols that had been put together by the prescribing nurses in areas such as bowel care, skin care, leg ulcer management and the treatment of infestations. Areas of clinical responsibility and referral indicators were established and treatment pathways agreed upon. Initially, the community and prescribing practice nurses decided to meet monthly to share experiences and iron out problems that had occurred with their new role. We elected to invite guests such as local pharmacists to these sessions who could give us useful insights into prescribing matters. When all parties were in consensus, the protocols were formally drawn up and distributed to all parties. It is generally considered good practice to review and update protocols at regular (say yearly) intervals to ensure that they remain relevant and reflective of best practice. The principle of group protocol use has now been endorsed by the first report of the second Crown review (DoH, 1998).

Prescribing in nurse led clinic situations

As more community nurses become involved in clinic based care for patients based on locally identified needs, the issue of their being able to prescribe for clinic patients, regardless of where they are registered, needs to be discussed. For example, many district nurses now run leg ulcer clinics in premises other than GP surgeries, although patients are usually referred by their GPs. One of the reasons for doing this is to make the clinics accessible to all patients from the area, regardless of who or where their GP is. In urban areas particularily, there may be several surgeries within a very small radius, and it is often a better use of resources and skills to hold clinics in convenient and 'neutral' community trust premises that can be accessed by a reasonable number of patients at set times in the week. In this environment, it makes sense for prescribing nurses to be able to write prescriptions for any patient receiving treatment at the clinic, rather than having to refer them back to their own practice to have prescriptions for nursing treatments generated by their GP.

Cover nurses

The pilot looked at the issue of providing 'cover' for prescribing nurses, and several district nurses and health visitors from neighbouring surgeries also attended the training course. Their effectiveness in providing cover was evaluated during the pilot and it was found that they had generally found little or no opportunity to prescribe during the year (Luker, 1997), and consequently felt less confidence in their prescribing role. Locally, the reasons for minimal use of cover nurses seemed mainly due to their difficulty in being able to release themselves from their own caseload responsibilities in order to take on the extra work involved with cover prescribing. The problem seemed to stem from the issues surrounding the need to assess each patient prior to issuing a prescription, and the time constraints that this imposed. Cover nurses were not usually familiar with the treatment needs of the demonstration site patients, and their own pressure of work did not allow them the time to take on the extra responsibility. This did create some degree of frustration among the cover nurses at not being able to develop their prescribing skills. However, as nurse prescribing is further implemented all these community nurses will be in position, after any necessary updating, to use their knowledge in their own practice areas.

In the event of the absence of the local prescribing nurse, the system tended to revert to the pre-pilot method of generating prescriptions. This entailed the nurses having to write a request for the prescription item, leave it with the receptionist, who would then enter it on the computer, print it out, leave it for the GP to sign (allowing 48 hours for this) and then arrange for its collection and dispensing. Using this system, patients rarely received their prescription items in less than 3 or 4 days and it was not uncommon for errors or misunderstandings to arise due to the number of hands that the prescriptions went through. If the patient needed the prescription urgently the nurse could obtain one by returning to the practice and waiting outside the GP's door in order to have a prescription signed. All of this took valuable time out of a busy working schedule and was only possible if there was a doctor available in the building. Consequently, when the prescribing nurse was absent and staff had to revert to the old way of generating prescriptions, the benefits of nurses being able to prescribe became graphically highlighted to all members of the practice team.

Prescribing generically

General guidance on the prescribing of medicines from the Joint Formulary Committee of the British National Formulary advises that where non-proprietary ('generic') titles are given, they should be used in prescribing. This allows the pharmacist to dispense any suitable product, and thus save delay for the patient and possible expense to the Health Service (BMA/ RPSGB, 1997). It has been agreed that exceptions can be made 'where bioavailability problems are so important that the patient should always receive the same brand, in such cases the brand name or the manufacturer should be stated' (BMA/RPSoGB, 1997).

Although the idea of generic prescribing is generally agreed to be sound, it did present some problems for prescribing nurses. The use of generic names in the case of several nurse prescribable items (wound care products in particular) was found to be unwieldy and impractical. The generic name for Elastoplast, for example, is 'vapour permeable waterproof plastic wound dressing BP', which takes up most of a prescription page when hand-written. Another problem that soon became apparent was that prescribing by generic name meant that patients would not necessarily always receive the product that was best for them. Many generic wound care items have several different products. For example, 'permeable non–woven synthetic adhesive tape' has four product alternatives, and 'vapour permeable adhesive film dressing BP' has five alternatives. There may be several reasons why a nurse may consider one particular item more suitable than another, ranging from patient comfort, patient sensitivity, ease of application or adherence, to product size and cost-effectiveness. Several nurse prescribers worked round the problem by specifying the product name after the generic name or by writing the product name only. Some pharmacists also reported finding it helpful to have specific named products on the prescriptions as they were not always familiar with the generic names and could also find the range of products confusing. This problem was highlighted in the evaluation of the demonstration sites and the authors suggested that 'problems surrounding generic prescribing should be reviewed before setting the policy framework for nurse prescribing' (Luker, 1997).

THE NURSE PRESCRIBERS' FORMULARY

Does it reflect practice?

The district nurse prescribers generally found that the Nurse Prescribers' Formulary reflected much of the 'bread and butter' of their practice and, on the whole, felt that many of their patients benefited from the nursing prescriptions that could be issued to them. The health visitors and the practice nurses did not find that the formulary was as responsive to the needs of their patients and consequently did not find as many opportunities to prescribe as the district nurses (Luker, 1997). The areas broadly covered in the formulary are listed in Box 8.2.

How could it be improved?

Nurse prescribers currently have to work from three different publications when prescribing: the Nurse Prescribers' Formulary, the British National Formulary and the Drug Tariff.[1] This arrangement is unwieldy and often duplicatory. It could be rationalised into something more manageable. In an office situation it may be possible to work from three books, but not

---

Box 8.2 Areas covered in the Nurse Prescribers's Formulary

◆ Urinary catheters and appliances

◆ Laxatives

◆ Local anaesthetics

◆ Wound management products

◆ Disinfection and cleansing preparations

◆ Skin preparations

◆ Mild analgesics

◆ Treatments for threadworms

◆ Diabetic reagents and appliances

◆ Treatments for scabies and headlice

◆ Drugs for the mouth

◆ Elastic hosiery

◆ Fertility and gynaecological equipment

◆ Stoma care products

The eight prescription only medicines that were added in January 1995 were wound care products, laxatives, anthelmintics and antifungal treatments.

---

[1]Although the Nurse Prescribers' Formulary is listed in the back of the BNF, it is without all the necessary prescribing information.

desirable. In a community situation, when the nurse is visiting people in their homes and carrying equipment and paperwork around with her, it is almost impossible. As nurse prescribing becomes more established, hopefully attempts will be made to make the nurse prescribing publications more 'user-friendly'.

In terms of what nurses were able to prescribe, there were anomolies in some of the items included. Some were rarely used in current practice and others were not included, even though they were frequently needed (for example water for injection and lubricating jelly). At the end of the initial pilot in 1995, the nurses who had been involved in the demonstration sites were asked to put together a 'Wish List' of items that they would like to see included in a future nurses' formulary. This gave nurses the opportunity to identify items that they felt would enhance patient care and nursing practice by making the formulary more responsive to the nursing needs of patients. It was also an indication of where nurses felt the boundaries to be in prescribing terms. Some nurses felt that there were areas of their work that could be improved by a widening of the formulary. Many practice nurses have, for example, taken a leading role in chronic disease management and family planning, and some of these nurses felt that the inclusion of items to reflect this aspect of their work would be useful. For example a practice nurse involved in a demonstration site who ran an asthma clinic felt that it would be helpful to be able to prescribe devices like peak flow meters (Sadler, 1995). The RCN also recognised the limitations of the existing formulary in relation to the fact that the GP contract had resulted in an increase in the number of practice nurses involved in the running of clinics, including those for asthma and diabetes (RCN, 1995).

There is a considerable body of opinion that the nurses' formulary is too limiting and does not reflect changes in nursing practice in recent years (Luker, 1997). Mayes's study of nurse practitioner prescribing under protocol (Mayes, 1996) identified items most routinely prescribed. These are listed in Box 8.3 (see also Ch. 11).

ACCOUNTABILITY ISSUES

There has been some discussion of whether it would be appropriate to have sections of the formulary accessible only to nurses trained in specific clinical areas, for example a nurse trained in asthma management with an ENB qualification, who would then be able to prescribe specific asthma treatments from a separate section of the formulary. Opinion is divided on this, with some feeling that it could be undesirable and unnecessary to subdivide the Nurses' Formulary and create rigid parameters for prescribing accessibility. As in all their areas of practice, nurses work within the clearly defined guidelines from the UKCC code and scope of practice. Prescribing nurses are no exception to this. These guidelines, when applied

Box 8.3 Items most routinely prescribed by nurses (Mayes, 1996)

◆ Vaccines

◆ Contraceptives

◆ Antibiotics

◆ Menopause and female medicine (including HRT, treatment for vaginal infections, premenstrual tension, and menstrual disorders)

◆ Asthma (including inhalers, peak flow meters, spacers etc)

◆ Diabetes (including insulin, hypoglycaemics, syringes, needles, reagents, etc.)

◆ Creams and ointments

◆ Analgesics

◆ Ear, eye and nose drops

◆ Antihypertensives

◆ Others grouped under miscellaneous (treatments for seasonal allergic reactions, laxatives, nutritional supplements, wound treatments and dressings, scabicides, and repeat prescriptions for a large range of medicines).

to nurse prescribing, should provide sufficient protection for both the public and the nurse. It has been argued that as nurses are accountable for their own practice and professional judgement, based on a coherent preparation for the role, they should be able to access the whole of the British National Formulary in the same way as medical practitioners (Jones and Gough, 1997).

In the same way as medical practitioners, prescribing nurses are legally and professionally accountable for their actions. If a nurse has not had adequate preparation in any area of practice and does not have the knowledge or expertise to ensure competent and safe treatment and care for patients then that nurse 'must acknowledge any limitations' in his or her 'knowledge and competence and decline any duties or responsibilities unless able to perform them in a safe and skilled manner' (UKCC, 1992a). Nurses must also 'ensure that no action or omission . . . on their . . . part, or within . . . their . . . sphere of responsibility, is detrimental to the interests, conditions or safety of patients and clients' (UKCC, 1992b).

Prescribing doctors are bound by the same constraints of accountability. All medical practitioners can technically prescribe from all areas of the

British National Formulary, but in practice they do not. They could not possibly be familiar with all areas of the formulary, or have the requisite in-depth knowledge of all medical specialities to enable them to prescribe safely in all circumstances for all patients. The same is true for prescribing nurses. Arguably, accountability renders prescribing self-limiting, therefore defining boundaries should be unnecessary.

Prescribing for patients

When considering prescribing treatment for a patient, knowledge of the item to be prescribed is only one part of the equation. Other factors to be taken into account include:

- The patient's circumstances, including current medication
- The patient's past medical history
- The patient's current and anticipated health status
- Thorough knowledge of the item to be prescribed – its therapeutic action, side-effects, dosage and interactions
- Thorough knowledge of alternatives to prescribing
- Frequency of use in a variety of circumstances (ENB, 1994).

The evaluation of the demonstration sites found that some prescribing nurses had, as the pilot progressed, become more cautious about what they would be comfortable to prescribe. This appears to be linked to a greater awareness of the complexities and responsibilities of prescribing (Luker, 1997). From the author's experience it would be true to say that having one's name on the bottom of the prescription pad does concentrate the mind in terms of responsibility and accountability. Nurses have previously always been able to, in effect, hide behind the doctor who wrote the pre-scription for them; this is not the case if they are themselves the prescriber.

Nursing expertise has, in many areas, outstripped that of most medical practitioners, wound care being just one example. The undoubted skill and knowledge of many community nurses in wound care is, for the most part, recognised and welcomed by the GPs they work with. Community nurses frequently work virtually autonomously in this area, assessing the patient, planning the care and treatment and taking full responsibility for their nursing decisions. It is anomalous in this situation for the nurse to then have to ask the medical practitioner to 'rubber stamp' their decision by signing the prescription for the wound care products identified by the nurse as being necessary for the patient's treatment. The fact that many GPs rarely see the wounds that they write the prescriptions for, and often have a limited and outdated knowledge of wound care highlights the anomaly further. It could be argued that this brings into doubt the advisability of medically prescribing in this type of context.

The next step, and one that was being addressed by pilot nurse prescribers, is doing away with the 'medical permission' and allowing nurses to take responsibility for the whole of the nursing process, including the actual prescribing. It sounds a small step, but it is for many nurses a large one, and in some instances leads nurses to express concern and disquiet about entering the prescribing arena. Stilwell (1988) thought that this might be: 'because nurses are unsure of their ability to make decisions. Nurses' history of subordination to medicine and its hierarchical traditions in education and management militates against their acquiring easily the confidence to make decisions and to be accountable for them.'

GP reactions to nurse prescribing

The supremacy of medicine, historically, gave rise to the 'handmaiden' role of nurses, who traditionally have been educated to follow instructions from doctors. For nurses trained in this way the idea of autonomy, whether in practice generally or prescribing specifically, is understandably often threatening and frequently results in negativity and resistance. The same can sometimes be said of medical practitioners. Traditionally trained doctors often have a somewhat stereotyped image of nurses and the role they expect them to fulfil. In the case of nurse prescribing initial reactions from GPs was very mixed. Dr Halpin from Staffordshire, whose practice took part in the pilot site, felt that: 'nurses are professionals in their own right, they have their own body of knowledge' (Cooper, 1994), whereas others such as Dr Twiston-Davis from Jersey felt: 'That "15 hours of very tough distance learning, followed by a two day course and an exam" can now be felt adequate to allow an individual limited prescriptive rights would suggest that drugs have become simpler, the teaching is better or that nurses are much brighter than we were' (*Daily Telegraph*, October 1994).

Fellows reports a reasonably positive view from the British Medical Association in his chapter (see Ch. 2), and most GPs seem to appreciate that nurse prescribing is a natural and common-sense approach to streamlining and improving community patient care. The recent shift in the focus of health care to being primarily in the community, and the NHS being primary health care led, has meant that everyone involved in primary health care teams has had to look carefully at who does what, where and when. They have collectively had to make a concerted attempt to try to rationalise and improve services and ways of working in order to be able to meet the ever increasing demands being made upon them. Dr Saul, another pilot site GP from Bolton, said: 'We have always had good relations with our community unit and we saw the scheme as a way of improving co-operation between us and improving patient care' (Dinsdale, 1994).

The concern of some GPs who felt threatened by possible role erosion by nurses, mainly due to sharing previously exclusively held prescribing rights, is also real but largely unfounded. There is a realisation by most GPs at the sharp end of community care delivery that there are not enough of them to go round, that traditional ways of working are not going to enable the increasing work load to be met, and that as they cannot be 'all things to all men' they have to look at ways of sharing the workload with other members of the primary health care team (PHCT).

COLLABORATIVE WORKING

A collaborative approach is increasingly seen to be fundamental to making primary health care work and is one of the cornerstones of nurse prescribing. Without it there could be inherent risks in nurses prescribing. Good communication and joint decision making are essential to ensure that patients receive the most appropriate treatment from the most appropriate person, and that everyone is aware of what care the patient has received. As Harrison (1993) stated, 'Effective collaboration would be essential to avoid either duplication or omissions in prescribing.'

As previously discussed, one of the ways we attempted to address this problem was by drawing up protocols as a primary health care team. These clarified boundaries and built in triggers for referral and agreed lines of communication and record keeping.

Record keeping

With regard to record keeping, the Crown Report recommended, in Sections 14 and 19 that:

• Good communication between health professionals and patients, and between different professionals, is essential for high quality care. All health professionals empowered to prescribe for a patient should have access to the relevant patient records.

And that

• Patients' personal record cards showing the timing and dosage of all medication, and other relevant information, should be completed by each professional who prescribes for the patients and updated to show any changes. They should be available to doctors and nurses treating the patient, and to pharmacists issuing medicines. Patient-held records should be used wherever possible (DoH, 1989).

All the nurses in the author's practice always had access to patients' medical notes. Although patient-held records were being discussed as a community trust initiative at the time of the pilot, they were not in use, and so we had to look at ways of using existing documentation to record prescribing information. The protocol drawn up by the Ipswich pilot site PHCT covered these areas by agreeing that:

- Details of nurse prescriptions would be recorded contemporaneously
- In the case of DNs and HVs, prescription details would be recorded in the nursing notes, the computer records and/or medical notes within 2 working days
- In the case of PNs, prescription details would be recorded in the medical notes and the computer only
- Adverse reactions would be reported immediately to the patient's GP and a record made in the medical and nursing notes.

On the whole this worked well. Occasionally it was difficult to access the medical notes if they were out in the system, but we found a way round this by using the deputising stickers used by GPs to record medical information for out of hours visits to patients from other surgeries. We recorded the prescribing information onto these when the notes were not available, and the receptionists then attached them to the notes when they were returned for filing. This meant that nurses did not waste time looking for notes that were not immediately available and were less likely to forget to enter the information at a later stage when they had reappeared.

Prior to the pilot the district nurses had to some extent streamlined practice prescribing by entering the prescriptions they wanted for patients on the computer, which meant time saving for both the receptionists (who had hitherto copied the nurses' handwritten requests for items onto the computer), and the GPs, who then only had to sign the prescription forms. This had worked well up to a point, especially when the nurses had a terminal in their office, but there were still the inherent time delays waiting for routine signing, and the problems surrounding accessibility and availability for patients.

We expected that for the purposes of the pilot there would be an increase in the amount of paperwork involved, due to the demonstration sites being so closely monitored. It was generally accepted that in order to test the benefits of nurse prescribing the extra paperwork was a necessary burden to be endured. For the purposes of evaluation, each nurse generated prescription had to be tracked through the Prescription Pricing Authority, to enable analysis by the researchers. Each prescription therefore had to be hand-written, on the appropriate pad, having been stamped with the prescribing nurse's details. This meant that we could not use the much more efficient printed computer roll prescriptions that were used by the GPs, which would have recorded the items prescribed, the dosage instructions, the amount requested and their date of issue. As it happened, the nurses had to hand-write the prescription and then enter it onto the practice computer for practice records, which was a duplicatory process. This was highlighted in the evaluation and the suggestion was made that 'If nurse prescriptions could be computer generated then this may save time, in terms of writing the script and recording in the medical notes' (Luker, 1997).

The potential problems with extra paperwork had been identified by management consultants Touche Ross in 1992. The firm had been commissioned by the Department of Health to undertake a cost–benefit analysis of nurse prescribing; in their report they had warned that time saved through nurses having prescribing powers could be taken up with extra paperwork created by its introduction (Tattam, 1992). However, as nurse prescribing becomes established these problems, having been identified, should be addressed and resolved relatively easily as part of practice administration processes.

RELATIONSHIPS WITH DRUG AND APPLIANCE MANUFACTURERS

A concern frequently expressed prior to the start of the demonstration was that the new nurse prescribers would be targeted by representatives from pharmaceutical firms and appliance manufactures keen to promote their products by trying to influence their prescribing decisions. It was felt that many nurses could find this an added and unwelcome pressure and might have difficulty coping with the situation. The ethical questions surrounding nurses' relationships with drug and appliance companies were examined in some detail in both the open-learning pack and the training course, and nurses were encouraged to look at and question their attitudes and views in this area. It would probably be true to say that nurses are somewhat ambivalent in their attitudes to drug companies and their representatives. On the one hand they are aware that representatives can often be a source of useful information and updating on products. They will also often sponsor educational initiatives, either by organising study days or funding places for courses and conferences, all of which are often difficult for nurses to access otherwise, due to inevitably restricted training budgets. On the other hand, nurses are aware that ultimately the aim of the company representative, however helpful, is to increase the company profits.

The ethical dilemma arises when the nurse allows a professional decision on patient care to be influenced by other pressures or considerations. Legally, also, the position is clear in regard to nurses being under pressure from pharmaceutical companies to prescribe particular products. This often applies especially to nurses whose posts are sponsored by private companies, for example stoma nurses. Guidance was given on this by Professor Dimond, a barrister-at-law, who wrote.

> *The sole criterion in deciding what product, if any, to prescribe must be the patient's best interests. Where the practitioner is under pressure, for what ever reason, there is a duty for that pressure to be resisted. This can cause difficulties where a pharmaceutical company is actually paying for the costs of the nurses'*

posts. However, it would be contrary to the professional standards of the practitioner to be influenced by that fact. (Dimond, 1995)

The fears of new demonstration site nurses being swamped by sales representatives eager to influence their new found prescribing status proved to be generally unfounded. Although there was interest from companies about the pilot, there was no increased feeling of being targeted or pressurised. Nurses in the community, in the same way as GPs, often see representatives in the normal course of their work. It is not a new concept. Pharmaceutical companies have known for a long time just how influential nurses often are in many areas of medical prescribing decisions, and have consequently increasingly focused their attentions on nurses as well as doctors. However, with the advent of nurse prescribing, it would be naive to think that nurses will not be subjected to even greater scrutiny.

In a pharmaceutical marketing supplement, *PharmaMarket Letter*, companies were advised that:

Nurses have always influenced prescribing – from behind the scenes at least. Now nurses' influence is growing, driven by the world-wide trend towards nurse prescribing, primary health care surveillance clinics and nurse specialists. These changes present the pharmaceutical industry with a new challenge: how to integrate nurses into a marketing mix traditionally focused on physicians. Those companies that fail to meet the challenge may be left behind.
(PharmaMarket Letter, 1995)

Many nurses may feel somewhat concerned about being the target of attention, but the situation does not necessarily have to be one-sided or out of nurses' control. The RCN, for example, has held conferences with pharmaceutical companies to discuss constructive ways of approaching the prescribing situation. Joint educational initiatives have been discussed, looking at ways of developing the existing sponsorship system, and enabling a more structured and controlled approach to be considered. With the backing of company money, it was felt that nurses' and subsequently their patients could benefit from educational programmes, and the pharmaceutical companies could benefit from gaining valuable market insights from nurse educationalists and a direct line of communication to the nursing profession (PharmaMarketletter 1995).

At a local level, nurses have to make their own decisions about how to respond to drug company representatives. If the degree of drug company interest in community nurses is expected to rise with the advent of widespread prescribing, nurses will have to be aware of the need to set ground rules to avoid constant interruptions to their pattern of work. Most sales people make it their business to know when and where they are most likely to be able to access doctors and nurses. Most community nurses have a regular time for meeting during the day. This is usually valuable time spent in organising caseloads, discussing and delegating work and making telephone calls. It is also often a time that other members of the primary health care team or patients know that they will be contactable. It is rarely used as free time for lunch. There is no reason that this time could not be used to meet sales people, but we felt, in our locality, that the parameters had to be drawn to guard against intrusive 'cold calling' and over-long, unscheduled meetings. Most company representatives are aware that nurses, like doctors, have to work to very tight schedules and that their time is restricted, but they do still on occasion, 'pop in on the off-chance'. Sometimes this pays off, and is mutually beneficial, but sometimes nurses are caught unawares and find themselves agreeing to see representatives at inappropriate or inconvenient times. This tends to breed resentment and frustration and does nothing for relationships between the two parties. The obvious solution is the development of mutually agreed and understood guidelines about accessing nurses' time. This approach is often adopted by GPs and clarifies the boundaries.

Nurses are arguably often not as good as doctors at telling represent-atives that they cannot see them or that they only have a very short time available. They usually appreciate that the sales force have a difficult job to do, and often feel sympathy for them. They are also aware of the need to keep abreast of new products and developments, but their time is increas-ingly pressurised, and impromptu, unscheduled visits are increasingly inappropriate. GPs, or their practice managers, usually manage their time with representatives more efficiently, for example surgeries often have a diary set aside specifically for seeing representatives. The receptionists hold the diary and the sales people make the appointments with them. It is a system that nurses can easily adopt, and is one that representatives are already often familiar with. It discourages the casual callers, who 'pop by' to talk about new products but who can often, unwittingly, disrupt valuable office or team planning time.

Another alternative, and one which is often most attractive to representa-tives, is to encourage them to book appointments through locality managers or team leaders. This is a way of accessing larger numbers of nurses, as managers will often have responsibility for several teams and can organise the attendance of a wider audience, making it more worthwhile for the representative. Nurses can schedule the session in their diaries and arrange their work around it. It also means that if a nurse is unable to attend for some reason there will probably be several others attending who can pass on the information.

Local interest groups are also an area that increasingly offer a forum for drug companies to participate in. Study days that are organised by groups interested in wound care, for example, are often relatively local and therefore more accessible and frequently attract nurses from a variety of backgrounds. These educational initiatives are usually arranged by members from the group, and are often self-funded on very small budgets. The groups are non-profit making and exist mainly to disseminate knowledge and encourage professional development. By sponsoring initiatives such as these, drug companies can help a wide number of nurses improve their knowledge and patient care and have a local opportunity to pass on information about their products. It also gives both parties the opportunity to share ideas and gain insight into each others' roles, which should aid constructive and mutually beneficial working relationships.

The emphasis on health care being evidence based and grounded in research and reflection is generally accepted as good practice. Nurse prescribing is no exception to this. Although there may be concerted efforts on the part of companies attempting to influence nurses' prescribing decisions, nurses should never allow these pressures or persuasions to sway them. Nurses may listen to the claims regarding products and look at the studies that manufacturers may have carried out, but they should always adopt an objective, critical and judicious approach to the information that is presented to them. The development of nurses' powers of analysis, reasoning and understanding of research are essential to enable them to base their decision making on firm foundations and in the patient's best interest.

IS NURSE PRESCRIBING USEFUL?

Over the period of the pilot and subsequently, there have been many examples of how it has benefited patient care and improved practice. Some anecdotal examples of case studies will probably illustrate this more effectively than abstract discussion (see Boxes 8.4 to 8.7).

One of the benefits of nurse prescribing has turned out to be the opportunity to combine prescribing with health education and advice. In the case of treating patients with constipation, for example, although nurses can and do prescribe laxatives, the issuing of a prescription should always be accompanied by a full assessment which looks at the patient's general condition including diet, fluid intake, mobility and medical history. By establishing the cause of the constipation the nurse can then take steps, in collaboration with the patient, to prevent its recurrence. The steps taken might be in the form of prescribing medication, but should also incorporate advice on diet, fluid intake, the constipatory effect of certain types of analgesia for example, and the importance, where possible, of exercise.

The pilot evaluation concluded that both nurses and patients felt that there was a difference in information given by nurses compared to GPs. 'Reasons given for this were that nurses had more time to spend with patients, who were often more at ease with them because they knew them better and because the consultation was taking place at home, rather than in the practice' (Luker, 1997). Many patients also thought it was easier to

Box 8.4 Case study: Mrs S

Mrs S takes her 8-week-old daughter to see the health visitor at the baby clinic. The session is held not in the doctor's practice but in the community trust premises, which are local for the family and more easily accessible by foot. The family does not have a car. The baby has developed oral thrush and her mother has come for advice and treatment. The prescribing health visitor is able to examine the baby, talk to the mother, whom she already knows, and diagnose the condition. She can then issue a prescription for the baby, give it to the mother together with instructions on how and when to use it, and arrange for a follow-up visit to make sure the treatment has been effective. She can also combine the session with health education and advice as necessary. Mrs S takes the prescription to the local chemist, has it dispensed immediately and starts the treatment when she gets home the same evening. The baby responds well, and is almost fully recovered when the health visitor sees her at the next clinic.

If the health visitor had not been able to prescribe, although she would have examined and diagnosed the condition, she would have then had to refer the mother and her baby to see the GP for a prescription. This would involve the mother having to make another appointment at the practice, a bus ride away, and possibly for 1 or 2 days hence. This would mean that the baby would have had a delay in starting treatment, resulting in prolonged discomfort and a possible worsening of her condition, and an increase in distress and anxiety for her mother. It would also involve the GP in seeing an extra patient and the taking up of practice appointment time.

speak to nurses about certain issues because they were considered to be more approachable.

These findings would imply that prescribing nurses are in a position to improve patient compliance, and therefore outcomes, although further studies would be needed to establish this conclusively.

CONCLUSION

Nurses at the original demonstration sites have now been prescribing since October 1994. Since then the prescribing pilot has been extended to enable evaluation of whole communities (Bolton initially, and subsequently a larger number of areas over England and Scotland). In December 1996, the Department of Health announced, as part of its primary health care plans, that nurse prescribing would be rolled out nationally from April 1998. In

Box 8.5 Case study: Mr G

Mr G was discharged from the local hospital on Friday afternoon following surgery and the subsequent drainage of an abscess. He has an abdominal wound which requires daily dressing, and the district nurse has been asked to visit. When she calls on Saturday morning, she finds that Mr G has been discharged home with no dressings (as per local agreement, dressings for 3 days should be sent home with the patient, but the system does fall down quite frequently). As the district nurse can prescribe, she issues Mr G with a prescription for items that she needs to continue his care. She agrees to call again later, after she has visited some more patients, which enables Mrs G to collect the prescription from the pharmacy. The district nurse returns later and carries on with the patient's treatment.

If the district nurse had not been able to prescribe, there could have been a problem accessing dressings. As many surgeries only open on Saturday mornings, or have deputising services, there is often a problem finding a GP to issue prescriptions. The district nurse would probably have spent some time trying to find a doctor, and then, if successful, would have had to take the prescription either back to the patient or to the pharmacy to have the items dispensed. Either way, there would have been a great deal of wasted time and mileage and an increase in anxiety levels for the patient, his family and the district nurse. If the nurse had been unable to find the doctor, he or she would have been in the difficult position of having to provide treatment without the right equipment. Many nurses, in an attempt to cope in this typical type of scenario, carry some dressings and equipment with them in the car, which they have gleaned from other sources. But it is far from ideal and is all too often crisis management in a difficult situation.

reality the 'roll out' was delayed for a few months, but we are getting there!

This move is welcomed by prescribing nurses everywhere, who know that nurse prescribing is beneficial to patients and health professionals alike.

The 'grass-root' feeling from community nursing prescribers is that nurse prescribing works, and works well. The benefits envisaged by the Crown Report in 1989 have all been realised, together with several others. They are that nurse prescribing:

• Enables patients to be treated speedily and effectively by nurses at home and in clinics/health centres

> **Box 8.6** Case study: Mr J
>
> Mr J has just been discharged from hospital having had a urethral catheter inserted after he had developed urinary retention. He is now on the waiting list for a prostatectomy, and should be admitted in 10–12 weeks for surgery. In the meantime he will be looked after at home by his district nurse and GP. It is not hospital policy to send patients out with spare catheters or equipment. He has a leg bag on and has brought home one non-drainable night bag. The district nurse is asked to visit to establish that Mr J and his family are coping and to identify any problems. The prescribing district nurse gives Mr J's son a prescription for a spare catheter, night and day bags and lignocaine gel. She has brought a pack for Mr J to keep in the house which contains everything else that would be needed for a catheter change. The prescription is dispensed that afternoon and Mr J is then equipped to cover most eventualities. If the catheter blocks in the middle of the night, for example, a duty doctor has everything he might need in order to change the catheter at home.
>
> If the district nurse had not been able to issue a prescription, there would have been considerable delay in accessing the equipment needed. Much more time would be taken up in requesting a prescription from the practice, waiting for the GP to sign it and arranging for it to be collected and dispensed. During this time the patient would have had problems with only having one night bag, and if the catheter had blocked at night, not having a spare one would have meant that he would have probably had to be readmitted for re-catheterisation. This would have been distressing for all concerned and a waste of resources.

- Reduces patients' and carers' anxieties
- Gives greater patient satisfaction
- Gives nurses greater autonomy
- Increases nurses' job satisfaction
- Helps to improve the planning and evaluation of care
- Enables GPs to concentrate on seeing patients in need of medical intervention rather than validating a nursing decision
- Gives a more cost-effective use of nurses' skills
- Results in less travelling, saving time and money
- Provides a service that is immediately responsive to patients' needs
- Results in less wastage of resources and more appropriate treatment
- Enables the nurse to combine prescribing with health education and health promotion

Box 8.7 Case study: an insulin dependent diabetic

The practice nurse works with the duty doctor on Saturday mornings, holding a clinic for urgent appointments. The practice is open from 9 a.m. until 12 midday, after which time it is shut for the weekend. The duty doctor is called away from the practice on an emergency visit at 11.45 a.m. The practice nurse is still seeing her last patient. The patient is an insulin dependent diabetic and needs a further supply of reagent strips for monitoring his blood glucose levels and blood lancets.

As the practice nurse is a nurse prescriber she issues a prescription to the patient, which is dispensed and collected on his way home.

If the practice nurse had not been able to prescribe the items, the patient would have had to return to the practice later the following week, having allowed 2 working days for the prescription to be generated and signed, and would only then have been able to access the items he needed.

- Results in better team working through clarification of professional responsibilities, through the use of protocols
- Encourages better collaborative care between all members of the primary health care team.

QUESTIONS FOR DISCUSSION

- Nurse prescribing cannot be viewed in isolation or simplistically. What are the major issues surrounding its implementation?
- How could nurse prescribing benefit community health care delivery and patient care?
- Who should prescribe – and why?
- Should the Nurse Prescribers' Formulary be extended? Who or what should set the boundaries?
- Autonomous practice – what are the issues surrounding this in relation to nurse prescribing?
- How should prescribing nurses be prepared for practice? What are the issues surrounding training and education?
- Accountability – what are the issues and implications in relation to nurse prescribing?

Further reading

Luker, K. (1997) Research teams of Liverpool and York Universities. Evaluation of nurse prescribing. Final Report. Executive Summary. January. [Unpublished. Copies available for consultation at University of Liverpool.]

Report on the findings of the joint research team set up by the Department of Health to evaluate the nurse prescribing demonstration sites.

Dimond B. (1995) The legal aspects of nurse prescribing. Primary Health Care, **January** (Supplement).

A comprehensive survey of the legal issues surrounding nurse prescribing, written by an academic barrister-at-law.

Department of Health (1989). Report on the Advisory Group on Nurse Prescribing (Crown Report), Department of Health, London.

Report to the Department of Health on the findings of the committee on nurse prescribing led by Dr June Crown. The report gives recommendations and proposals for its introduction and implementation and suggests anticipated benefits.

Cumberlege J.(1986) Neighbourhood Nursing – A Focus for Care. Report of the community nursing review, London, HMSO.

Initial report which identified the need for community nurses to have limited prescribing rights and the seed from which nurse prescribing grew.

REFERENCES

Brew, M. (1994) Teaching nurses to prescribe. *Nursing Times*, **90(21)**, 32–34.
British Medical Association/Royal Pharmaceutical Society of Great Britain (1997) *British National Formulary*. No. 33, March.
Cooper, C. (1994) Weighing up options in nurse prescribing. *Doctor*, **8 September 1994**, 46.
Department of Health and Social Security (1986) *Neighbourhood Nursing – a Focus for Care. Report of the community nursing review*. (Cumberlege Report.) London: HMSO
Department of Health (1989) *Report on the Advisory Group on Nurse Prescribing*. (Crown Report.) London: Department of Health.
Department of Health (1994) Press Release, 24 April 1994. *Nurse Prescribing to Become a Reality*. Richmond House: London.
Department of Health (1998) *Report on Prescribing, Supply and Administration of Medicines*. London: Department of Health.
Dimond, B. (1995) The legal aspects of nurse prescribing. *Primary Health Care*, **January**.
Dinsdale, P. (1994) GPs welcome nurse prescribing. *Monitor Weekly*, **12 October**.
English National Board for Nursing, Midwifery and Health Visiting (1994) *Nurse Prescribing. Open learning pack*. London: ENB.
Harrison, A (1993) Job prescription. *Nursing Times*, **89(24)**, 50.
Jones, M. & Gough, P. (1997) Nurse prescribing – why has it taken so long? *Nursing Standard*, **11(20)**, 39–42.
Luker, K. (1997) *Evaluation of nurse prescribing. Final Report and Executive Summary*. Liverpool: University of Liverpool and Univerity of York.
Mayes, M. (1996) A study of prescribing patterns in the community. *Nursing Standard*, **10(29)**, 34–37.

Morris, J. (1994) Demonstration sites for nurse prescribing. *Nursing Times*, **90(21)**, 31.

Ogilvie, A. (1995) Protocols – get it down in writing. *Practice Nurse*, **9(8)**, 608.

PharmaMarket Letter (1995) Nurses' evolving role: new communications challenges and opportunities for pharmaceutical companies. *PharmaMarket Letter*, **22(25)**, 19 June 1995.

Royal College of Nursing (1995) *Whose Prescription?* London: RCN.

Sadler, C. (1995) Stretching the limits. *Health Visitor*, **68(10)**, 403–404.

Stilwell, B. (1988) Should nurses prescribe? *Nursing Times*, **84(12)**, 31–34. .

Tattam, A. (1992) Time-consuming procedures may negate prescribing gains. *Nursing Times*, **88(46)**, 7.

Twiston-Davis, C. (1994) Letters to the Editor. *Daily Telegraph*, **4 October**.

United Kingdom Central Council for Nursing, Midwifery and Health Visiting Register (1994) Prescribing by Nurses, No. 15, **Autumn**, 3.

United Kingdom Central Council for Nursing, Midwifery and Health Visiting (1992a) *The Scope of Professional Practice*. London: UKCC.

United Kingdom Central Council for Nursing, Midwifery and Health Visiting (1992b) *Code of Professional Conduct*. London: UKCC.

Winstanley, F. (1992) Extract from supporting letter for application to take part in the prescribing demonstration.

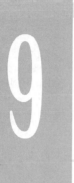

9 ·Nurse prescribing

Practice nurse opinions

Ann Ogilvie

Key issues

- Practice nurse perceptions of nurse prescribing.

- Strategies adopted by practice nurses to facilitate the supply and administration of prescription only medicines in the absence of prescribing rights.

- Suggestions for the extension of prescribing rights to practice nurses.

- Critique of the suitability of the nurse prescribers formulary.

INTRODUCTION

Having worked as a practice nurse for 10 years now, I have experienced the frustration of trying to get prescriptions signed for patients for such items as dressings when the doctor is busy or not available. Standing outside consulting room doors waiting for the opportunity to pounce, while feeling like an eavesdropper, has become an occupational hazard. Surely there must be an easier and more efficient way to prescribe? After all, how many times do doctors read the prescription you have written anyway? These feelings led me to look more closely at the issue of practice nurse prescribing. Graduate research study offered the ideal opportunity. After completing a comprehensive literature review, it was clear that practice nurses used various methods to procure prescriptions, but there were no published research findings to quantify them. This chapter describes the work undertaken with practice nurses in an attempt to appreciate their real feelings about nurse prescribing.

Beginning the study

Having identified the gap in the research, a focus group was set up consisting of myself and five practice nurses from outside my health authority. The aim of the group was to 'thrash out' ideas regarding the layout and content of a questionnaire which was being developed to ascertain practice nurses' views. The focus group held discussions around the following areas:

- The use of counter-questioning
- Maximum number of questions to be included
- Areas to be covered
- Identifying current methods of 'unofficial' prescribing
- Determining questions that would elicit what practice nurses would like to see happen in the future with regard to prescribing
- Possible use of rating scales, i.e. the Likert scale (Oppenheim, 1992)
- Whether to conduct a retrospective or prospective study.

Following the focus group recommendations and research objectives (as outlined below), and the results of the pilot study, a final draft questionnaire was developed based on the McColl framework (McColl, 1993). A retrospective convenience sample survey was then carried out which targeted practice nurses within the local health authority. The questionnaire was then posted to 84 practice nurses, obtaining a 45% response rate which is an acceptable figure for this method of data collection (Polit and Hungler, 1995).

RESEARCH OBJECTIVES

1. To determine the extent of current practice nurse prescribing with regard to the range of items prescribed and the number of prescriptions issued.

2. To determine the current level of practice nurse education and identify what they would like to see as the minimum level of education for prescribing practice nurses.

3. To determine the extent of prescribing using group protocols.

4. To determine the time taken by practice nurses to obtain GPs' signatures on prescriptions they have issued.

5. To determine the frequency and methods of prescribing used.

6. To determine the number of practice nursing hours worked per week.

7. To determine the level of interest in practice nurse prescribing.

8. To determine the level of willingness to undertake further study (pharmacology/prescribing) and perceived problems in undertaking this.

9. To determine practice nurses' views on being excluded from pilot projects unless they have a district nurse or health visitor qualification.

10. To determine what practice nurses would like to see included in the Nurse Prescribers' Formulary.

11. To determine practice nurses' perceptions of outcomes if all practice nurses were allowed to prescribe.

Following receipt of the completed questionnaires, the data were analysed manually; the results are as follows:

RESULTS

Current practice nurse qualifications

Question 1 – *What qualifications do you have?*

– All respondents replied to this question. The qualifications of practice nurses within the health authority are diverse, but mainly revolve around chronic disease management, family planning and health promotion. As can be seen in Table 9.1, all practice nurses are registered general nurses (RGNs) although two initially trained as enrolled nurses.

Table 9.1 Practice nurse qualifications			
Rank	Qualification	Number of nurses	Percentage
1	Registered general nurse	38	100
2	Asthma diploma (or equivalent)	24	63
2	Family planning certificate (ENB 901)	23	60
3	Diabetes diploma (or equivalent)	20	53
4	Diploma in practice nursing	19	50
5	Registered midwife	8	21
6	Teaching certificate (ENB or City & Guilds)	7	18
7	Cytology certificate	4	11
8	District nurse certificate	3	8
9	COPD diploma	3	8
9	Health education certificate	2	5
9	Health visitor diploma/certificate	2	5
9	Orthopaedic nursing certificate	2	5
9	State enrolled nurse	2	5
10	BSc in nursing	2	5
10	ENB 124	1	3
10	ENB 941	1	3
10	ENB endoscopy certificate	1	3
10	Family planning instructor	1	3
10	Lay tutor	1	3
10	PWT certificate	1	3
10	Registered sick children's nurse	1	3
10	RSA in counselling	1	3

Number of prescriptions issued by practice nurses

Although it is appreciated that in the truest sense of the word 'prescribing' is an act undertaken by an individual authorised to sanction the supply or administration of a prescription only medicine – generally a doctor – for the purpose of this study, 'prescribing' is taken to mean the practice nurse taking a decision or acting in a way as to lead to the supply or administration of such a medicine.

Question 2 – *How many times a week do you personally issue a prescription and then get the doctor to sign it without him/her seeing the patient?*

– All respondents replied to this question (see Fig. 9.1). Only one practice nurse stated that she did not prescribe. As the responses to this question were grouped (i.e. 1–5, 6–10, etc.), it was difficult to establish the actual number of prescriptions issued by the sample group per week, therefore an average was calculated. The average number of scrips issued per sample per week is 484, which is an average of 13 per nurse per week. Knowing that the number of practice nurses working within the health authority is 107 (personal telephone communication, May 1998), it can be extrapolated that 1391 scrips are generated by practice nurses per week in one health authority alone. Knowing that there are 100 health authorities in the UK (Binley's Directory, 1998), an average of 7 233 200 prescription per year are generated by practice nurses in the UK. As the actual number of practice nurses employed per health authority will vary, this figure could in reality be much higher.

Time taken by practice nurses to obtain GPs' signatures on prescriptions

Question 3 – *How much time do you spend in a week getting doctors' signatures on the prescriptions you are issuing?*

– All respondents replied to this question, although four said they did not spend any time getting GPs' signatures on prescriptions. One said she never personally prescribed, and the other three said they gave their

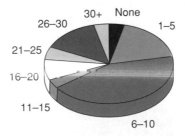

Fig. 9.1 Number of prescriptions (scrips) issued by practice nurses per week.

prescriptions to the receptionists to get them signed. From the remaining answers given (n = 34), the average time taken per nurse per week was 42.65 minutes. Extrapolated to the study population, this totalled an average of 3955.0766 hours per year. If the average hourly rate of practice nurses is £9.53 (Medeconomics, 1998), then this incurs a cost of £37 691.88 per health authority per year. Extrapolated to the whole of the UK, this comes to a staggering £3 769 187.90 per year! If the average practice nurse works 26.875 hours per week (see Question 12), this money would be enough to employ an extra 283 part-time or 204 full-time nurses.

Frequency and differing methods of prescribing

The replies to Questions 4, 7, 8, 9 and 10 have been grouped together in Figure 9.2.

Question 4 – *Are you ever left with blank signed prescriptions to use at your discretion?*

Question 7 – *Do you ever obtain 'prescription only' items from the chemist for which you provide a prescription at a later date?*

Question 8 – *Do you ever personally prescribe items for a patient and keep the excess items for stock?*

Question 9 – *Do you ever prescribe for a patient who no longer receives nursing care and keep the items for stock?*

Question 10 – *Do you ever issue a patient with items/medication given to yourself or the GP by pharmaceutical companies?*

– All nurses replied to these questions except the one nurse who did not 'prescribe'.

It can be seen from Figure 9.2 that 5% of nurses are left with pre-signed, blank prescriptions on a daily basis, and 18% on an occasional basis. 34% obtain stock items by over-prescribing for patients they have seen, and 18% by issuing prescriptions for patients they have not seen. 52% will issue items/medication given to them by pharmaceutical representatives, and 50% of nurses obtain items from the chemist for which they provide a prescription at a later date. One practice nurse commented that the GPs wanted to leave her with blank, pre-signed prescriptions, but she declined.

Items prescribed by practice nurses

Question 5 – *Which categories of items do you prescribe?*

– The question was followed by a list of categories which included dressings, asthma medication, oral contraceptives, etc. Respondents were

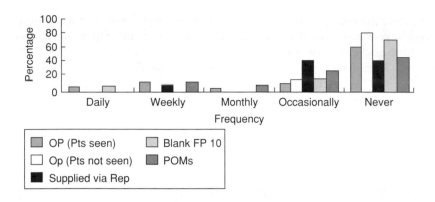

Key:
OP (Pts seen) = Over-prescribe for patients seen and keep excess items for stock
OP (Pts not seen) = Over-prescribe for patients who have not been seen in surgery
or at home, and keep excess items for stock
POMs = Prescription only items obtained from the chemist without a prescription
(which will be forwarded to the chemist at a later date)
Blank FP10 = Nurse left with pre-signed blank prescriptions to use at her discretion
Supplied via Rep = Patient issued with items/medication which have been given to the
practice by pharmaceutical representative

Fig. 9.2   Frequency and methods of prescribing.

asked to indicate all categories that they personally prescribed from. There
was also room on the questionnaire to indicate categories that were not
included in the list. All respondents replied to this question except for the
one nurse who stated she did not prescribe. A total of 230 responses were
obtained from the 38 respondents, averaging six categories per nurse. The
results are given in Table 9.2.

Items 'prescribed' using group protocols

Question 6 – *From the list identified in Question 5, which would you prescribe
using a group protocol? (A group protocol is defined as 'a locally agreed statement
defining the standard management of certain categories of patients which has been
agreed by all relevant health professionals').*

37 nurses responded to this question. The remaining nurse stated she did
not prescribe. Although items supplied or administered under group
protocols are not strictly 'prescribed' by the practice nurse (as the GP who
signs the protocol takes responsibility), this question was devised to
identify the extent of use of such protocols. The results are given in Table
9.3.

Table 9.2 Categories of items 'prescribed' by practice nurses

Rank	Category	Number of nurses	Percentage
1	Vaccinations and immunisations	31	82
2	Asthma devices (spacers, PEFR meters, etc.)	29	76
2	Inhaled asthma medication	29	76
3	Diabetic monitoring equipment	25	66
3	Oral and injectable contraceptives	25	66
4	Dressings	24	63
5	Diabetic medication	18	47
6	Oral asthma medication	11	29
7	Hypertension medication	10	26
8	Antibiotics	6	16
8	Eye, ear and nose drops	6	16
8	Parasiticidal treatments	6	16
9	Analgesics	3	8
10	Laxatives	2	5
10	Hormone replacement therapy	2	5
11	B_{12} injections	1	3
11	Thyroxine tablets	1	3
11	Vaginal thrush treatments	1	3
12	Stoma care products	0	0

Are group protocols widely used?

Figure 9.3 shows the top five categories of items prescribed by practice nurses. The darker area shows the percentage of the total prescribed using

Table 9.3 Categories of items 'prescribed' under group protocols

Rank	Category	Number of nurses	Percentage
1	Vaccinations and immunisations	11	30
2	Inhaled asthma medication	9	24
3	Asthma devices	7	19
3	Diabetic monitoring equipment	7	19
3	Oral and injectable contraceptives	7	19
4	Diabetic medication	6	16
5	Hypertension medication	3	8
6	Parasiticidal treatments	2	5
6	Dressings	2	5
6	Hormone replacement therapy	2	5
7	Antibiotics	1	3
7	Eye, ear and nose drops	1	3
7	Oral asthma medication	1	3
7	B_{12} injections	1	3
7	Thyroxine tablets	1	3

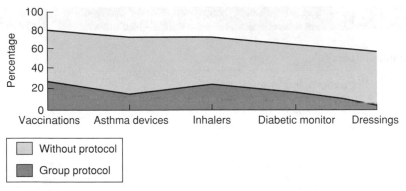

Fig. 9.3 The use of group protocols.

group protocols. It is quite clear from the figure that group protocols are severely under-used. No more than 30% of the practice nurses surveyed used group protocols for 'prescribing'.

Prescribing by other means

Question 11 – *Do you prescribe by any other means than the methods listed above (i.e. as outlined in Questions 4, 7, 8, 9 and 10)?*
– 37 nurses replied to this question: 21 (57%) nurses ·answered 'no'; one (3%) said they administered asthma medication via a nebuliser in emergencies; one (3%) said they supplied wound care items in emergency situations; 13 (35%) said they advised patients about purchasing appropriate medications from the chemist; and one (3%) said they re-issued repeat items already added to the practice computer system.

Practice nursing hours worked per week

Question 12 – *How many hours do you work per week?*

– 32 nurses (84%) replied to this question. Their replies are charted in Figure 9.4. It can be seen from the figure that plotting the number of hours worked per week produces a normal distribution curve which is positively skewed. This leads us to expect that mode < median < mean. Calculating these figures, this proved to be correct:

• Median = 26.25 hours
• Mean = 26.875 hours
• Mode = 30 hours

With skewed distribution curves, the most accurate measure of average is taken to be the mean (Bowers, 1996), therefore the average number of hours worked per nurse per week·is 26.875.

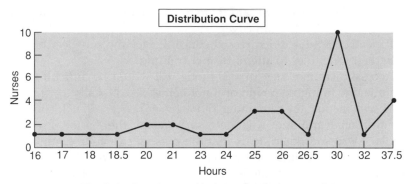

Fig. 9.4 Practice nursing hours worked per week.

To prescribe or not to prescribe

Question 13 – *Would you wish to prescribe (i.e. sign your own prescriptions) if the opportunity became available?*

– An overwhelming majority of 94.7% (n = 36) replied 'yes' to this question. The 5.3% (n = 2) who said 'no' gave the following reasons:

'GPs would expect more, and this is not what I became a nurse for.'

'I do not want the responsibility.'

Out of the remaining 36 respondents who wished to prescribe, 94.4% (n = 34) were willing to undertake further study (**Question 14** – *Would you be willing to undertake a programme of further study to be eligible to prescribe?*), while 5.6% (n = 2) were not. Both these respondents stated that they had already completed a prescribing module as part of their Diploma in Practice Nursing course (**Question 15** – *If you answered 'No' to Question 14, please state briefly why*).

Perceived problems of further study

Question 16 – *If you answered 'Yes' to Question 14, please state briefly any difficulties you may see with undertaking a further programme of study.*

– 18.4% (n = 7) of nurses failed to reply to this question, 5.3% (n = 2) had already completed a prescribing module and 7.9% (n = 3) did not see a problem with undertaking a further programme of study. Of the 26 others who replied to this question, two nurses listed four possible problems, and three nurses listed two problems. The remaining 17 respondents only listed one problem each. This gave a total of 35 responses which fell into four categories:

1. Finance: 51.4% (n = 18) said there was a concern over funding, either for the course itself or locum cover.
2. Time: 22.8% (n = 8) expressed concern over the prospect of finding time in their schedules to attend further training.
3. Access to course: 8.6% (n = 3) thought it would be difficult to access the course due to high demand or it not being based locally.
4. Miscellaneous: the remaining 17.1% (n = 6) covered such concerns as why additional training was necessary when the Nurse Prescribers' Formulary was so limited, fears that the prescriber's course might be too in-depth for practice nurses needs, fear over possible litigation, the fact that GPs would have to accept the issue of nurse prescribing before agreeing to study leave, and the fact that the prescriber's course would be out of date by the time we were allowed to prescribe anyway!

Feelings regarding practice nurses being excluded from the pilot projects unless they hold a district nurse or health visitor qualification

Question 17 – *How do you feel about practice nurses not being eligible to participate in the prescribing pilot projects unless they have a district nurse or health visitor qualification?*

– 97.4% (n = 37) of nurses answered this question. One nurse stated that she did not have a problem with practice nurses being excluded, but she happened to have a district nurse certificate anyway. Of the remaining 94.7%, 48 responses were received, indicating an average of 1–2 replies per respondent. All remaining replies were distinctly negative towards the exclusion (see Table 9.4).

Preferred minimum level of education for practice nurses eligible to prescribe

Question 18 – *What do you think the minimum qualifications/level of education should be to enable a practice nurse to be eligible to prescribe?*

– All nurses answered this question (n = 38). Most responded with a combination of two or more qualifications/level of education. Each individual response was then broken down into its component parts (i.e. individual qualification), which amounted to 50 single responses. These were then charted (see Fig. 9.5).

Four qualifications/levels of experience appeared to be what most practice nurses thought should be the minimum level to be eligible to prescribe: these were a registered general nurse at degree or diploma level with extra qualifications in their area of practice (e.g. asthma/diabetes diploma, family planning certificate, etc.) who had also undertaken a module in prescribing.

Table 9.4 Comments on exclusion from prescribing of practice nurses who are not qualified as district nurses or health visitors

Rank	Comment	No of nurses	Percentage
1	Some PNs have higher qualifications than HV/DN and are still excluded – why?	6	16
2	It's not fair	4	11
2	Disgusted	4	11
3	It's ridiculous	3	8
3	If a PN feels competent and has experience, she should be able to prescribe	3	8
3	Can't understand it now we have the diploma in practice nursing	3	8
4	We should be included as we prescribe anyway	2	5
4	We are the most likely group of nurses to benefit	2	5
4	We are always seen to be less important	2	5
4	Most PNs are more up to date than HV/DNs, so why are we excluded?	2	5
4	It's not fair	2	5
5	PNs with a dipoma in practice nursing should be included	1	3
5	Frustrated	1	3
5	Annoyed	1	3
5	I've been in post longer than DN/HV colleagues – it's not fair	1	3
5	NPF is so limited it would be of no use anyway	1	3
5	I feel like a second class practitioner	1	3
5	It's a great oversight by the 'powers that be'	1	3
5	Mixed feelings	1	3
5	Unacceptable	1	3
5	Totally unjust	1	3
5	It's stupid	1	3
5	OK	1	3
5	It's not a problem as we have easy access to GPs to get scrips signed	1	3
5	It makes me feel undervalued	1	3
5	Inappropriate answer (misread question?)	1	3
5	Non-responder	1	3
5	Can't see the logic in it	1	3

What should be included in the Nurse Prescribers' Formulary?

Question 19 – *What do you think should be included in the Nurse Prescribers' Formulary?*

– Four nurses failed to reply to this question. Figure 9.6 shows the number and percentage of nurses that suggested categories for inclusion in the Nurse Prescribers' Formulary. It can be seen that the most popular

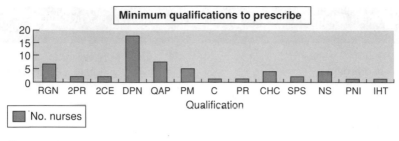

Key:

RGN = Registered general nurse
2CE = 2 years community experience
QAP = Qualification in area of practice
     e.g. asthma/diabetes diploma
PM = Prescribing module
PR = Professional responsibility
SPS = Specialist Practitioner Status
PNI = Practice nurse induction course

2PR = 2 years post-registration
DPN = Diploma in Practice Nursing
C = Competence
CHC = Community Health Care Nursing
     Degree
NS = Not sure
IHT = In-house training

Fig. 9.5   Minimum qualifications to prescribe.

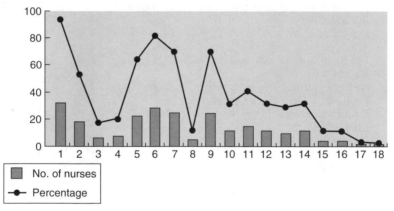

Key:

1 - Asthma inhalers
2 - Oral contraceptives
3 - Antibiotics
4 - Ear drops
5 - Travel vaccinations
6 - Diabetes monitoring items
7 - Asthma devices/monitoring items
8 - Non-responders
9 - Dressings

10 - Diabetes medication
11 - Wide range of contraceptives
12 - Oral asthma medication
13 - Analgesics/antipyrexials
14 - Anti-paraciticidal treatments
15 - Hypertension medication
16 - Laxatives
17 - Stoma care items
18 - Anti-diarrhoeals

NB: Item 11 did not include IUCDs, IUSs or Norplants.
232 responses were obtained from the study group (n = 34). This gave an average of 6.8 categories per nurse.

Fig. 9.6   What should be in the Nurse Prescribers' Formulary?

categories for inclusion are asthma inhalers, travel vaccinations, diabetic monitoring items, asthma devices/monitoring items (e.g. spacers, PEFR meters, etc.) and dressings.

Perceived benefits of practice nurse prescribing

Question 20 – *What do you think the benefits/positive aspects would be if all practice nurses were able to prescribe?*

– Three nurses failed to reply to this question. From the remaining 35 nurses, 75 responses were received, giving an average of two categories identified per nurse. These 75 responses fell into 24 categories (see Table 9.5).

These results were then grouped into four main categories:

1. Time saving – 42.66%
2. Better patient care – 26.66%

Rank	Category	No of nurses	Percentage
	Table 9.5 Perceived benefits of nurse precribing		
4	Less time waiting for scrips to get signed	4	11
3	Increased job satisfaction	5	14
5	More total patient care given	3	9
4	Less pressure on GPs	4	11
4	Less time consuming for patients	4	11
6	More free appointments with GPs for people who really need them	2	6
7	Immediacy of treatment commencement	1	3
7	More responsibility towards cost	1	3
1	Will save time for all concerned – doctors, nurses, patients	20	57
2	Improved patient care	6	17
5	No reply to question	3	9
3	Increased autonomy	5	14
6	Stronger position as a more accountable practitioner	2	6
7	Extend role	1	3
7	Patients would benefit from more careful and appropriate prescribing	1	3
5	Cost saving through more appropriate prescribing	3	9
7	Increased personal and professional development	1	3
7	Would bring us in line with DN/HVs	1	3
7	Would help us provide a seamless service	1	3
7	Better continuity of care	1	3
7	Increased responsibility	1	3
5	Better holistic care	3	9

3. Increased professional standing – 22.66%
4. Cost saving – 4%.

Of course, saving time could be construed as saving money, but with practice nurses it is more likely that they would be able to better utilise the hours they work rather than reduce the hours worked per week.

Perceived problems of practice nurse prescribing

Question 21 – *What do you think the problems/negative aspects would be if all practice nurses were able to prescribe?*

– Three nurses failed to reply to this question. The remaining respondents listed a total of 22 comments totalling 45 separate responses indicating an average of 1–2 responses per nurse (Table 9.6). It was intended to group these responses, as with the previous question, but all answers pointed to a degree of apprehension regarding this extended role. As indicated previously, the majority (94%) of nurses were eager to prescribe, but the results here reflected their awareness of the need for careful preparation prior to prescribing.

Table 9.6 Perceived problems

Comment	Number of nurses
Fear of litigation	6
Patients may see a nurse when they should see a doctor	1
Limited formulary, therefore limited benefit	3
Resistance from some GPs	3
Addressing costs	3
Increased responsibility	2
Risk of over-prescribing	3
Generic prescribing	1
Ill-prepared for role	3
Risk of nurses not keeping up to date	4
Problem with nurses only prescribing in their area of skill	1
Human error	1
No problem	2
Increased paperwork and record keeping	2
GPs!	1
Less patient involvement by GPs	1
Patient may perceive Rx by nurse as less important. Poor compliance?	1
Some HV/DNs may feel undermined	1
GPs may take advantage of nurses being able to prescribe	3
Risk of some nurses prescribing just to pacify patients	1
Time-consuming	1
Not being paid according to responsibility and level of practice	1

General comments

Question 22 – *Are there any other comments you would like to make about nurse prescribing?*

– 66% (n = 25) of respondents did not wish to make any comment. Of the remaining 34% (n = 13), comments ranged from the need for a larger pilot study prior to the national roll out of prescribing to the need for clear guidelines. Some of the comments coincide with possible negative aspects of prescribing, such as possible abuse of the system. The main concern, however, was why prescribing was taking so long to be implemented.

DISCUSSION, RECOMMENDATIONS AND IMPLICATIONS FOR PRACTICE
Response rate

Response rates to postal surveys of this kind usually vary from anything between 20% and 50% (Polit and Hungler, 1995). Anything above this is considered an exception. Low response rates for such surveys can be due to a number of variables, such as low motivation, subject matter of little interest, busy lifestyle/working environment, etc. (Parahoo, 1993; Polit and Hungler, 1995). The main hurdle in practice is ensuring that the questionnaire actually reaches the person intended. Even though all questionnaires were sent in sealed envelopes marked 'Private', it is known from personal experience and discussions with peers that other members of practice staff often open all incoming post first. If this is the case, then it is unlikely that all practice nurses received their questionnaires. Another reason is that some may simply have gone astray in the post. Although positive steps were taken to encourage a good response, perhaps the results would have been more meaningful if a larger sample had been targeted (i.e. practice nurses working in two or three health authorities). In this instance, however, this would have proved too expensive and time-consuming. Nevertheless, what we have is an accurate reflection of the perceptions of at least one group of practice nurses.

Qualifications

Comparing the qualifications of practice nurses at present with what practice nurses would like to see as the minimum levels for prescribing nurses, the only major shortfall is the module in prescribing/pharmacology. 55% of practice nurses already hold a diploma in practice nursing or a degree, all are RGNs, and 53–63% have extra qualifications in their areas of practice (e.g. asthma/diabetes/family planning, etc.). 68% of practice nurses identified potential problems in undertaking further study, their main concerns being funding and securing time away from the practice. A substantial sum of money would need to be made available to cover course and locum fees. As this is currently provided by the health authority, this agreement would need to continue if the situation is to be resolved. It seems that practice nurses views on minimum qualifications to prescribe are not dissimilar to those of the RCN (see Chs 1 and 15).

While searching the relevant literature, it was noted that a number of individuals had made derogatory comments regarding the current training for prescribing nurses. If nurse prescribing is to go ahead on a national level, issues such a course content, method of study (distance learning versus formal teaching), length of course, etc. need to be addressed. From personal experience, distance learning is the preferred method, as it offers a higher degree of flexibility and is less likely to cause disruptions within the working environment. However, a good support/tutor network is needed if this method is to succeed. One possible drawback of this method of learning, may be that nurses would be expected/encouraged by their practices to undertake the module of study at home in their own time. Again from personal experience and discussion with peers, work may already be eroding free time; many work-related meetings and study days are held in the evening or at weekends. Expecting even more of practice nurses in this way may well lead to 'burn–out', and should not be asked of them.

The literature suggested that 15% of practice nurses held either a district nurse or health visiting qualification (Atkin *et al.*, 1993; Practice Nurse, 1994). This research confirms the finding, with 13% of the sample group holding one or other of these qualifications. If current guidelines remain, this would mean that 87% of practice nurses would not be eligible to prescribe.

Do practice nurses wish to be granted prescribing rights?

Taking into account the results from Questions 13 and 17, the answer to this is a resounding 'Yes'. Virtually all practice nurses feel bitter towards the fact that few practice nurses have been able to take part in the pilot projects, and feel that practice nursing is one, if not *the* domain which is likely to benefit most from the prescribing initiative.

'Prescriptions' issued by practice nurses

Although practice nurses cannot yet officially prescribe (except those in the pilot sites), it is clear from this piece of research that practice nurse prescribing does happen, and on a large scale (7.2 million prescriptions per year in the UK). With 3955 nursing hours per year taken up by waiting outside consulting rooms and hunting down elusive GPs to sign scrips, another 23 730 patients could have been seen (basing appointment times at 10-minute intervals). This time could also be utilised to enable such activities as practice profiling, which helps to identify local and practice-specific health care priorities, an activity strongly endorsed by the Department of Health (DoH, 1996). These are just examples of how this time could be utilised if all practice nurses were granted prescribing rights.

The Nurse Prescribers' Formulary

Comparing items prescribed now by practice nurses (Table 9.2) and what practice nurses would like to see included in the NPF (Fig. 9.6), there is little difference. However, if these two results are compared with what is currently included in the NPF, only three categories are the same (laxatives, ear drops and limited dressings). This suggests that the current NPF would need comprehensive restructuring if practice nurses and their patients were to obtain maximum benefit from prescribing rights. As suggested by Jones (1994) and Anderson (1997), perhaps allowing practice nurses to prescribe from the British National Formulary (within their range of competence), would be a suitable alternative.

Group protocols

It can be seen from the results that group protocols are grossly under-utilised. It is possible that practices actually have protocols and they are just not used. With the increasing involvement of practices in such initiatives as the King's Fund Organisational Audit and 'Investors In People', a higher use of group protocols was expected. In 1995, the RCN stated that group protocols had become the norm. This research has shown otherwise.

For years, group protocols have attempted to cover the grey areas surrounding supply and administration of medication, and their legal standing was never made clear. Following the recent report from the Crown review body (DoH, 1998), practices are now being encouraged to re-evaluate current protocols in line with the report's recommendations (Cresswell, 1998; Parker, 1998; Saunders, 1998). Health secretary Frank Dobson has now promised to address any ambiguities in the law for health professionals using group protocols, following recommendations from the Crown Review (Community Nurse, 1998).

Methods of prescribing

As well as prescribing in the usual manner (i.e. during a one to one consultation), a number of other methods were identified (Questions 4, 7, 8, 9, 10 and 11). Practice nurses, on occasion, will administer emergency medication (e.g. nebuliser therapy). No specific question was included in the questionnaire to identify the frequency of such activities and whether these are undertaken using group protocols. Only one nurse identified such a situation in her reply to Question 11. It is envisaged that such activities will be more widespread. The same applies to practice nurses giving advice regarding over-the counter (OTC) medications.

The replies to the other questions mentioned above lead to a number of unanswered queries, such as:

• Is over-prescribing for patients (whether they have been seen or not) to maintain surgery stock a legal activity?
• How many patients actually know that prescription items in their name are being kept at the surgery as stock?
• Where does both the practice and the pharmacist legally stand if prescription only items are being supplied without prescriptions (even though they are provided later)?
• Do any current guidelines exist regarding the above?
• How often do GPs refuse to sign prescriptions initiated by a practice nurse?

These questions identify the need for more research in these areas.

52% of practice nurses will at some time supply a patient with items/ medication given to them by pharmaceutical representatives. Although this is not strictly prescribing, guidelines should exist surrounding this issue. Practice nurses should remain aware that free gifts, promotional materials and free samples are used to hopefully increase sales. Decisions to use such items should always be made with the patient's best interests in mind.

23% of practice nurses are left with pre-signed, blank prescriptions (5% on a daily basis). As mentioned previously, this is an illegal practice and should not occur. One nurse mentioned in her questionnaire that she had refused to accept pre-signed blank prescriptions, despite her GP's encouragement to use them. More practice nurses should follow her example and protect themselves (and patients) from unsound practice. It is possible that some nurses do not realise the implications and potential repercussions of this, and perhaps awareness should be raised. It would prove difficult to solve this dilemma using other methods, as practices would not be willing to be identified as using illegal methods.

Practice nursing hours

Practice nursing at present is a predominantly part-time occupation. Whether this is through individual choice or financial restrictions on the part of practices is not known. Perhaps with the increasing emphasis on primary care, this trend will change; it remains to be seen.

It must be borne in mind when looking at the results for the number of prescriptions issued by practice nurses, the time taken to obtain signatures on these prescriptions and so on that in most cases the nurses are part-time. Obviously if they were full-time, the results would be even more astounding.

Benefits versus problems of practice nurse prescribing

Many of the perceived problems revolve around legal issues and poor preparation for this extended role. Careful planning (including protocol development) and training will go a long way to diminishing such fears. The perceived benefits of time/cost saving, better patient care and increased professional standing would far outweigh the possible problems encountered. Both the Crown Report (DoH, 1989) and the evaluation by the Universities of Liverpool and York (Luker, 1997) support this. The original groups of patients perceived to benefit (see below), would be dramatically increased, with the added potential of all patients registered with a GP benefiting from practice nurse prescribing.

Main groups of patients to benefit from nurse prescribing (DoH, 1989)

- Patients with a postoperative wound and/or varicose ulcer
- Patients with stomas or catheters
- Homeless individuals and/or families who may not be registered with a general practitioner.

Study design

The majority of the results are based on averages, as the questionnaire was using retrospective information. More accurate results would have been obtained if this had been a prospective study. However, this was not deemed possible in this particular instance. Perhaps research of this kind could be undertaken at a later date.

The majority of questions were reasonably straightforward to analyse, but as suggested by Parahoo (1993), the data collected from open-ended questions has proved difficult. Many variables exist which could have affected the respondents' replies; these include having the opportunity to confer with colleagues and the problem of articulation, as individuals differ on how they formulate written responses.

Due to restricting the number of questions used in the survey, it was not possible to ascertain the reasons why certain prescribing activities take place. Time and money permitting, it would have proved valuable to perhaps interview the sample group (although confidentiality would have been an issue), or at least determine a method to elicit such information.

GPS' VIEWS ON THE RESULTS

A copy of the results was given to a small number GPs within my health authority. The GPs were asked to express their views. Some commented on the fact that they did not realise practice nurses prescribed from such a wide formulary. This was surprising as it was they who signed the prescriptions, and therefore this seemed to confirm the fact that not all doctors actually read what they were signing. One particular GP said that this piece of work had brought to their attention certain aspects surrounding the issue of nurse prescribing that they had not thought of before and were particularly alarmed by the high costs incurred by practice nurses waiting to get doctors' signatures on prescriptions. After reading the full research document, they were much more in favour of extending nurse prescribing than they had been before. Although some GPs seemed keen for nurse prescribing to be extended, the majority still have reservations. Perhaps they view this extended role as erosion of their medical domain, or perhaps they feel that increasing nursing knowledge on the issues of prescribing and phar-macology will help to highlight their own knowledge gaps and see this as threatening? Who knows? But until such insecurities have been straightened out, the success of extending nurse prescribing hangs in the balance.

PRACTICE NURSES' VIEWS ON THE RESULTS

Following a number of informal discussions with colleagues, two main issues were raised:

1. The number of scrips written by practice nurses, and the time taken to obtain GPs' signatures appeared to be much less than most nurses anticipated.

2. Smiles appeared on a number of faces when they discovered how much the current system was costing the health authorities. Comments were made such as 'Maybe they'll do something about it now it has been turned into pounds!'

Perhaps if a similar prospective, rather than retrospective study was undertaken, the results would be even more astounding.

Achievement of objectives

Referring back to the 11 objectives at the beginning of the chapter, this piece of research has managed to achieve them all. Although, as indicated previously, further research would be beneficial in this particular area of nursing practice, it is hoped that these results will in some small way help to bring a national implementation of nurse prescribing nearer to becoming a reality sooner rather than later.

QUESTIONS FOR DISCUSSION

* Do practice nurses have a good case for the extension of prescribing rights to them?

* Are the means used by practice nurses in the study to 'prescribe' drugs simply a reflection of their desire to provide the best possible care in the absence of true prescribing rights, or are they risking their registration and endangering patient safety by 'prescribing' in the ways identified?

* Why is it that GPs seem happy to collude with practice nurse influence on their prescribing habits?

* Is it feasible to establish competency criteria as a marker for practice nurses' eligibility to prescribe and how could this be done?

* How should the nurse formulary be expanded to encompass the needs of practice nurses?

At the time of writing, the Crown Report 2 had not been published. The author is aware that further measures have now been implemented to extend nurse prescribing.

REFERENCES

Anderson, P. (1997) News. Formulary must go, says RCN. *Community Nurse*, **3(7)**, 6.
Atkin, K., Lunt, N., Park, G. & Hirst, M. (1993) *Nurses Count: a national census of practice nurses.* York: University of York Social Policy Research Unit.
Binleys Directory (1998) *Binleys Directory of NHS Management,* Spring edition. Appendix XV. Corringham: Binleys.
Bowers, D. (1996) *Statistics From Scratch: an introduction for health care professionals.* Chichester: Wiley.
Community Nurse (1998) Dobson to address legal protocols ambiguities. *Community Nurse*, **4(5)**, 8.
Cresswell, J. (1998) Group protocols and the law. *Community Nurse*, **4(5)**, 37–39.
Department of Health (1989) *Report of the Advisory Group on Nurse Prescribing.* (Crown Report.) London: HMSO.
Department of Health (1996) *Primary Care: the future.* London: HMSO.
Department of Health (1998). *Review of Prescribing, Supply and Administration of Medicines: a report on the supply and administration of medicines under group protocols.* London: HMSO.
Jones, M. (1994) Scripted by nurses. *Primary Health Care*, **4(9)**, 8–11.
Luker, K. (1997) *Evaluation of Nurse Prescribing. Final Report.* Liverpool: University of Liverpool and University of York.
McColl, E. (1993) Questionnaire design and construction. *Nurse Researcher*, **1(2)**, 16–25.
Medeconomics (1998) Database. *Medeconomics*, February, **19(2)**, 32.
Oppenheim, A.N. (1992) *Questionnaire Design, Interviewing and Attitude Measurement*, 2nd edn. London: Pinter Publications.
Parahoo, K. (1993) Questionnaires: use, value and limitations. *Nurse Researcher: Questionnaire Design*, **1(2)**, 4–15.
Parker, S. (1998) Protocols are good for nurses. *Practice Nurse*, **15(10)**, 575–577.
Polit, D.F. & Hungler, B.P. (1995) *Nursing Research: Principles and Methods*, 5th edn. Philadelphia: J.B. Lippincott.
Practice Nurse (1994). News. Budget-minded nurses prepare to sign scrips. *Practice Nurse*, 7, **1–14 June**, 539.
Saunders, D. (1998) The protocol of protocols. *Practice Nursing*, **9(10)**, 3.

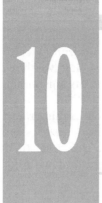

Nurse prescribing

Alternative approaches

Pauline Emmerson   Penny Lawson

Key issues

♦ Health issues facing homeless people.

♦ Nursing formulary development.

♦ Practice development.

INTRODUCTION

This chapter describes the development of a nursing formulary by the Three Boroughs primary health care team (PHCT). The team provides primary health care services to homeless people in south London. The barriers to access and health issues facing this population are significant and formed the rationale for developing a formulary so that a comprehensive service could be delivered to patients at the point of contact with the team.

This chapter will consider some of the facts about homelessness and highlight the difficulties that are faced by homeless people trying to access health care, and those planning and providing services to meet their needs. The environment of care within which services are provided and the patient characteristics of the people seen by the PHCT are described, and we discuss the stages of development of the PHCT formulary and the process used by the team to provide regular examination of practice and patient care.

The project involved people from a range of disciplines working to provide a tool that enables patients to receive immediate treatment by nurses. The recurrent work involves ensuring the formulary remains relevant to the patient group and that practice within the team is evidence based and audited. These processes have been enabled by an acceptance and ownership of the formulary both locally by the PHCT nurses, and at an organisational level by Lambeth Healthcare Trust (now Community Health South London NHS Trust). The challenges and obstacles that we have encountered have not come from a lack of professional or organisational will; it was often the incidentals that puzzled us most.

The purpose of this chapter is to describe how all the facets of this project came together and to highlight some of the challenges and puzzles we encountered in the work. The PHCT experience provides a rich case study for examining nurse prescribing and practice development and we offer the story as a contribution to the continuing debate.

HEALTH CARE FOR HOMELESS PEOPLE
The size of the problem

Several difficulties are encountered when attempting to count the number of homeless people within a locality; the task becomes even more complex when attempting to agree a national figure. In order to count a population there needs to be agreement about who is to be included, and clarity about how many times they have been counted.

Towards a definition of homelessness

When it comes to describing the homeless population, a range of definitions are used by different agencies throughout the UK. The literature on homelessness provides definitions that encompass a simple definition of 'homeless and rootless' to broader statements that consider the concept of home, and the state of potential homelessness that is a reality for so many people in our society (Stern, Stilwell and Heuston, 1989; Greve and Currie, 1991).

The people seen by the PHCT are a varied population. They are not just the stereotyped homeless men who roam the streets or the young drug user begging at the station. They are teenagers who have left homes where they were abused, or who have been in care and are now no longer the responsibility of the state. The people we see may have had mortgages repossessed and be left wondering what happened to their lives; or they may be asylum seekers who do not understand the language let alone the health care system and who are surviving on food handouts in an overcrowded hotel.

There are no official statistics kept on single homeless people (Everton, 1993), although many local surveys are undertaken. However, as these often use different definitions and are not centrally collated they can differ widely in their findings. An example of the discrepancies that can arise is evident when comparing the figures from the 1991 Census and those from the Salvation Army. The 1991 Census included a head count of homeless people sleeping rough. In Birmingham the results from the Census showed no people recorded as sleeping out. This conflicts with the Salvation Army count for the same area that yielded 61 people sleeping out on one night (Standing Conference On Public Health, 1992). Head counts of people sleeping rough provide 'guesstimates' and exclude those staying in hostels, squatting or staying with friends and family. Homeless people will only appear in local authority figures of people accepted for housing if they come into one of the categories of priority need. If you are a well person between 17 and 60 years old, with no dependant children or diagnosed mental illness, then you will not be accepted for local authority housing.

As well as demonstrating a priority need, people have to show that they have a local connection to the area in which they are applying for housing, and that they are not intentionally homeless. This last category can include people who have incurred rent or mortgage arrears, or who have left or turned down offers of housing without good reason.

Homeless people may stay in one area and use services within other local authority or health authority boundaries or they may use several agencies across a wide area, and can accrue a plethora of case records and temporary GP registrations. Work has been undertaken that provides guidance on how to count homeless populations; recent research recommends a longitudinal survey as a way of obtaining a meaningful picture (Crane, 1997). Information about the number of homeless people in an area is only part of the picture. It needs to be supplemented by information about the availability of resettlement services for homeless people and their effectiveness in preventing relapse.

HEALTH PROBLEMS OF HOMELESS PEOPLE

Being homeless is bad for your health. Just how bad depends on a variety of factors such as the type of accommodation available or lack of it, the level of income or benefits received – with significant numbers of people receiving no financial support at all (Murdock, 1994; Refugee Council, 1997) – and the amount of information and support that is accessible. The average age of death amongst homeless people is 47 years (Keyes, 1992).

Bines (1994) national survey of single homeless people found that the physical and mental health of people was considerably worse than that reported in the general population and that many had multiple health problems. The information on presenting health problems of people seen by the PHCT shows a similar pattern of high presentation of musculoskeletal, dermatological, respiratory and mental health problems (Table 10.1).

Developing a response

While health may often be of significant concern to homeless people, many patients have difficulties in accessing mainstream services. This may be due to structures within health care systems such as appointment

Table 10.1 Health problems of people seen by the PHCT Source: PHCT 1993/94 data

Medical problems of clients contacting services	Number of contacts
Trauma	588
Dermatology	578
Respiratory	412
Musculoskeletal	360
Mental health	356
Endocrinology	241
Gastrointestinal	166
Cardiovascular	120
Neurology	86
Gynaecology	63
Haematology	48
GUM	44
Family planning	27
Opthalmic	25
ENT	12
Total	3101

systems, the need for an address, or distance to services. Negative experiences or perceptions by both users and providers of services can also affect access.

The health needs of homeless people cannot be met by a single agency approach. The complex interrelation of housing need, health problems and social exclusion need a web of services working together in order to provide a comprehensive 'safety net' service for homeless people. There is continuing debate about the best way to provide health services for homeless people, with both support for providing specialist services that are located in the world of homelessness (Leddington, 1993), and arguments that separate services perpetuate the isolation and stigmatism of homeless people (Williams and Allen 1989; Bayliss 1993).

Recent developments in services for homeless people have been attempting to encourage a whole system response as an approach to meeting the needs of homeless people. Projects that bring together a diverse range of agencies under one roof have the potential to provide an accessible and flexible response to complex problems.

THE THREE BOROUGHS PRIMARY HEALTH CARE TEAM

The team was established in 1992, and provides services within the London boroughs of Lambeth, Southwark and Lewisham (LSL). The aim of the team is to provide direct access primary health care to homeless people and to assist people with access to 'mainstream' health services (LSLHA, 1992).

The practice of the PHCT has been to develop integrated services wherever possible by working within mainstream and voluntary services both as a resource for information, advice and training as well as providing clinical services directly to patients. Bayliss (1993) suggests that this model can provide a more comprehensive service to people without a home base, as it reaches beyond specialist centres, which are limited to people who categorise themselves as homeless.

The PHCT team was formed around a nursing team that had been working with homeless people in the area for nearly 10 years. There is now an established multidisciplinary service provided by people with a range of skills. The core team, shown as the shaded area in Figure 10.1, is managed by Lambeth Health Care Trust; some of the podiatry and the dental service are separately managed by other community and acute trusts. The GP facilitator is funded via LSL Health Authority and is responsible for incorporating the medical services both as clinical services to patients and as a support to the wider team.

These services are coordinated by the nursing team to ensure that they are placed to maximum effect and work closely with other primary health care and mental health services.

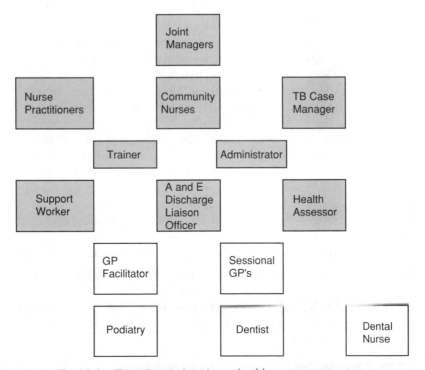

Fig. 10.1 Three Boroughs primary health care team structure.

Environment of care

The team provides walk-in clinics for homeless people in hostels and day centres. The people using these services are more likely to be from the mobile homeless population and least likely to have contact with mainstream services. Contact is maintained with mainstream colleagues via joint working and liaison with a variety of statutory and voluntary services, both in specialist sites and mainstream services. The clinical services provided by the PHCT nurses take place within hostels and day centres which are used by homeless people for their daily needs of food, shelter, advice and social contact. Placing services in these centres provides an accessible access point to health care services within a familiar environment. Direct access nursing services are run from 15 voluntary sector agencies. In each of these centres a surgery room is provided and the number of nursing sessions will range from one to four a week. In five of the centres a GP provides a weekly visiting session and doctors will see patients within their own surgeries. Other GP practices are linked to the team by providing points of referral for the nurses or by joint working with the practice team.

WHY DEVELOP A FORMULARY?

The idea of developing a nursing formulary as part of the clinical response to the physical problems that patients presented to the team came about during a time of organisational change and new developments in nursing practice. The transfer of organisational management and the establishment of new operational structures took place at the same as nurse practitioner skills first became available within the team. The process of discussions and story telling that the team used to describe their practice and experiences to the new managers was accompanied by willingness on behalf of the organisation to examine how new skills could be incorporated into practice.

The puzzle that arose for the nurse practitioners and community nurses was how to provide treatment for homeless people within the parameters of individual skills, professional accountability and legal requirements. The skill mix of the team allowed the nurses to offer a high level of clinical intervention which was hampered, in effect, by the lack of prescriptive authority.

The following questions arose from the discussion and debate that ensued:

- What were the most commonly presenting ailments or illnesses which it was felt the nurses should and could be treating?
- What treatments were the nurses providing?
- What were the legal and professional constraints to practice and how were they interpreted?
- What were the moral dilemmas that the team needed to consider in this area?

- Who needed to be consulted to ensure that advice was sought from the appropriate sources?
- How to develop acceptable procedures and protocols to govern the issuing of medication to patients?
- What would be the knowledge base and training requirements for all team members?
- Structural considerations: how would the drugs be supplied, what needed to happen to meet transport and storage requirements?
- How would the formulary be monitored and evaluated?
- How to organise ongoing changes to the development of the formulary?
- Where would we find our main support?

The formulary was developed from the discussion ensuing from these questions.

The evidence

Patients presented to the nurses with a variety of complaints that matched other national and local research (see Table 10.1, above). A third of the people seen by the PHCT did not have contact with a primary health care service and they often needed immediate or fairly urgent treatment (Table 10.2). Research undertaken within Lambeth had shown that registration with GPs was problematical for people sleeping out or moving frequently between accommodation (Stern *et al.*, 1989).

Table 10.2 Number of people in contact with another health care agency (Source: PHCT 1993/94 data)

Other agency contacts by clients	n = 3533
No medical contact	965
Accident and Emergency	251
Outpatients department	173
General hospital	198
Alcohol service	151
GP	125
Mental health team	146
Other homeless service	56
Community nurse	49
Drug service	39
Dentist	25
Other	26
Psychiatric unit	16
Optician	15
Chiropodist	2

Of the people seen by the PHCT, 70% were sleeping out or living in hostel accommodation (Table 10.3). These people moved frequently, both between hostels and on and off the streets. Temporary GP registration rates were high in this group and they were more likely to complain of health problems (Bines, 1994).

The nurse practitioners within the PHCT had all completed the RCN nurse practitioner diploma and had been educated and assessed as potential prescribers. They all held a community nursing qualification and were eligible to apply for inclusion in the nurse prescribing pilot sites that the Department of Health was establishing at the time. When this option was considered, the nursing team concluded that very few of the treatments contained within the Nurses' Formulary would be useful in treating the commonly presenting problems seen by the PHCT. It was highly frustrating to have gathered the evidence of need and to have the skills available to provide differential diagnosis and treatments, yet be unable to put the two together in practice.

Although we were technically frustrated in being able to provide drug therapies for the patients, a range of inventive responses were identified when the nurses addressed the question, what happens when people present needing prescription treatments?

What treatments were the nurses providing?

A general amnesty was declared and all the nurses were asked to reveal the contents of their cupboards! A variety of medications had been acquired from different sources to enable immediate treatments to be provided.

Table 10.3 Accommodation status of people seen by the PHCT (Source: PHCT 1993/94 data)

Accommodation used by clients	n = 2934
Sleeping out	1058
Hostel accommodation	1001
Council flat	491
Housing association	143
Night shelter	98
Staying with family	59
Resettlement unit	39
Hostel or B&B	31
Residential home	4
Squat	7
Staying with friends	2
Other	1
Owner occupier	0

Discussion about what the drugs were used for and in what circumstances revealed a high level of knowledge and expertise. There was also a firm belief that although the practice was clearly contravening professional guidelines, and in some cases was probably illegal, it was morally justified in order to provide an acceptable service to the patients.

As well as squirreling drugs away, other practices were identified that included obtaining verbal orders via pharmacists, before a GP had been identified to act as a prescriber. Some of the nurses had agreements with individual GPs that they would provide treatments for certain conditions, for example infestations or skin infections. In these cases bulk prescriptions had been written by the GPs against a named patient.

All the nurses acknowledged that most of the practices being used to obtain treatments had to stop immediately. This left a tension for the team, as it was perceived that there would be less flexibility in the responses available for patients seeking help from the nurses. As a way forward we decided to draw up a 'wish list' of treatments alongside examples from our clinical practice that described the situations where it was felt appropriate to be able to provide medications. This would then be used as a basis for the discussion with the trust's principal pharmacist about the content of the PHCT pharmacy stock and the legal constraints that applied to practice in this area.

The dialogue

At this point the team had a list of conditions and scenarios that, in their experience, benefited from an immediate and flexible treatment response. We also had several qualms about opening up the discussions with other people, as this meant revealing previous practices and being held account-able for our actions. How would this be received?

The initial meeting between the trust pharmacist, the health authority pharmacist, the nurses and the GP facilitator was not the scene of recrimi-nation and accusation the we had feared. It was clear form the case studies that there was a need to provide immediate treatments, there was recog-nition of the skills and knowledge of the nurses and acknowledgement that the initial list of drugs provided appropriate responses to the conditions identified. However, there was no easily available answer of how to provide this service via a nurse led team.

The nurse prescribing pilot sites were being developed at the same time as the PHCT were trying to solve this puzzle. There was some hope that this initiative would enable the PHCT to find a way forward by applying to become a pilot site. However, the Nurse Formulary did not contain the majority of drugs that the PHCT needed to provide. It was obvious that this route would not solve the puzzle.

The way forward came about more by accident than design. At one of the

Box 10.1 Exemptions from the controls on retail sale

Hospitals and Health Centres
The restrictions on the sale or supply of prescription only medicines do not apply to the sale or supply of any such medicine in the course of the business of a hospital where the medicine is sold or supplied in accordance with the written directions of a doctor or dentist. The written directions need not satisfy the requirements for a prescription given in the prescription only order.
Section 1.4 Medicines, Ethics and Practice No 11. 1993

meetings the HA pharmacist produced a supplementary document supplied to the profession as an aid to interpreting the Medicines Act. The guidance notes and the clause that they related to in the Medicines Act 1968 (shown in Boxes 10.1 and 10.2) had set her thinking about how the directions of a doctor were interpreted. The pharmacists saw this as away of being able to supply the PHCT with medicines as the written directions of a doctor did not need to be on an FP10 prescription. A document that gave the appropriate directions for the issuing and administration of medicines, signed by a doctor, would meet the legal requirements.

Seeking help from other agencies

At this point we sought further advice and guidance. Did the activities of the PHCT relate to the business of a hospital or a health centre when they took place outside of trust premises? What was the opinion of the UKCC if the nurses were to develop a protocol to provide treatments? What information would need to be included in a protocol?

The team consulted with the Royal Pharmaceutical Society (RPS) and the UKCC. The advice we received from the RPS was that the work of the nurses constituted the business of the trust, not the premises. The UKCC

Box 10.2 Medicines Act 1968 Part 3

55(1) The restrictions imposed by sections 52 and 53 of this act do not apply to the sale, offer for sale or supply of a medicinal product . . .
(b) in the course of a business of a hospital or health centre, where the product is sold, offered for sale or supplied for the purpose of being administered (whether in the hospital or health centre or elsewhere) in accordance with the directions of a doctor or dentist.

drew our attention to the Scope of Professional Practice (UKCC, 1992b) and the Standards for the Administration of Medicines (UKCC, 1992a). They also reminded us that all the legal requirements for the dispensing of medicines must be met by the protocol. Naturally the agreement of the trust management was sought and given, initially in principle. The management wished to consult with the trust solicitors and risk management team as the protocol neared completion. A list of organisations and professionals the PHCT consulted is given in Box 10.3.

THE FORMULARY

The next step was to sit down and write the protocol. We started by setting down why we wanted to provide treatments, how we were going to do it, and what we were going to do. This gave us a document that contained the policy, procedures for issuing the medication, and a protocol for each condition to be treated which was then signed by the medical director and the GP facilitator. The formulary was intended to provide medication for immediate and necessary treatment of conditions listed within the protocol to the homeless population who are seen by the team. The conditions identified were ones that may become more serious if left without intervention, or where it was considered appropriate for the nurses to be able to offer an intervention (for example skin infestations or vitamin supplements). An example of the protocol is given in Table 10.4.

Initially two formularies were drawn up, one for the use of the nurse practitioners and one for the use of community nurses. The intention was to identify the conditions where physical examination skills were needed to provide a differential diagnosis (for example chest infections). It was

---

Box 10.3 Organisations and professionals consulted

♦ Trust pharmacist

♦ Health authority pharmacist

♦ GP facilitator

♦ Medical director

♦ Director of nursing

♦ Royal Pharmaceutical Society

♦ UKCC

♦ Risk management committee

Table 10.4 Extract from formulary protocol

	Drug	Indication	Assessment	Cautions	Dosage	Further Action
ENT	Sodium bicarbonate Ear drops GSL	Removal of ear wax	ENT History Examination of ear Evidence of ear wax	Discharge from ear No evidence of ear wax Red ear drum	2-3 drops 3-4 times daily	Patient to return in 1/52 for further exam. May need ear syringe if wax still evident.
INFECTIONS	Amoxycillin PoM	Otitis media	ENT History Examination of ear Palpation of mastoid process Pain, red, bulging eardrum Purulent effusion. Amber eardrum, serous effusion, perforated membrane	Penicillin hypersensitivity	250 mg every 8 hours for 5 days	Refer if no improvement
	Flucloxacillin PoM	Skin infections	Assessment of skin/wound. Pain, offensive odour, purulent discharge, cellulitis underlying cases or cause of wound.	Penicillin hypersensitivity	250 mg every 6 hours for 5 days	Wound swab Refer if no improvement. If folliculitis is florid or repeated consider immune suppression.Consider spread of disease in impetigo etc.

thought that this would provide guidance to nurses when they were using the formulary. Subsequent evaluation showed that it was confusing and difficult to work and the second edition therefore contained one formulary for the use of all the nurses in the team, with nurses being accountable for having the relevant skills and knowledge about the drugs and conditions that they treat.

The patients presented to the team with two main medication needs. First, a need for new medication, which it may or may not be within the remit of the nursing team to provide, and second, with a request for repeat medication that was needed urgently, such as anti-epileptic treatments.

The first problem was met by the protocol. If the drugs required were beyond the scope of the protocol, the patient had an appointment arranged with a GP or dentist, or a hospital referral, according to urgency of the presenting problem. The second problem was solved by exploitation of a clause in the Medicines Act 1968, which allows a pharmacist to supply a limited quantity of medicines to a patient who is in immediate need of medication and when it is in the interest of the patient. The PHCT would help patients to make a request to a community pharmacist. This involved contacting the previous prescriber to establish the correct drug and dose where necessary and ensuring that the patient had a means of identification.

This part of the protocol was removed less then a year following its development. The main reason was that when the patient needed to present to a pharmacist stating what was required, the local pharmacists had an agreement with the team that a script would be provided within 72 hours by the GP facilitator. This meant that once again doctors were signing a prescription for a patient they had not seen and this was felt to be poor practice. This part of the document was abandoned and directions added for the provision of medicines not included in the formulary (see Box 10.4).

Record keeping and documentation

The team agreed to use the SOAP documentation model (Box 10.5) for recording consultations that involved issuing a drug from the formulary. This would ensure that details were recorded of the history given by the patient, physical findings on examination, and the assessment of the problem, as well as a plan of action. It also provided a consistent framework that could be audited.

Training

The nurse practitioners in the team had completed a pharmacology module for nurse prescribing during the course. The community nurses, however, were not trained in pharmacology to the same level, and all members of the

---

Box 10.4 Provision of treatments not included in the formulary

In order to facilitate provision of treatments not included in the formulary the practitioner should undertake one of the following routes:

◆ Refer to GP if the identified problem is beyond the agreed treatment remit of the nurse or if symptoms other than those in the agreed range are noted, or if further advice is thought necessary.

◆ Use of A&E – if referral to a GP is not possible and/or treatment is considered to be immediately necessary.

◆ Use of community pharmacist – if the medication required has been previously prescribed the community pharmacist can provide an emergency supply at the request of a patient. This service is available at the discretion of the pharmacist.

◆ Verbal order – see local drug policy.

---

team wanted further training on the supply and administration of medications. The team also wanted to be able to debate the implications for their accountability when using the formulary.

To develop an appropriate training event for the team, advice was sought from a member of the Nurse Prescribing Education Committee. Help was provided to develop a self-directed learning pack for the PHCT

Box 10.5 SOAP model of record keeping

S = subjective information from the patient

O = objective information
history given by the patient
findings from any physical examination
results of any investigations performed
relevant information received from third parties (e.g. other health practitioners)

A = the nurses assessment of the problem to be treated, including the differential diagnosis where appropriate, and the rationale for issuing any medication

P = the intervention plan agreed with the patient. This should include the name of any medication, the dose and quantity

and to plan and deliver a study day. Issues covered included legal and ethical issues, accountability, pharmacology and record keeping, symptom analysis and patient information.

Evaluation

The trusts' service evaluation department audited the formulary during the first year. The process involved examining individual records for evidence of the SOAP model for documentation and other aspects of good record keeping. The auditors also interviewed the nurses about their understanding of the policy and its application to their practice. The evaluation raised certain areas that needed addressing.

Not all the record entries had a complete signature or clear date and some were written in inks of a variety of hues. The interesting point was that every nurse was sure that they would have dated and signed all record entries. A decision was made to re-audit this aspect in 3 months and check on the rate of errors.

The other area that was identified from the interviews was a degree of frustration among the community nurses about the different formularies for nurse practitioners and community nurses. The community nurses felt that they had an appropriate knowledge base to treat conditions such as wound infections and asthma but drugs for these problems were restricted to the nurse practitioners' formulary. On reflection the team realised that this structure prevented the community nurses from taking decisions about their own knowledge base and skills, so a single formulary list was introduced. A clause was inserted into the document outlining the individual's accountability for his or her practice as described in the UKCC Scope of Professional Practice (UKCC, 1992b).

Audit and evaluation of the formulary takes place throughout the year, with different aspects being examined each quarter and an annual report. The process is one of peer review facilitated by the service evaluation department. The report includes a review of the notes in relation to the standards for record keeping, an analysis of the appropriateness of drugs issued for particular conditions, identification of drugs not issued in the year, and critical incident reporting. The results and recommendations are made available to the Drugs and Therapeutics Committee as part of the ongoing risk assessment. They also enable decisions to be made about the addition or removal of drugs from the formulary.

The process of peer review has been an important factor in raising the standard of record keeping as well as providing a platform for case study presentations where nurses assessment and decision-making processes are discussed. The drugs we use do change. We did have some medications that were never used and others which we had left off which really should have been on the formulary. For instance, the formulary did not include adrenaline, which is part of the anaphylaxis shock pack. Although this was provided for by the anaphylaxis policy within the trust, we thought that it should also be included in the formulary protocol as good practice.

As a result of case study discussions, post-coital contraception was added to the formulary and a decision was taken not to add tetanus toxoid. We did back this decision up with research which showed that most of our patients have had well over the necessary amount of tetanus toxoid needed for protection. The case studies illustrate how the formulary is used (see Boxes 10.6 and 10.7).

HURDLES AND OBSTACLES

As we tell the story of developing the PHCT formulary, we are struck by how few obstacles we faced along the way. Selling the idea and getting people on board proved easier than we had anticipated. Perhaps this was because the need was so obvious to all concerned. Everyone involved in this project was supportive and constructive. Whether they were involved

---

Box 10.6 Case study: Brian

Brian is 42 years old and sleeps on the streets. A generally fit man, he drinks alcohol occasionally. Smokes 20 cigarettes per day. He was a regular visitor, but seldom saw the nurse practitioners except for his 'flu vaccination. He came to the surgery complaining of severe earache, which had started about 2 to 3 days ago and seemed to be steadily worsening.

On examination, his right ear was normal. His left drum, however, was obscured by wax. He had pain on palpation of the tragus, but no mastoid pain. Otitis media was diagnosed, he was treated as per the formulary with amoxycillin 250 mg t.d.s. There was no sensitivity to penicillin. Brian was told to return to the clinic or see another one of the nurses or local doctors if the pain worsened. He was told the antibiotic would take 2 days to start to work. He was also given paracetamol for pain.

He returned the following week feeling much better. He then said that he had been deaf in the left ear for months. This was hardly surprising as it was blocked with wax. I suggested he waited another week and then had some sodium bicarbonate ear drops for 1 week. He had a successful ear syringing about 3 weeks following the initial infection. His hearing was restored and he was a highly satisfied patient. He remains without a GP by choice.

Box 10.7 Case study 2: George

George is 49 years old. He has been street homeless for many years and he is alcohol dependent. He came to see the nurse with trauma to his head following a fall. He had quite a large gash to his forehead, which had been seen in casualty by a doctor, but George did not wait to have the wound dressed. The wound was now 2 days old, dirty, oozing greenish yellow pus and inflamed. During the examination George was found to have virtually no sensitivity to sensation, soft or sharp, below the mid shin of both legs. This is often caused by alcohol. His BP, pulse and blood sugar were all within normal range.

George was asked about his wishes regarding his alcohol intake and his options were discussed with him. He did not want to stop drinking.

His treatment was:

1. Kaltostat dressing to forehead, to review the following day.

2. Flucloxacillin 250 mg q.d.s. for his infected wound. There were no contraindications.

3. Multivitamin capsules and thiamine 100 mg to ameliorate the paraesthesia caused by his high alcohol intake.

in the original thinking or contributing advice or opinions, the consensus was one of achieving the aim of providing this service for the patients.

Critical to the success of this project was the support given by key professionals. The team had extensive support from the principal pharmacist of the trust and the pharmacist at the health authority. These experts took us through the legal requirements and helped us explore the possibilities we could achieve within a legal framework. The format of the protocol was enhanced by the work of our pharmacist colleagues. The pharmacists were also sympathetic to the nurses' desire to provide well-rounded patient care as well as developing our own nursing skills.

The GP facilitator and the medical director of the trust were the next pillars of support. They were the people who would be signing the protocol and were accountable as prescribers. Our medical colleagues gave not only their signatures but were actively involved in the whole process. The work of the team's GP was invaluable. He gave advice, discussed which drugs to add to the list and which to take out, and contributed his extensive knowledge and experience of working with this group of patients. He also helped us to develop a rationale for the provision of the drugs in the formulary.

The nurse academic who helped us to devise the training programme challenged us to think critically about the process and the meaning of the terms in the formulary. These discussions often ended with the reflection that we knew what was meant, but we could see that the meaning could be interpreted in more than one way. This process helped to clarify several ambiguities in the draft document and gave us confidence in the final document.

Multidisciplinary working can be a major challenge due to the different perspectives of the professions involved. However, it never occurred to any of the group that the views of any one individual or profession would take precedence over others. Each person would be accountable for some aspect of the formulary, as signatories to the document, by dispensing the medications, or by issuing the drugs to the patients. The atmosphere at the meetings was one of trust and respect for each other's knowledge and skills. There was willingness to learn from each other, as we all felt equally uninformed at the beginning of the project. The outcome could have been very different if people had taken defensive positions that prevented full and frank discussion.

A further potential obstacle was the organisation accepting the role of the nurse practitioner. Our experience was quite the opposite, with the trust encouraging us at all times to fulfil the full potential of the role and supporting us in our continuing development.

The major obstacle that we did face was the amount of time it took to develop the formulary. It took the team 2 years to produce the final document and complete the training – we had thought it would take about 6 months. In the beginning, the objective was to provide our manager with a list of substances that the team would need supplied from the pharmacy and to set a budget for these items. As the idea for a formulary grew, it never occurred to us to consider the amount of administration time the project would need. Meetings needed to be arranged with a group of people who already had full diaries and time seemed to expand when waiting for replies to the letters that we wrote. It came as quite a shock to realise that typing the formulary was up to the nurses, as we did not have an administrator at the time. One hurdle that we overcame was learning how to master the computer and set out the tables for the protocol.

Once we had the protocol in place, the pharmacist had to arrange for the drugs to be dispensed in the appropriate quantities. Packaging the drugs was not a problem, but getting the labels sorted out was another matter altogether. The amount of information that was needed to meet the legal requirements for dispensing meant that the labels were too big for the packaging. This was one problem that we would never have anticipated.

Once we had the formulary completed and the drugs in the clinics, the team presented their work through publications, speaking at conferences and as finalists in the 3M Pathfinder's Awards. It was felt necessary to disseminate this work widely and to inform as wide an arena as possible, as we were aware that there might be some disagreement as to our interpretation of the Medicines Act. We also felt that many nurses were in a similar position to us, though with different groups of people, and we felt that our work could easily be adapted for other patient groups.

This was the really difficult bit: it meant not only speaking in public, but also opening up our practice and decision making to critical examination. We felt it was important to do this with a wide range of agencies, as the development of this level of drug provision for patients was – at the time – ground breaking. This kind of protocol is now more common, although open to much more scrutiny.

CONCLUSION

Nursing is undergoing rapid change and development. Nursing skills and knowledge base, and the capacity to create change for the greater health good of the population are unrecognised. This formulary is an example of creative nursing work, evolved for the continued benefit of the patient. It demonstrates professional and accountable nursing practice. It is dynamic and responsive to change, both to patients' needs and research findings. It is hoped that soon there will be no need for the nurses to depend on this protocol, but rather they will be granted prescriptive rights to enable them to deliver a well rounded package of care in a truly creative and cost-effective manner.

Whilst there are those who may either doubt the ability of nurses to undertake a more holistic and less task orientated approach to health care, and others who may question the legality of this formulary, it must be recognised that there is a real need for nurses to be able to prescribe within the bounds of their own practice and knowledge base. This is not nursing as medicine, but rather nurses focusing their skills to problem solve in a safe and professionally astute way. As we write, the Department of Health is producing guidelines for group protocols used by nurses. This is to be welcomed as the current situation is confusing and ambiguous. It has resulted in nurses feeling that they need to break the law in order to provide adequate care for their patients; the consequences of this for both nurses and patients are unacceptable.

Our experience has been one of continual support from our colleagues and employers as we attempted to provide a flexible and seamless service for homeless people. We are aware that this is often not the case, and that nurses can become embroiled in power struggles when they attempt to advance their practice.

The patients seen by the PHCT have benefited by receiving appropriate and timely interventions. Having the formulary to use as a tool for patient care has not resulted in escalating costs, nor have people been denied access to mainstream health services. Care and consideration are taken by the nurses when using the formulary and the patients report satisfaction at having one less hurdle to overcome. In our view the challenge has been worthwhile.

QUESTIONS FOR DISCUSSION

- Do the access to health issues facing homeless people justify a response such as the formulary described in this chapter?
- What are the ethical issues that face nurses when undertaking prescribing?
- Should the drugs used in the PHCT formulary remain limited to those needed to treat urgent conditions?

FURTHER READING

Fisher, K. & Collins, J. (1993) Homelessness, health care and welfare provision, London, Routledge.

This book gives a comprehensive analysis of the issues facing homeless people in our society.

Shelter (1991) Left Out: Sleeping Out in Severe Weather Conditions, Shelter, London.

Shiner, P. & Leddington, S. (1991) 'Sometimes it makes you frightened to go into hospital ... they treat you like dirt.' Health Service Journal, 7 November, 21–24.

These texts give a vivid description of the circumstances that homeless people face each day.

REFERENCES

Bayliss, E. (1993) Models of health care provision. In *Homelessness, Health Care and Welfare Provision*, ed. Fisher, K. & Collins, J. London: Routledge.
Bines, W. (1994) *The Health of Single Homeless People*. York: Centre for Housing Policy, University of York.
Crane, M. (1997) *Homeless Truths. Challenging the myths about homeless people*. London: Crisis/Help the Aged.
Emmerson, P. (1994) Get in on the Act. *Community Nurse*, **October**.
Everton, J. (1993) Single homelessness and social policy. In *Homelessness, Health Care and Welfare Provision*, ed. Fisher, K. & Collins, J. London: Routledge.
Greve, J. & Currie, E. (1991) *Homelessness in Britain*. London. Joseph Rowntree Memorial Trust.
Keyes, S. (1992) *Sick to Death of Homelessness: an investigation into the links between homelessness, health and mortality*. London: Crisis.
Lambeth, Southwark and Lewisham Family Health Services Authority (1992) *Roots To Health. A strategy for the development of health care services for homeless people*. London: LSL FHSA and South East London Health Authority.

Leddington, S. (1993) *What Homeless People Say About General Practice*. London: Simon Community.

Medicines Act 1968. London: HMSO.

Murdock, A. (1994) *We are human too. A study of people who beg*. London: Crisis.

Refugee Council (1997) *Just Existence: a report on the lives of asylum seekers who have lost benefits in the UK*. London: Refugee Council.

Standing Conference on Public Health (1994) *Housing, Homelessness and Health*. London: Nuffield Hospitals Trust.

Stern, R., Stilwell, B. & Heuston, J. (1989) *From the Margins to the Mainstream. Collaboration in planning sevices with single homeless people*. London: West Lambeth Health Authority.

Three Boroughs PHCT (1993/4) Annual General Report. [Unpublished].

Three Boroughs PHCT (1995/6) Annual General Report. [Unpublished].

United Kingdom Central Council for Nursing, Midwifery and Health Visiting (1992a) *Standards for the Administration of Medicines*. London: UKCC.

United Kingdom Central Council for Nursing, Midwifery and Health Visiting (1992b) *The Scope of Professional Practice*. London: UKCC.

Williams, S. & Allen, I. (1989) *Health Care for Single Homeless People*. London: Policy Studies Institute.

Nurse prescribing

Alternative approaches: protocols in practice

Mary Mayes

Key issues

♦ How nurses currently prescribe.

♦ Which nurses need to prescribe in practice.

♦ Protocols used in different types of practice.

♦ Results of research into nurse practitioner prescribing.

INTRODUCTION

Many nurses need to prescribe as part of their practice. For some this will only happen once or twice a month, for others many times a day. Unfortunately the law does not allow them to do this and alternative means of obtaining prescriptions have to be found. The time and effort in doing this is described. Some nurses working autonomously have developed protocols with doctors and pharmacists to overcome the current legal restrictions which do not allow them to sign for items they have decided need to be prescribed for patients. Examples are given of protocols used in different nursing situations and developed jointly by nurses, doctors and pharmacists. Qualified nurse practitioners in the community frequently decide upon prescrition items for patients. Research showing the groups and types of medications 'prescribed' by the nurse practitioners is discussed. As most of the drugs that nurses are prescribing are not in the Nurses' Formulary, the need for a wider formulary is considered.

As doctors have always taken the responsibility for writing prescriptions, why should nurses also need to? This is a question which can be readily answered by most community nurses and many of the doctors who work with them. Since nurses are not currently able to sign prescriptions, the time wasted by nurses, patients and doctors must be costing both the

National Health Service and private health care dearly. Care giving by nurses involves frequent nurse/patient contact, while doctor/patient contact time is often much less. When patients are unable to self-medicate (e.g. if the medication is administered intramuscularly, or if it is a particular wound dressing), this will be done by a nurse. As a result of this contact, the nurse will be able to observe the effects of the medication and will often be aware of the need to change either the dose or type. In the community, doctors and nurses rarely see the patient together. Any change in the prescribed medication cannot be written by the nurse as, by law, the general practitioner has to sign the prescription to enable the patient to obtain the medication from the pharmacist. This can then involve the nurse tracing the doctor, who writes the prescription, which has to be delivered either back to the patient or direct to the pharmacist for dispensing. If the nurse had been able to write the prescription immediately, the patient would have received the medication sooner and the doctor and nurse would have been able to spend the time wasted by these delays with other patients.

Every day thousands of nurses are making decisions about prescription medicines which they know are appropriate for their patients' care, but the doctor has to sign the prescriptions because this is what the UK law demands: the district nurse whose patient needs a particular wound dressing will have to travel to the GP's surgery to obtain the necessary prescription; the diabetes specialist nurse who wishes to change a patient from oral medication to insulin has to obtain a signed prescription from a doctor; the family planning nurse who has made the decision on the size and type of contraceptive diaphragm and the appropriate spermicide for the patient to use will have to wait until a doctor is free to sign the prescription; the health visitor who suggests a particular cream for a baby's nappy rash; the practice nurse who administers prophylactic vaccines to clients prior to foreign travel; the Macmillan nurse who wishes to alter the analgesic dose for a patient terminally ill with cancer; the nurse practitioner who prescribes an antibiotic for a man with sinusitis – all of these nurses have made decision on appropriate medication, all have to wait for the doctor to sign the prescriptions before the medication can be dispensed.

The community nurses who need to prescribe will include the following:

- Nurse practitioners
- Practice nurses
- District nurses
- Health visitors
- Midwives
- Mental health nurses
- Specialist nurses in:
  - oncology

- diabetes
- continence care
- respiratory care
- family planning
- dermatology.

It would also be appropriate for nurses in accident and emergency departments of hospitals and nurses in nurse led units.

District nurses often visit patients who need nursing care but do not need a high medical input. These nurses frequently give wound care and make decisions on the appropriate dressings for these. They will advise on nutritional supplements, skin and mouth care, aperients, catheter care and many other areas of nursing care. If a wound swab indicates the need for a specific antibiotic, the appropriately trained district nurse could instigate this.

Health visitors are often the first health care professionals consulted by mothers about a baby who has a skin rash, or a toddler with sticky eyes, head lice or scabies. Some health visitors administer vaccines to babies. Health visitors who have an elderly caseload may also need to prescribe skin care treatment, aperients and dietary supplements.

Specialist nurses will be knowledgeable about the medication used in their field of practice and will prescribe appropriate treatment within that area of expertise. The respiratory nurse specialist may wish to add or alter doses of existing asthma medications. Family planning nurses may need to prescribe emergency contraception when there is no doctor on the premises to sign for this.

Practice nurses have a very varied job. As specialist practitioners they would need the ability to prescribe vaccines and wound dressings at the very least, and those who have completed specialist courses in respiratory disease, diabetes, family planning, etc. may then wish to prescribe items in these areas.

For all of these nurses, it is important that their education in pharmacology includes the physiological effects of medication, its side-effects and interactions. It is also vital that the nurse is aware of any allergic reaction that a patient has had to previous medication. Access to computer dispensing records held at the patient's surgery would ensure safety in this area.

Nurses have specialist skills

A great deal of the benefit derived from medication is dependent on its correct use and other factors used in conjunction with it. Nurses are good at giving the appropriate health education as part of their treatment, for example a woman who has cystitis needs to understand trigger factors for this – personal hygiene, sexual intercourse, low fluid intake and aggravating factors such as bath oils. Advice, such as drinking cranberry juice, may reduce the incidence and the number of prescription medicines the patient has to take. This advice, backed up by an appropriate information leaflet, should accompany any necessary prescription. How the prescription works and possible interactions and side-effects should be explained. Patients perceive nurses as having more time than doctors and are more likely to ask nurses about their medication. If the condition persists after treatment, the nurse must be aware that further investigations may be necessary.

Initially, nurses working in the community will need prescribing rights. Not all nurses will wish to take on this role and only those who wish to do so should. Before taking on the role it is essential that nurses have undertaken nationally recognised, adequate education in pharmacology and prescribing. They should also have an appropriate level of nursing education, either at degree or postgraduate diploma level, which qualifies them in the area of nursing in which they wish to prescribe. To fully reflect the autonomy of their practice they also need to sign their own prescriptions, and take full responsibility for doing so. All nurses are accountable for their practice and all must be accountable for the care they give.

Many specialist nurses see patients on hospital wards, hospital outpatient departments and in patients' homes. They are in an appropriate position to assess the patients' ability to use their medication and the probable compliance level with different types of medication. Allowing them to add or alter medication, without first consulting a doctor, would save both patients' and professionals' time.

NURSE PRACTITIONERS

The nurse practitioner movement is comparatively new in the UK; the first nurses to complete the graduate programme qualified in 1992. However, nurse practitioners have been working in the USA for over 30 years. Nurse practitioner training involves a module on pharmacology for prescribing at degree level 3. This gives the appropriate skills to enable the nurse to use prescription medications as part of her consultation, if it is necessary. The consultation with the patient will involve history taking, physical examination, arranging investigations such as blood tests, diagnosing and prescribing treatment. Often this will be lifestyle advice, such as rest, or dietary advice. Sometimes a written prescription will be given, or the use of over-the-counter (OTC) medication, which the patient may purchase without a prescription written by a nurse or doctor, will be advised.

Most states in the USA have passed legislation to enable nurse practitioners to prescribe. The formularies they work from vary. Some use the same formularies as the doctors. In states with a large rural population and a shortage of doctors the nurses' formularies tend to include a large range of items. In some states where there is no shortage of doctors there can be more limited formularies. This means that some nurse practitioners who work in speciality areas such as care of patients with HIV may not use the formulary, as it contains little of relevance to that client group. When looking at a formulary for nurses in the UK, it is important that we learn from such situations, which may not have worked well in other countries.

INTERNATIONAL EXAMPLES OF NURSE PRESCRIBING

Some research has been done into nurse practitioner prescribing in the USA. Munroe *et al.* (1982) described research done with primary care NPs (nurse practitioners) in Detroit. One thousand prescriptions were analysed over a 6-month period. The nurses prescribed from 3 groups of medication:

1. Primary prevention:
    Comfort, maintenance of activities of daily living, family planning and nutrition
2. Secondary prevention:
    Infection
3. Chronic disease management:
    Arthritis, chronic lung disease, congestive heart failure, coronary artery disease, gout, hypertension, seizure disorders and diabetes mellitus.

They conclude that primary care nurses who had received appropriate education could prescribe appropriately. The formulary used by the nurses was quite broad.

Since 1994, district nurses in Sweden have been able to prescribe; available data indicate that the first year of this scheme has been successful (David and Brown 1995). These Swedish nurse precribers have attended an 8-week course on pharmacology and drug treatment. They are not allowed to issue the initial prescription. They have a formulary of 230 brands of products to be used for 60 specific indications. These include the following areas:

- Oral care
- Bowel care
- Nutrition
- Wound care
- Breast care
- Dermatology
- Infection
- Incontinence.

Walt and Wield (1983) describe the situation in many 'third world' countries where health service provision may be more limited than in more affluent nations. Medical assistants working in rural areas have a training more basic than nurses are given in Western countries but are given limited range of medications to use with patients. They are in effect prescribing for their patients. An example of this was the village health worker, introduced after independence in Mozambique. The health workers received a 4–6 month training and were allocated drugs to prescribe by the health service. These were used as they considered appropriate and the patients paid for the drugs.

In the late 1960s, as a newly registered nurse, I worked on a voluntary basis in Malawi, Central Africa, in a bush hospital with 100 beds, with five European registered nurses and 18 nursing students. For 6 months a doctor worked in the hospital, but for the next 6 months the nearest doctor was 40 miles away with no telephone link. The pharmacy mainly contained medication sent from Europe and generally good supplies of treatment for infections, parasitic worms, malaria, tuberculosis, leprosy etc. Unwritten protocols were used for the administration of these medicines. As there was frequently no doctor present, the nurses were the only prescribers. There was no legislation to restrict this, as the alternative would have been no access to essential 'Western' medicines for the majority of the population. The only alternative health care was from the local witch doctor and a herbalist, and most patients had tried this approach before attending the hospital. If we had not been able to administer antibiotic treatment for malaria, TB, hookworm, leprosy etc., the mortality would have been even higher than it was (at the time it was 70% in under 2-year-olds). We worked to informal protocols and taught these to the nursing students. Once qualified, they would be working in villages with very basic facilities. They were then given a limited range of medication to prescribe for their patients, as they would be working some miles away from the nearest doctor.

PROTOCOLS

In the UK some prescribing protocols have been agreed and written in by doctors and the nurses intending to use them. This enables them to select prescription only medications (POM) appropriate for their client group. These nurses have been educated in how to prescribe and have appropriate training in the mode of action, interactions and adverse reactions of the drugs they prescribe.

Examples of protocols

Research into prescribing by clinical nurse specialists in family planning at the Margaret Pyke Centre in London, for 15 months in 1993–4, appeared successful. An initial prescription for the contraceptive pill was written by a doctor. Patient checks, as laid out in a protocol, were conducted by the nurses. The nurses assessed the patients at each clinic visit. Those with observations within the limits laid down in the protocol and who had no new medical conditions were given repeat prescriptions by the nurses (Wedgewood, 1995).

Nurse only family planning clinics are also held in Louth, Lincolnshire. The nurses work to a protocol agreed with the district community pharmacist, the senior nurse manager and the head of the FP service. The nurses issue repeat prescriptions of contraceptive pills, PC4 – the emergency oral contraceptive – and all barrier forms of contraception (Ross, 1996).

Many practice nurses have protocols for the administration of vaccines. A document signed by their general practitioner employers is used to enable the nurses to administer the vaccines from stock. Thus an individual prescription does not have to be signed prior to giving a vaccine to the patient, for example (see Fig. 11.1).

Another example of a protocol is one used by nurses working in a minor injuries department in a community hospital (see Fig. 11.2). There are nursing staff on duty and general practitioners give medical cover. The doctors are only occasionally on the premises, but can be contacted by pager. In this case it is often necessary for nurses to give first aid care, before the doctor arrives to see the patient. The protocol was devised by the nurse managers, general practitioners and the hospital pharmacist. Details of the training and responsibilities for the nurses are given in the protocol and include informing the duty doctor of the use of any medications.

An American paediatric nurse practitioner working for the US Airforce, in Suffolk, England, continues to prescribe from the airforce formulary, as she would in the USA. However, as formularies for nurses in the USA tend to be out of date before the law to permit them is passed, she believes that nurses in America often resort to the use of protocols written for medication they need in their immediate practice (Parkinson, 1996).

A respiratory nurse specialist attached to a hospital in the south of England has a written protocol for drug administration (see Fig. 11.3). The consultant in respiratory medicine is responsible for the operation of the protocol. The protocol allows the nurse to administer drugs to seek out any reversibility of existing respiratory disease and to aid in the diagnosis of any such disease. The nurse is allowed to alter the type, dose or route of any such drug on the treatment card of any in-patient, and supply the most effective and appropriate respiratory drugs to patients attending the outpatients department. The drugs which have been agreed with the consultant will be supplied by the hospital pharmacist. For some patient groups specific medications are excluded. The protocol indicates that all prescriptions filled must be carefully documented in the patient's medical and nursing records.

Form authorising delegation of immunisations and vaccinations used at the
Seaview Road Surgery, Canterbury

We hereby certify that Ann Smith has been fully instructed in the administration of the
below-named immunisations and vaccinations:

Cholera vaccine
Typhoid vaccine
Poliomyelitis vaccine
Tetanus vaccine
Diptheria, tetanus and pertussis vaccine
Diptheria and tetanus vaccine
Measles, mumps, rubella vaccine
Rubella vaccine
Influenza vaccine
Hepatitis A and B vaccines
Japanese encephalitis
Rabies vaccine
Meningitis vaccine
Gammaglobulin
Hamophilus influenzae b (Hib)
Hib/diphtheria/tetanus/pertussis
Meningococcal
Pneumococcal
Tic-borne encephalitis

She is competent in administering the vaccines and has a good knowledge and
understanding of the indications for their use, the recommended dosages,
contraindications and the side-effects.

We therefore give authorization for her to administer these vaccines in accordance with
the guidelines that are provided in '1996 Immunisation against Infectious Disease'
HMSO.
The above named vaccines, with the exception of tetanus, should only be given while a
medical officer is on the premises and adrenaline must be readily available, which may be
administered by Ann Smith if necessary.

Dr. T. PINT   _____

Dr. C. SIX   _____

Dr. M. O'LEARY   _____

Dr. V. APPLE   _____

Dr. J. MUNSTER   _____

Dated the _____ day of _____1997

I, _____ hereby agree that I have received adquate instructions for the
above procedures and am willing to perform this duty.

Fig. 11.1 Protocols of administering vaccines.

Items which may be prescribed:
The following non-prescription only medicines
Antiseptic agents
Medicated and non-medicated dressings
Emollients
Topical anti-pruritic preparations
Desloughing agents
Topical circulatory agents
Anti-fungal agents
Tincture of mixture of ipecacuanha
Oral antihistamine
Paracetamol

The following medicines, including those classified as prescription only to be used within specific criteria:
Flamazine cream
Hydrocortisone cream 1%
Chloromycetin/chloramphenicol eye drops/ointment
Oxybuprocaine 0.4% minims
Adrenaline 1 in 1000 injection
Ibuprofen
Chlorpheniramine injection
Glucagon injection
Salbutamol nebuliser solution
Ipratropium, bromide nebuliser solution
Glyceryl trinitrate spray
Tetanus vaccine and human tetanus immunglobulin

Fig. 11.2   Protocol for nurse led minor injuries unit.

NURSE PRACTITIONER PRESCRIBING

Nurse practitioners generally work to prescribing protocols which have been agreed jointly by the doctor who signs the prescription and by the individual nurse practitioner. Nurse practitioners working in different settings will use different amounts and types of medications. However, research has shown that they tend to prescribe very similar items (Mayes, 1996).

The author's research into the prescribing habits of qualified, community based, generalist nurse practitioners was undertaken 3 years after the first UK graduates completed their course at the Royal College of Nursing in London (Mayes, 1996). These were all very experienced nurses before taking the course. Their prescribing rates and types of medication were affected by the factors listed in Box 11.1.

In socially deprived areas, a high percentage of patients are entitled to free NHS prescriptions, therefore items such as mild analgesics and skin creams were prescribed on FP10 forms. In areas where a larger proportion of the population paid the full prescription cost, these items were not written on prescription forms. Patients were advised what medications to purchase, without a prescription, as the cost of these was often cheaper than a prescription charge.

The clinical nurse specialist in respiratory medicine has the authority to alter in-patient prescriptions for respiratory drugs when a written referral has been made. This will include the type, dose, frequency and delivery system.

Drug details and dosage are as in the British National Formulary, No. 26, section 3 and section 6.3.

Section 3.1.1.1 Selective beta2 adrenoceptor stimulants
All drugs in this section excluding:
Fenoterol hydrobromide
Pirbuterol
Reproterol hydrochloride
Tulbuterol hydrochloride
Section 3.1.1.2 Other adrenoceptor stimulants
All drugs in this section excluding:
Ephedrine hydrochloride
Section 3.1.2 Antimuscarinic bronchodilators
All drugs in this section
Section 3.1.3 Theophylline
All drugs in this section (please see under limitations)
Section 3.1.4 Compound bronchodilator preparations
Only Duovent and Combivent to be given from this section
Section 3.1.5 Peak flow meters and inhaler devices
All from this section
Section 3.2 Corticosteroids
All from this section
Section 3.3 Cromoglycate and related
All from this section excluding:
Ketotifen
Section 6.3 Corticosteroids
Only prednisolone is to be used from this section (see limitations)

Limitations of use
Before any drugs from sections 3.1.3 and 6.3 are issued to a patient, their case will be discussed with the consultant in charge of their care.

Fig. 11.3 Protocol for respiratory nurse.

City and rural dwellers can encounter different health problems. Pollution levels vary, injuries and allergies can be different. Some minority ethnic groups have higher incidence of diseases such as diabetes and heart disease (Allen and Phillips, 1997).

Nurses with a high caseload of elderly people will prescribe more:

- Aperients
- Skin creams
- Treatments for rheumatoid and arthritic conditions
- Diabetic treatments
- Hypotensive agents

Those with a high paediatric caseload will use more:

- Asthma treatments
- Vaccines

> **Box 11.1** Factors affecting prescribing habits of nurse practitioners (Mayes, 1996)
>
> Nurses were affected by:
>
> ♦ The area where they were based
>   - affluent or deprived areas
>   - rural, suburban or city
>   - ethnic group
>
> ♦ The types of client seen
>   - all ages both sexes
>   - mainly children
>   - mainly the elderly
>   - mainly female
>   - mainly adolescent
>
> ♦ The individual nurse's previous experience and interest
>   - paediatric
>   - female medicine
>   - respiratory disease
>   - general practice
>   - chronic disease management
>   - accident and emergency.

- Skin creams
- Treatments for upper respiratory tract infections
- Infestation treatments

Those with a high female caseload will use more:

- Contraception
- Hormone replacement treatment
- Treatments for vaginal infections
- Thyroid disorder treatments
- Treatments for urinary tract infections
- Treatments for menstrual problems.

The current Nurse Formulary used by some district nurses and health visitors in the nurse prescribing pilot sites (as discussed in Chapter 7) includes a very limited group of medications which broadly are:

- Skin creams and lotions
- Shampoos
- Catheters and their care solutions

- Aperients and enemas
- Mouth care solutions
- Urine testing strips
- Hypodermic equipment
- Incontinence and stoma appliances
- Wound dressings
- Film gloves and hosiery.

Research into prescribing by the first group of qualified nurse practitioners in the UK, all of whom work in the community, mostly in general practice, showed that very few of their 'prescriptions' were covered by this formulary. Forty-three nurse practitioners recorded their prescribing for 1 month. The items were grouped into 11 categories. Examples of each are given in Figure 11.4.

The research did not include medications which had been previously prescribed by the NP (nurse practitioner) and which the patient received on a repeat prescription basis. Repeat prescriptions are given to patients who will be taking a particular medication on a regular basis for a long time, such as diabetic or asthma drugs. Most practices simplify the system with patients being given a card containing the medication required and the number of times it can be repeated before a check is due with the doctor or NP. This card is handed to the receptionist in the general practice surgery. The receptionist writes out the prescription, the doctor signs it and the patient collects the prescription. This practice means that research into NP prescribing will not show the many repeat medications that patients use regularly, as the NP will only write the initial prescription. Therefore the data does not show the full amount of medication taken regularly by patients which the NP was initially responsible for prescribing. Bearing this in mind, the research showed that the percentages of prescriptions written in these 11 groups were as depicted in Figure 11.5.

A Vaccines: Routine children's, adult and travel vaccines, diphtheria/tetanus/pertussis, typhoid, polio
B Contraception: Combined oral contraceptive pill, diaphragms, PC4, spermicides, progesterone only pill
C Antibiotics/antibacterials: Amoxicillin, trimethoprim, penicillin
D Female medicine: All types of HRT, menstrual problems, (e.g. mefenamic acid), vaginal infections (e.g. canesten)
E Asthma: All inhalers, devices and steroids – salbutamol, peak flow meter, prednisolone
F Diabetes: Gliclazide, insulin, Diastix
G Creams and ointments: Hydrocortisone cream, Diprobase, Fucidin cream
H Analgesics: Paracetamol, ibuprofen, lignocaine
I Ear, eye, nose drops: Fucithalmic eye drops, Otosporin ear drops, sodium chloride nasal drops
J Hypertension: Bendrofluroside, Tenoret, captopril
K Miscellaneous: Lyclear, Zocor, Piriton

Fig. 11.4   Examples of each category of items prescribed by the first group of qualified nurse practitioners.

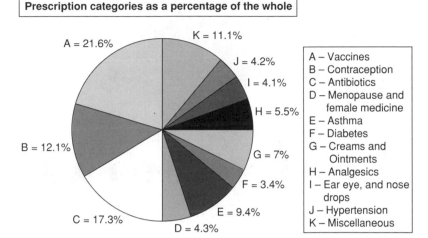

Fig. 11.5 Percentages of different medication prescribed by nurse practitioners.

Each NP will prescribe according to the clients' needs. The client caseload depends on the demographic spread of the population the NP works with and the NPs particular skills or expertise, which in turn determine which patients consult that NP. Prescribing decisions are also dependent on the make-up of the team in which the NP works. NPs generally work with other nurses in the team who will do most of the dressings and vaccinations, therefore the NP will infrequently prescribe these items unless colleagues are asking for advice in a specific area. If the NP sees many patients categorised as 'considered urgent' patients (i.e. patients with a problem that cannot wait for a routine surgery appointment and must be seen by a health professional the same day, e.g. an acute ear infection), a higher rate of antibiotics will be recommended than would be the case for the NP who sees mainly routine problems. If working with mainly male medical colleagues, then a female NP will have a high proportion of 'women's health' cases (e.g. contraception, hormone replacement therapy, gynaecological problems and vaginal infections).

Figure 11. 6 compares the prescribing patterns of three NPs, showing the variation associated with their differing work practices. All work in the community. Figure 11.7 shows a list of 1 month's prescribing by one NP working in general practice, and Figure 11.8 shows a list for one NP working in an accident and emergency department in a hospital.

Seasonal factors will affect the prescribing pattern:

1. Increased antibiotics prescribing for respiratory tract infections in the winter.

2. Asthma inhaler use is greater in the winter for some patients, and for others in early summer with pollen production.

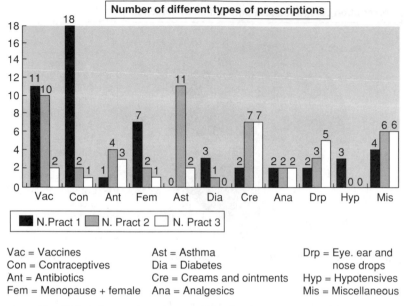

Number of different types of prescriptions

■ N.Pract 1   ▨ N. Pract 2   ☐ N. Pract 3

Vac = Vaccines	Ast = Asthma	Drp = Eye. ear and
Con = Contraceptives	Dia = Diabetes	nose drops
Ant = Antibiotics	Cre = Creams and ointments	Hyp = Hypotensives
Fem = Menopause + female	Ana = Analgesics	Mis = Miscellaneous

Fig. 11.6 Comparison of prescribing by three nurse practitioners.

3. Antihistamines are used more in spring and summer.

4. Mild trauma wounds are more frequent in the summer.

5. Treatment for urinary tract infections is more commonly needed in hot weather.

Some of the prescriptions written by NPs will be repeat prescriptions of items previously prescribed by a doctor or another NP. An example of this is one NP working in general practice who wrote 114 prescriptions in 1 month, of which 97 were for items originally prescribed by her, and seven were for items prescribed by the doctor.

PRACTICE FORMULARIES

Many general practices in the UK have a practice formulary. This includes items agreed by the practitioners who make prescribing decisions. It helps to provide some consistency in items prescribed by using medication of proven efficacy. The use of generic drugs also helps to keep the prescribing costs as low as possible. For example a practice formulary might consider that:

1. For the treatment of hypertension this should include: specific diuretics, beta blockers, ACE inhibitors, calcium channel blockers.

2. For non-insulin dependant diabetics: one sulphonylurea, one biguanide will suffice.

Vaccines

1 Hepatitis B
2 MMR
1 Hepatitis A
1 Typhoid

Contraception

8 Microgynon
2 Mercilon
2 PC4
2 Trinordiol
3 Marvelon
2 Ovranette
1 Logynon
1 Femodene
1 Cilest
3 Micronor

Antibiotics antibacterials

1 Flucloxacillin
2 Trimethoprim
4 Amoxycillin
1 Co-Amoxiclav
1 Augmentin
1 Erythropod
1 Metronidazole

Menopause and female medicine

1 Premique
1 Evorel
3 Tibilone
1 Tisequens
2 Prempak-C
1 Nuvelle
1 Estracombi
1 Premarin
1 Climaval
1 Kliofem
1 Gamelonic acid

Asthma

3 Salbutamol
1 Peak Flow Meter
1 Becotide
1 Becotide Forte

Diabetes

2 Gliclazide
1 Metformin
2 Diastix

Creams and ointments

2 Hydrocortisone
1 Oilatum
1 Aqueous
1 Lamisil

Analgesics

1 Lignocaine
1 Brufen
1 Co-codamol

Eye, ear, nose drops

3 Fucithalmic
1 Sofradex
1 Beconase

Hypertension

2 Ramipril
1 Bendrofluazide

Miscellaneous

1 Modalim
1 Dioralyte
1 Thyroxine
1 Beconase
2 Hydroxocobalamin

Dressings

0

Fig. 11.7 List of items prescribed by nurse practitioner in general practice in 1 month.

Some health authorities give guidelines on the specific medications to use. They will include the antibiotics to use for first line prescribing for general infections (e.g. wound infections and pneumonia).

Specific formularies are very useful as guidelines, but will not cover every case. The doctor or nurse prescribing must have access to other medication for a number of reasons:

1. Patients who have been on one brand or variety of treatment may not respond as well to a generic alternative, so should be prescribed the treatment which is most effective.

2. Patients who have been prescribed a specific medication whilst in hospital often need it repeated; these items may not be in these restricted formularies.

Vaccines	Contraception	Antibiotics antibacterials
11 Tetanus	7 PC4	11 Penicillin
1 Rabies		11 Flucloxacillin
		5 Amoxycillin
		1 Metronidazole

Menopause and female medicine	Asthma	Diabetes
0	0	0

Creams and ointments	Analgesics	Eye, ear, nose drops
0	11 Lignocaine	Sofradex
	8 Co-dydramol	
	2 Naproxen	
	2 Voltarol	

Hypertension	Miscellaneous	
0	6 Prochlorperezine	

Fig. 11.8 List of items prescribed by nurse practitioner in an accident and emergency department in 1 month.

3. Patients who move from one doctor to another, after taking a particular drug for a long time, may not respond well to a change.

4. A patient may be resistant to, or have had an allergic reaction to a particular medication in the past.

Therefore, the ability to utilise the wider range of medications listed in the British National Formulary is still necessary.

The use of a Nurses' Formulary – similar to that currently in existence – will not cover all the treatments used by nurses working with different groups of patients. This is borne out both by nurse practitioner prescribing patterns already discussed above and by Luker's evaluation *Nurses' and GPs' Views of the Nurse Prescribers' Formulary* (Luker, 1997). This paper showed that the range of nurse prescribing and the changing role of nursing practice require a broad formulary. All prescribers, therefore – both doctors and nurses – should be able to access the whole of the British National Formulary (BMA and RPSGB).

CONCLUSION

In reality, nurses have been prescribing for many years; many are now doing this to agreed protocols. Nurses working in different specialities prescribe very different medications. Compare, for example, the family planning nurse, respiratory nurse specialist and the generalist nurse practitioner. All nurses are required to take responsibility for working within the limits of their own competency (UKCC, 1992), and this applies no less to their making prescribing decisions than to other aspects of practice. The only formulary which is appropriate for nurses is the same one that doctors use – the British National Formulary. Nurses, like doctors, are professionally accountable and should use the items from the formulary which they have a knowledge of and fully understand. The alternative is an unworkable nightmare of many different formularies for each speciality, and a plethora of different education and certification systems for nurses who wish to use items from different formularies. Giving nurses the power to sign their own prescriptions for medication from the BNF would be a tremendous saving in time and money for the health services in the UK.

QUESTIONS FOR DISCUSSION

- Why should nurses need to prescribe medication?
- What information should be included in a protocol for a specialist nurse who needs to prescribe?
- What type of formulary is appropriate for nurses?
- What education should a nurse receive before becoming a prescriber?
- What safeguards exist to prevent nurses prescribing inappropriate medication?

REFERENCES

Allen, K.M. & Phillips, J.M. (1997) *Women's health across the lifespan*. Philadelphia: Lippincott, 375.
British Medical Association & Royal Pharmaceutical Society of Great Britain (ongoing serial publication) *British National Formulary*. London: BMA & RPSoGB.
David, A. & Brown, E. (1995) How Swedish nurses are tackling nurse prescribing. *Nursing Times*, **91(50)**, 23–24.
Luker, (1997) Nurses' and GPs' views of the nurse prescribers formulary. *Nursing Standard*, **11(22)**, 33–38.
Mayes, M. (1996) A study of prescribing patterns in the community. *Nursing Standard*, **10(29)**, 34–37.
Munroe, D., Pohl, J., Gardner, H. & Bell, R. (1982) Prescribing patterns of nurse practitioners. *American Journal of Nursing*, **10**, 1538–1542.
Parkinson, C. (1996) An American nurse prescriber in Britain. *Community Nurse*, **Nov/Dec**, 14.
Ross, G. (1996) Nurse only family planning clinics. *British Journal of Family Planning*, **21**. (Reproduced in *National Association of Nurses for Contraception and Sexual Health*, Summer edition, No. 32, 86–88.)
United Kingdom Central Council for Nursing, Midwifery and Health Visiting (1992) *The Scope of Professional Practice*. London: UKCC.
Walt, G. & Wield, D. (1983) *Health Policies in Mozambique*. Case study 3 U204. Third World Studies series. Buckingham: Open University Press, 27.
Wedgewood, A. (1995) The case for prescribing the pill. *Nursing Times*, **91(50)**, 25–27.

Nurse prescribing

Auditing the prescribers

Gabby Fennessy

Key issues

♦ Audit can be used as a tool for checking the quality of practice and prescribing.

♦ Audit is more than just checking what is happening; it can also lead to quality improvement.

♦ Improving practice is a team effort which requires ownership and sharing of results so that things can move forward.

INTRODUCTION

In his discussion of medicines management (see Ch. 13), Chapman challenges the nursing profession as to whether we are sufficiently well equipped to manage the prescribing process. In rising to this challenge, a major part of our endeavour will be to demonstrate the ability to audit prescribing practice. This chapter provides the essential background to developing an audit process through which it is envisaged that nurse prescribers will be able critically to analyse and evaluate their work, so demonstrating the benefits to patients and clients.

COMMENCING THE AUDIT PROCESS

Thinking about what we do and how we do it should be a fundamental part of nursing. But how do we do this? Audit can be one way of checking to see if we are doing the right things at the right time, and to help us reflect on our work in a systematic way. Audit can help nurses find out what is happening in relation to prescribing activity by providing information about practice, and then assisting them in meeting good practice. By looking at prescribing activity and promoting good practice, nurses can not only find out whether they are prescribing appropriately, but also if they are doing so in a cost-effective way.

There is a range of definitions for clinical audit and a number of reasons why health practitioners should get involved. Audit can mean different things to people in health care, ranging from a data collection exercise to a tool for improving patient care. By the time you have finished reading this chapter, it is hoped you will be in the second category.

Audit is not a new term, but the concept of measuring and comparing practice has been around for a long time; this concept may also be described as quality improvement, quality assurance or continuous quality improvement. This chapter aims to explain the audit process, the steps involved in auditing practice, and how audit might be used by nurse prescribers.

Defining clinical audit

Audit has been described many times. The most popular definition is that from the Department of Health (1989): 'Clinical audit is the systematic and critical analysis of the quality of clinical care, including the procedures used for diagnosis, treatment and care, the associated use of resources and the resulting outcome and quality of life for the patient.'

Clinical audit in the UK is widely understood as a team activity; these sentiments are described by Batstone and Edwards (1994) as 'multi-disciplinary professional, patient focused audit, leading to cost-effective, high quality care delivery in clinical teams'. The emphasis is on health care professionals working together to develop the quality of care received by patients.

Clinical audit has also been emphasised and discussed by a range of government documents in implementing and checking evidence based practice and clinical effectiveness and, more recently, as an integral part of clinical governance.

Different ways of understanding the term 'audit' have arisen from the fact that many different projects and initiatives have been funded by audit money, for example research projects. The difference between audit and research is that research generates new knowledge, while audit is a way of implementing knowledge or making sure that it is being applied in practice.

Different approaches to clinical audit

The approach to audit described in this chapter is criterion based audit, that is, based on the development of specific criteria. There are several other ways of auditing practice; these include:

• Peer review mechanisms within an audit framework which focus on specific practice episodes allowing detailed problem solving and action planning.
• Benchmarking and national sentinel audits where practitioners compare their practice across organisations and learn from those achieving excellence.
• Care pathways and the Teler system used as mechanisms for planning and documenting care so that outcomes can readily be used for clinical audit.

The criterion approach to audit is also one that should sit within a wider framework for quality improvement where ownership for clinical audit projects rests with the staff involved. In order to sustain a programme of clinical audit, it cannot be imposed. The involvement of the multi-professional clinical team must be nurtured by good training, facilitation and support from the wider organisation. If practice is to change, clinical audit must be led by the clinical staff involved with the issue under review, in collaboration with managers, audit staff and patients.

THE AUDIT CYCLE

Carrying out an audit consists of four different phases, each of these phases also includes small steps that need to be taken before you can move onto the next phase. These steps include those shown in Figure 12.1.

Defining best practice

In the first stage of the audit, defining quality, the focus of the group is on writing a standard. This involves five steps:

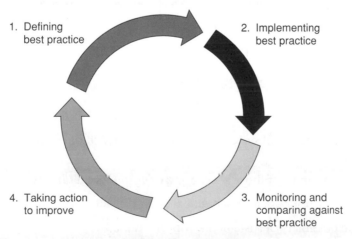

Fig. 12.1   The audit cycle.

1. Identifying an area for quality improvement
2. Clarifying the purpose and rationale
3. Determining the evidence base for standards and criteria
4. Agreeing standards and criteria
5. Implementation into practice.

Identifying an area for quality improvement

The first step in the defining phase is to identify an area for improvement; this should address important aspects of practice or concerns about quality of care. In this chapter we concentrate on the development of locally based standards. However, there may be occasions where nationally or externally developed standards are available to you. Local interpretation of these standards is essential to ensure that they relate to your organisation's needs and that they are *reliable, achievable, desirable and can be monitored*. Your reasons for choosing a topic might include those shown in Box 12.1.

Choosing an area for developing standards involves identifying an issue which is a source of concern and one which is presenting problems in practice (see Example 1 in Box 12.2). For example, an acute surgical unit may want to introduce a patient controlled method of analgesia or a community unit may want to create a system of patient held medical records. The development of standards in these new areas would enable a systematic and structured approach to the process of change.

Box 12.1 Choosing a topic for quality improvement

♦ An area of high cost, volume or risk

♦ Where cost is an issue and resources need monitoring

♦ Evidence of a serious quality problem (e.g. patient complaints, infection rates)

♦ A review of the patients' perspective on quality of care

♦ The availability of systematic reviews of research or national clinical guidelines

♦ Requirements of those purchasing or commissioning care

♦ Requests for data from a national audit project

♦ The possibility of sustainable improvement

Box 12.2 Example 1: Selection of area for audit

A group of staff in a general practice may be concerned about the lack of consistent prescribing and documentation for patients experiencing pain, they select this as an area for quality improvement and audit.

Describing current practice

Now that a topic for audit has been decided it is worth taking stock and reflecting upon the state of practice before setting standards takes place. The purpose of collecting data at this early stage is to describe current practice in a way that illustrates the problems and areas for improvement. In building up a good picture of current practice you can then see any improvement. If data is not collected at this stage, there is a risk that improvement in practice may not be captured as experience suggests that much of the practice development happens as the criteria are implemented. Sections later in this chapter explain how to collect data through audit. You can then use this data as a baseline for your practice against which you can compare the effects of any changes you make.

There will be several existing sources of information which can be brought together in order to provide an overview of the aspect of care under review. These could include:

- Information from routine data sources including numbers of patients involved
- Letters from patients, complaints or comments from external agencies
- Direct observation of care
- Summaries of team meetings or grand round where the issue has been discussed
- Patient stories or feedback from focus groups
- Variance data from care pathways critical incident reports – where members of staff have described and analysed important concerns following one incident.

Documenting what is happening

Keeping a record of each stage of the audit cycle is an important part of the process. A number of pre-devised forms exist to document each part of the Dynamic Quality Improvement (DQI) system. These include the:

- Standard form
- Audit form

- Audit record
- Audit summary
- Action plan.

Other audit tools may also provide audit forms and checklists as a way of documenting what is happening. The forms outlined in this list will be shown throughout the chapter.

Determining the evidence base for standards and criteria

When developing statements of best practice, the first task of the group is to critically appraise the available evidence for the topic concerned. The term 'evidence' may include research findings, professional expertise and the preferences of service users. Research evidence is available from a number of sources. As well as searching the indexes in your local library, a number of national databases and sources of information exist, the details of which can be found at the end of this chapter. National clinical guidelines may exist for the practice issue you are addressing, in which case the task of the group is to appraise them and adapt them for local use.

Sometimes there will be no research on a clinical area chosen as the topic for audit. This might affect your decision to continue, as the amount of available evidence is one important consideration in choosing a topic. If you make the decision to proceed in the absence of research, because the area is a priority in all the other ways listed above, then you will need to consider other types of evidence, such as professional consensus and patient preferences.

Using research findings

Information found during a search for evidence must be critically appraised to make sure it is of a sufficient quality and current enough to be valid and reliable as a basis for practice. The findings of randomised controlled trials (RCTs), observational and experimental research can provide evidence of effectiveness, and critical appraisal must ensure that the research itself is well designed.

Obviously the more research that exists, the better able you will be to make informed decisions about effective practice. This may pose a problem, as it takes time and effort to locate and appraise all the information. More and more often, systematic reviews exist which have been constructed so that the evidence is brought together and appraised. Criteria for appraising research papers and systematic reviews are available from the critical appraisal skills programme and other similar programmes.

Using clinical guidelines

You may find national clinical guidelines available for the clinical audit topic you have chosen. These clinical guidelines could be presented in a format where the recommendations lend themselves to use as standards, either by forming statements of objectives or by incorporation as criteria. Guidelines need careful adaptation for use locally, so as not to undermine the research evidence on which they are based. Factors you will need to consider in the local interpretation of any nationally or externally developed guideline include:

- Is it achievable in your workplace?
- Is it achievable for the clients you work with?
- What needs to change to make it achievable?
- Are there options given for adaptation?
- Are the recommendations desirable for the clients and staff you work with?

A guidelines appraisal tool has been produced by a team coordinated by St George's Hospital Medical School (Cluzeau et al, 1997) to assist practitioners in appraising guidelines.

Using professional expertise

Where there is no research, there may be a current and accepted consensus of opinion; this should be based on a multi-professional group of experts in the field. There may also be consensus of opinion published through position statements. This should include the opinions and preferences of the user group they represent.

If there is no published expert consensus, best practice will need to be agreed upon by reaching professional consensus locally. This process can become time consuming as it involves ensuring that all the relevant groups are thoroughly consulted.

Incorporating the preferences of service users

Even if there are other types of evidence, it is important to include the views of the people who receive the services locally in order to determine best practice locally. The views of patients and clients can sometimes be found in research studies. However, you can also find out what patients value in care in a number of other ways, such as contacting local support groups concerned with the clinical issue under review, using focus groups, interviews or patient stories.

Learning from the experiences of others involved in clinical audit

It is useful to find out whether there are good audit projects by asking colleagues who have considered the topic in the past and are further around the audit cycle. It is often helpful to see how others have decided upon best practice and also to look at the tools and techniques they have used to monitor and develop their practice.

Writing the standard

Once the literature has been reviewed and the evidence brought together, the next step involves setting a standard. A standard needs to set out what is best practice and give some indication of how that is to be achieved.

What is a standard?

'A statement which outlines an objective with guidance for its achievement given in the form of criteria sets which specify required resources, activities and predicted outcomes' (Harvey, 1994).

In documenting the selected topic on the *standard form*, the quality issue identified by the group is classified at both a general and a more specific level. On a general level, the issue is classified under a *topic* heading; this relates to the broad category being addressed by the standard. The more specific issue being looked at is then described as the *sub-topic*. Each topic heading may contain a number of separate sub-headings.

The classification also takes account of the patient or client group for whom the standard is applicable.

The classification of the topic, the sub-topic and client group makes the standard specific to the situation the group is working in (see Example 2 in Box 12.3). On the standard form you will also see a number of additional

---

Box 12.3 Example 2: Standard for influenza vaccination

Topic
Vaccinations
Sub-topic
Selective influenza vaccination programme
Patient/client group
Adult patients
Standard objective
All patients over the age of 65 years will understand and have a choice of an annual vaccination

classification entries for the standard. These can be used to identify the *location* and the *author* of the standard (see Example 4 below, Box 12.6).

Clarifying the purpose and rationale

At this stage, you should also include the *rationale* underlying the standard. This is the reason for the standard. For example, in the standard on providing influenza vaccinations to older adults, the rationale would be that evidence from systematic reviews (Centre for Reviews and Dissemination, 1996) has shown evidence that those who suffer from chronic illness benefit from immunisation, which protects them from disease and helps to maintain quality of life.

In this chapter the term *standard* means the definition of best practice which may be expressed in terms of an objective and criteria (see Box 12.4). A standard includes both an objective and a set of criteria. The *standard objective* sets the goal for practice, and the *criteria* provide the more detailed and practical information on how to achieve the objective. Example 3 (Box 12.5) presents the standard objective written by a quality improvement group working in a general practice. It is the objective for the standard shown in Example 4 (see below, Box 12.6).

The group decided to look at providing assessment and information to adults within the practice, during the period October to November. This was seen as an area where improvements could be made, by helping to reduce the number of patients being adversely affected by 'flu and making them aware of the benefits of immunisation.

Formulating criteria

While the objective gives a broad indication of good practice, it does not provide much detail about how you reach this. This is the role of the *criteria*. These refer to the resources (*structure*) which you need, the actions (*process*) that must be undertaken, and the results (*outcomes*) you intend to achieve.

Structure criteria [what you need]. These are resources in the system which are necessary for the successful achievement of the objective under

---

Box 12.4 Standard objective and criteria: definition

Standard objective
A broad statement of good practice based on the best possible evidence
Criterion
An item necessary for the achievement of best practice

Box 12.5 Example 3: Practice standard objective

Practice nurses assess all patients over the age of 65 and provide information about the benefits of vaccination in reducing risk of influenza. Patients are provided with information leaflets to inform their decision.

review. This may include a consideration of staffing levels and skill mix, requirements for knowledge and expertise, organisational arrangements, and the provision of equipment and physical space.

Process criteria [what you do]. These are actions and decisions undertaken by staff, in conjunction with clients, in order to achieve the specified objective. These actions may include assessment, education, evaluation and documentation. Process criteria may refer to existing policies, procedures or protocols.

Outcome criteria [what you expect]. These describe the desired results of the project from the perspective of the recipient of the service. Outcomes are typically expressed in terms such as physical or behavioural response to an intervention, reported health status, and level of knowledge and satisfaction. (See Box 12.6.)

Some teams choose not to classify their criteria as structure, process and outcome, preferring instead to use unclassified lists of criteria or indicators. The advantage of separating the criteria in this way is that if an outcome is not achieved, the structures and processes necessary have already been identified and so the source of the problem should be obvious. If you only monitored outcomes, you could end up with insufficient information to develop an action plan for improvement.

You may find it helpful to adapt one of the forms to help the group identify the structure, process and outcome criteria for the objective they have identified. These are derived using the information collected in your search for evidence. You may also wish to consider:

- Beliefs and values about the practice issue held by team members
- Acceptability to patients/clients or user groups
- Existing policies, procedures and protocols
- Relevant strategies, initiatives and systems within the organisation.

When identifying criteria it is not expected that you will identify an outcome and a process for every structure criterion, as this is unnecessarily repetitive. There are times when it is difficult to determine into which area a particular criterion most naturally fits, but with experience this becomes significantly easier.

It is also important to make sure that outcomes are not merely processes stated in the past tense. Outcomes are the anticipated results of implementing

Box 12.6 Example 4: Standard form

STANDARD FORM

(Author: Practice nurses

Reference No:	PR/VAC/IN	**Implement-By Date:**	
Topic:	Individualised care	**Audit/Assessor Date:**	
Sub-Topic:	Influenza assessment and information giving	**Signature (1):**	
		Signature (2):	
Client Group:	Older adults	**Standard Date:**	

Rationale: Evidence has shown links between those who suffer from chronic illness and immunisation benefiting them by protecting them from disease and maintaining quality of life

Standard Objective: Practice nurses assess all patients over the age of 65 and provide information about the benefits of vaccination , to reduce risk of influenza and provide patients with information for decision making about vaccination.

STRUCTURE	PROCESS	OUTCOME
S1 Nurses have the necessary knowledge and skills to care for patients with chronic conditions	P1 The patients visit practice for health check and the initial assessment done by a practice nurse	O1 Patient shows an understanding of why vaccination is important to reduce risk of influenza
S2 The following resources are available in the practice: a. Mentorship b. Relevant teaching programme c. Multidisciplinary team d. Interpreter e.	P2a The patients' individual needs are identified, and a plan written with the patient if appropriate P2b From the assessment, the patient is referred to the appropriate member of the multidisciplinary team P2c Goals are set with patient managing condition and date for vaccination	O2 Patient states choice regarding vaccination Documented evidence of appropriate input from members of the multidisciplinary team
S3 Educational booklets are available to patients: e.g. 'You and flu vaccinations'	P3 The multidisciplinary team will continue with education and condition management	O3 Expected clinical goals have been met
S4 Completed care plan. Referral criteria for multidisciplinary team.		O4a Assessment checklist complete O4b Vaccination documented and re-visit time identified

structure and process criteria usually expressed in terms of patient behaviour, knowledge or signs of recovery. It may be useful to ask yourselves, 'What do you expect the patient to be able to do now that they could not do before the intervention of the health care team?'

Refining the criteria

Once the standard objective has been developed, you may find that the group can identify a large range of criteria necessary for the implementation of the objective. It is important to distil this list into its necessary components. This can be done by applying the mnemonic DREAM (Morrell, 1999). This asks whether the *criterion* you have developed is:

- Distinct – is it identifying something new, not repeating other criteria?
- Relevant – does it relate to practice locally?
- Evidence based – is the source of information clear?
- Achievable – is it realistic within current resources (staff and otherwise)?
- May be monitored – can it be monitored?

These may be the cause of some debate within the team. It is worth keeping your criteria as short and to the point as possible. This could mean referring to other documents that you have, or ones that need to be created. For example, your process criteria may list actions such as group protocols to be followed by nurses. It might then be appropriate to refer to protocols, policies, and procedures within the practice as this stage.

Implementing standards in practice

When the standard statement, with its structures, processes and outcomes defined, has been agreed by the team, the next stage is implementing the standard. Being able to get this stage right is important if you are going to use the standard and then move to improve practice. This includes the following stages:

- Communicating the standard
- Getting agreement from others to move forward with implementation
- Agreeing realistic target dates for implementation and audit.

Communicating the standard

During the whole process of discussing and writing about best practice, the group should be informing and involving those who are going to be affected by the standard and who are expected to implement and act upon it. This involvement will create a sense of ownership and should be shared by everyone, not just those who developed the standard. This sharing is part of the quality improvement approach to audit. Getting feedback from colleagues and getting them to comment on the standard will also give them a chance to feel that they have had involvement in what is happening. If the staff do not agree with the practices laid down in the standard, they are unlikely to implement them in practice. Ways in which the standard can be shared with colleagues and feedback can be sought include:

- Distribution of minutes at meetings
- Using existing staff meetings
- Placing standards in the front of the care plan

- Reminders
- Notice boards
- Newsletters.

Getting agreement for the standard

As well as communicating the standard to others, the group should seek formal recognition of the standard by getting the support of practice managers, team leaders or GPs within the practice. Their support can be recorded as a written signature on the standard form. However, it is important that this process is seen as supporting the standard, not just as a mechanism for vetting the standard.

Setting target dates for implementation and audit

The group should not assume that just because the standard has been written it will automatically be put into practice. In planning for implementation you will need to consider:

- Who is responsible for these changes
- How long they will take
- What changes should take place before the standard can be implemented in practice.

Working this out will involve systematically looking at the structures and processes which have been listed on the standard form. You may find that some of the things that have been set out do not currently exist, or have not yet been put into place. For example, in the standard on influenza vaccination information giving, one of the structures states that there needs to be a patient leaflet available to patients. Part of the implementation plan might be to develop such a leaflet if it is not already available in the practice. In this way, the standard is used as a type of action implementation.

Depending on the actions that need to be taken, including communication and obtaining agreement for the standard, the group should set itself a realistic date by which it aims to implement the standard. This date should be one where the agreed structures, processes and outcomes are in place. The group should also set themselves a date to carry out an audit of the standard. The goals need to achievable and realistic, that is they should be mainly short and medium term; such goals can be set within the following time-frame:

Standard implementation

Short term goals	:	less than 1 month
Medium term goals	:	1–3 months
Long term goals	:	more than 3 months.

PLANNING AN AUDIT

Once the area of care has been chosen and defined, the monitoring phase of the cycle can be undertaken. This is achieved through the process of *audit* and involves the following four steps:

- Developing an audit tool
- Collecting audit data
- Collating audit data
- Summarising audit data.

To help you plan how to monitor and compare practice with the agreed standard, an audit form can be used. The audit form provides a template for the decisions that you need to make before collecting data. A lot of the information you need to reach these decisions is provided in the standard that you have already developed. It is recommended that you complete the audit form immediately after agreeing the standard. Aim to complete the entire audit cycle for each sub-topic identified, rather than writing several standards and then deciding to audit them.

Developing the audit form at this stage has the advantage of allowing you to collect baseline data prior to implementing the standard. You then have a point of comparison against which to evaluate whether improvements occur as a result of implementing the standard in practice.

In planning the audit from the standard, it is useful to address the following questions:

- What should we audit?
- How should we audit?
- When should we audit?
- Who should conduct the audit?

What to audit

When addressing what to audit, two of the headings on the audit form are particularly important. These are the *audit objective* and the *target group* for audit.

Audit objective

This summarises the overall purpose of conducting the audit. In this way it is similar to the standard statement. In many cases, the audit objective simply represents the standard statement phrased as a question. The audit objective for the assessment of patients over the age of 65, and the provision of information on influenza vaccination is given in Example 5 (Box 12.7).

Box 12.7 Example 5: High Street Practice audit objective

Audit objective
Are practice nurses able to assess all patients over the age of 65 and provide information about the benefits of vaccination, in order to reduce risk of influenza and provide patients with information for decision making about vaccination?

Target group

The target group is the group you will need to use to collect data from for the audit. This involves looking at the structures, processes and outcomes listed on the standard form and identifying possible sources of information which will tell you to what extent you are achieving the standard. When planning the audit, data is collected from a number of different target groups in order to get as complete a picture as possible of how well you are achieving the standard.

The following groups may make up target groups: patients and clients, relatives and carers, and colleagues. You may also want to collect additional information about the environmental factors you identified as necessary to the achievement of the standard, described by structure criteria. For example, in the vaccination standard one of the structures specified that there would be a patient leaflet available on 'flu vaccinations; as part of the audit exercise you may choose to observe whether the practice makes this leaflet available to patients at the practice. In this case the target group would be defined as the practice environment.

The target groups from which information was collected during an audit of assessment and information for influenza vaccination are listed in the first column of the audit form illustrated in Example 6 (Box 12.8). You will see that three target groups were selected (practice environment, record review and patients) to provide information about whether this standard had been reached.

Staff and patient consent

The consent of all those involved in providing data should also be sought before data collection takes place. A system for ensuring that staff and patients are given the opportunity to opt out of involvement in audit is essential.

It is important to let staff know that data collection will be taking place so that they can ask questions and clarify any difficulties they may have. The usual communication channels can be used to this end – notice boards,

Box 12.8 Example 6: Audit form, influenza assessment and information giving

AUDIT FORM

Reference No:	PR/VAC/IN
Sub-Topic:	Influenza assessment and information giving
Audit Objective:	Are practice nurses able assess all patients over the age of 65 and provide information about the benefits of vaccination, to reduce risk of influenza and provide patients with information for decision making about vaccination?
Client-provider	5 nurses for 200 patients, seen over a 1 month period
Sample Context: Time-Frame: Auditors:	1 month
Form Date:	

Target	Method	Code	Audit criteria
Practice environment	Observe	S2	Are resources a–e available?
Record review	Check	S4 & 04b	Is care plan and documentation complete?
Practice environment	Observe	03 & 04a	Have clinical goals been met?
Patient	Ask/Observe	S3	Were you given a leaflet?
Patient	Ask/Observe	P1	Is the patient aware that a risk assessment has been made to establish suitability for vaccination?
Record review	Check	P2a	Is there evidence of assessment?
Patient	Ask/Observe	P2b	Is the care plan individualised?
Patient	Ask/Observe	P2d	Has the patient been referred to an appropriate member of the multidisciplinary team?
Patient	Ask/Observe	P2c(a)	Have goals and vaccination date been set?
Patient	Ask/Observe	P2c(b)	Does the patient know what they are?
Patient	Ask/Observe	P3	Is the education plan reflective of patient's assessment?
Patient	Ask/Observe	O1a	Is the patient aware of vaccination?
Patient	Ask/Observe	O1b	Is the patient aware of benefits?
Patient	Ask/Observe	O1c	Is the patient aware of risk?
Patient	Ask/Observe	O2a	Does the patient state choice for having/not having vaccination?
Record review	Check	O2b	Is evidence documented of input from team?

meetings, team briefing. If any staff members are anxious about having their practice scrutinised, it is important to take time to reassure them that audit is about the development of patient care and not the inspection or criticism of individual staff. As previously discussed, within a culture of trust and support clinical audit has the potential to empower and develop staff.

It is worth thinking about:

- What information is given to patients about quality improvement in your workplace?
- What could be done to improve it?

How to audit

Having broadly defined what you want to audit by agreeing an audit objective and specifying key target groups, the next issue to consider is how you will actually undertake the audit exercise. This involves thinking about the development of *audit criteria* and determining the *method* of data collection.

Identifying audit criteria

Audit criteria provide you with the main questions to ask during the audit. They are derived directly from the structure, process and outcome criteria you identified for the standard. However, to provide all the information you need to evaluate care, audit criteria often need to be broken down into a series of more direct questions. For example, you might use a standard on pain management to audit your practice as follows:

• The standard includes a structure criterion that states, 'Nurses have up-to-date knowledge of the assessment for pain.'
• The audit criterion asks, 'Do nurses have an up-to-date knowledge of pain assessment?'
• The person carrying out the audit (the auditor) has a set of more detailed questions asking about pain assessment; these are used to assess the nurses knowledge.

In the vaccination standard the audit criteria ask if patients have been assessed for being chronically ill or at risk. To find out whether the patients have been assessed and thus to audit this criterion, observations could be carried out and a record made of when patients are assessed and by whom. Such data collection gives a more accurate and detailed picture of what usually happens.

In some cases, and particularly when you begin an audit, you may decide to audit all of the structure, process and outcome criteria identified in the standard. On the *audit form*, in the column immediately before the audit criteria, you will see a space in which a *code* should be added. This is an abbreviated reference to the criteria of the original standard. For example, an audit criterion referring to the first process criteria is coded P1.

When planning the audit, it is helpful to group all the audit criteria that apply to a particular target group together. In addition, all those criteria that will be audited using the same method of data collection can also be grouped together.

Once you know the questions you want to ask (audit criteria), and know where you are going to collect the information to answer those questions (the target groups), you have to decide the most appropriate method by which to collect that information (data).

Methods of collecting data

The second column of the audit form is for recording the methods you will use to collect data to answer the questions of the audit criteria. Three possible methods of data collection can be identified, as outlined in Box 12.9.

None of these methods is perfect and each has benefits and disadvantages. Questionnaires are relatively quick and easy to administer but they are not easy to develop, they are not always reliable and they may not achieve a high response rate. Interviews are comparatively slow and more time-consuming to undertake but can reveal more in-depth data than a questionnaire. Observation allows direct evaluation to take place and is a useful technique when attempting to audit interpersonal aspects of the service. However, you should be aware that observer subjectivity or bias can occur. Record review is probably one of the quickest and most efficient audit techniques and is a useful method when evaluating whether specific actions have been documented, as stated by a standard. To rely on record review alone, however, would assume that written records are an accurate and full representation of what happens in practice. This is not necessarily the case. Some people fail to document what they do, others may document things they do not actually carry out in practice.

No single method of data collection is automatically infallible or better than another. It is important to select methods that are relevant and appropriate to the questions you are trying to answer. For example, if one of the expected outcomes of the pain standard is that patients are assessed for pain, then the most appropriate way to audit this is to ask the patient whether they have been asked about their level of pain, either verbally or looking at a pain chart. In the vaccination example previously described the group decided to use observation, record review and asking as methods

---

Box 12.9 Methods of data collection

♦ **Asking** may involve the use of either questionnaires or interview methods, both of which may use a structured or unstructured format

♦ **Observing** may be undertaken as by participant or non-participant. The data may be collected using a standardised format (quantitative) or may be descriptive (qualitative)

♦ **Record review** involves the retrieval of data from written documentation, either while service delivery is in progress (concurrent), or after the service encounter is complete (retrospective)

of data collection to audit how well they were achieving the standard in practice (see Example 6, Box 12.8 above).

The choice of method for your audit is therefore determined by:

- The target groups for data collection
- The questions you are asking, derived from the criteria with which you plan to compare your care.

The next stage of planning your audit is deciding when to carry out the audit. The timing of the audit is influenced by the sample size you need and any other variables that might affect the results, such as staff changes or seasonal variation.

When to audit

At this point it is essential to agree on the nature of the *audit sample* and define the time frame for conducting the audit.

Agreeing an audit sample

The entire set of people to whom your audit applies is called the *target population*. It is possible that your project applies to a small population, for example pregnant women who are rhesus negative, in which case it may be straightforward to collect data from the entire population. If the clinical topic is children with asthma you could have a very large population: collecting data from them all would take a long time and a lot of resources. To make audit feasible with large target populations, a *sample* can be taken. If the sample (or subset) are representative of the total population as a whole, we can generalise findings based on the responses of the sample to the total population.

For the purposes of an audit, therefore, it is important to have a sample which represents your usual patients or typifies the target groups from which you are collecting data. The sample should be planned to provide you with information about what normally happens in practice. In audit, the sampling procedure tends not be as intensive as that of a research study, but you should be satisfied that the conclusions you draw from the audit reflect a true picture of the service. (Sampling is described in more detail in the further reading section at the end of this chapter. It is also discussed extensively in texts on research methodology.)

A different sample might be required for each target group from which you plan to collect audit data. For example, if the target group is patients or clients, you need to decide how many clients would give you an indication of what is normal practice. The number of clients you can realistically include in the audit depends partly on the specificity of your standard. If you have focused on an aspect of care which arises infrequently (for example the care of women expecting to give birth to twins), this will limit the number of patients you have access to in a given period of time. In this case you may need to include every patient or client in the audit sample. If the issue focused on applies to all patients or clients (for example in a standard on patient held records), then you would have access to a large population. In this case it is useful to apply some form of sampling technique.

Deciding on a sample size and types of sampling

The validity of an audit project depends in part on how the sample is selected. There are two types of sampling method, known as probability and non-probability sampling. Describing at length the ways of sampling are beyond the scope of this chapter; it is recommended that you read more about the following types of sampling and ask a local expert for their advice on the issue:

- Probability sampling
- Systematic sampling
- Simple random sampling
- Stratified random sampling
- Non-probability sampling
- Purposive sampling
- Convenience sampling
- Quota sampling.

From these different types of samples it is suggested that, where possible, a probability sample gives us a more representative and therefore a more valid picture of the entire population. If a list of the population exists, then simple random sampling is the method of choice because systematic sampling can bias results. In addition, the sample should be stratified as well as random to ensure that it represents the characteristics of the population as a whole (e.g. ethnic groups, gender, age).

Probability sampling methods allow statistical tests of significance to be used, enabling the detection of true difference. This increases the rigour of an audit project. When making the case for change to be made on the basis of audit results, it increases the credibility of your case. However, available time, support and the reality of clinical workloads often outweigh the advantages of probability sampling.

Alternatively, your audit objective may require qualitative methods for data collection. In this case non probability sampling methods may be more appropriate to allow in-depth exploration about an experience rather than the generation of information which can be generalised to the population. Whatever methods are chosen by the team, they should be clearly stated with the rationale when reporting the project results to others.

Sample size

An important issue for all audit projects is how large a sample is needed for the audit to meet its aim. The idea is that the audit should be large enough for us to be able to have confidence about how well or otherwise our practice conforms to the standard set, or with the audit criteria, but not so large that it wastes effort and resources collecting unnecessary data. Sample sizes can be calculated or estimated using norms developed by researchers over the years, for example a sample of 100 is often suggested for patient satisfaction surveys (Lampling and Rowe, 1996). The question to ask when deciding on your sample size is how large does it need to be to represent what is 'normal' and to take account of expected, acceptable variation. Sample size calculations enable you to do this formally. You may find it useful to enlist the help of a statistician or researcher to work out the sample size you need. Calculation of sampling size is well described in good statistical texts. However, if the sample sizes recommended in the textbooks that you read are not realistic for your purposes, you may need to consult someone locally with the necessary expertise to help you decide whether reducing the confidence level or the tolerance would be acceptable within the aims of the project.

If you are using a qualitative approach to collecting data you are likely to be looking at non-probability sampling. For example, a project looking at uptake and duration of breastfeeding might wish to complement their data collection on breastfeeding rates with some focus groups looking at advice received and the factors influencing women's decisions. A random sample of those choosing to breastfeed and another of those choosing artificial methods could be approached and asked to join focus groups. Alternatively, volunteers to participate in focus groups could be found using local new parent newsletters. The sample would then consist of enough women to participate in focus groups to ensure that the range of views had been included from women choosing to breastfeed, choosing not to breastfeed and women from ethnic minority groups.

As well as considering issues relating to numbers and methods of selecting the sample, you also need to consider the period over which you are going to conduct the audit. This is referred to as the *time-frame* of the audit.

The audit time-frame

The specified time in which the audit takes place (the time-frame) influences the selection of the sample because it may determine the size of the population from which you can draw that sample. It may also affect the representativeness of the sample.

Imagine that you are auditing care against the influenza vaccination standard. The target group is all practice patients over the age of 65, which gives you a large population from which to select a random patient sample. You may therefore decide to carry out the audit on a particular day, over a typical work period of 8 hours. However, on that particular day some of the practice nurses are away, and staff have to be redeployed to ensure that clinics are adequately covered. You are unlikely to derive a representative picture of the information given in these circumstances. In the case of this audit, therefore, it might be more appropriate to take a smaller sample of patients on a daily basis over a period of 1 month.

A previous example described a standard for the care for women expecting twins. The time-frame for an audit of care for such women would have to be extended up to perhaps 6–12 months in order to achieve a large enough sample for meaningful results.

The time-frame has two key purposes:

1. It describes the time you may need to collect the sample
2. It ensures that the sample drawn is as representative as possible.

The issue of representativeness is central to much of the discussion on audit. However, it is important that the audit exercise remains both practical and feasible, emphasising the importance of discussing and agreeing the more detailed aspects of sampling and the timing of audit at a local level.

Who should audit?

Having defined the standard and completed the audit form, the standard setting group identify specific individuals to take responsibility for collecting and collating the audit data. This may be just one person or it may be a group of people (the *auditors*). In order for them to retain the ownership of the standard, it is essential that the group decides who should take on the role of auditor.

The auditor is the person who the group feels would be most appropriate to audit the standard. This obviously depends on the type of structures, processes and outcomes specified in the standard. For example, if one of the structures states that practice nurses possess an agreed level of knowledge and understanding about a particular subject area, the auditor has to be someone who is capable of assessing the knowledge levels and who is both acceptable and non-threatening to patients and staff.

Once nominated and having agreed to take on the role, the auditor assumes responsibility for collecting and collating the audit data.

Collecting audit data

Once the audit has been planned, the audit form completed, a person allocated to do the audit and a time-frame specified, the collection of data can begin. Data collection sheets are normally devised as the audit is planned. If you have access to specialist audit software packages these may be generated for you. Methods for analysis of data should be planned from the start of the project and may influence the way in which data are recorded. Audit records can also be generated using word processing packages and spreadsheet packages such as Microsoft Excel. Piloting your audit tool gives you the opportunity to check that your data collection sheets or audit records are set out appropriately with adequate space in each section for auditors to record the necessary information.

Data needs to be collected so that no individual patient or staff member can be identified (it needs to be anonymised). It may be helpful to devise a coding system known only to the auditors.

You may wish to set an expected compliance rate or target for how well you think your practice will meet the standard you have defined. You may have considered this already when you decided on the sample size for each target group. Comparing the actual with the expected level of compliance allows the auditor to see at a glance areas where achievement is good, or areas where the results are lower than expected.

You can use the *audit form* to collect responses to the audit criteria. Or the auditor can record the responses in written form on the audit record. It can be helpful to record the responses as 'Yes' or 'No' in the first instance. However, you may also need to record 'no reply' responses and additional comments which can add important qualitative information to the data. Data is recorded in this way until the pre-defined sample size has been obtained over the specified time-frame of the audit. The data record for the example standard is illustrated in Example 7 (Box 12.10).

Collating and analysing audit data

Once the audit data is collected, the next stage involves analysing the responses and collating the data in preparation for feedback. This is where a software programme such as the DQI Toolbox can provide invaluable support. However, if analysing the data manually, the auditor calculates the average response for each of the audit criteria and expresses this in the form of a percentage. These percentages are displayed in the audit record as the actual compliance to the standard.

To evaluate how close your practice comes to meeting the standard you set for care, you first need to compare what you are doing with the criteria that have been set in the standard. This is known as comparing the *actual compliance rate* with the rate you expected (the *expected compliance rate*). The expected compliance to the standard is normally 100%. This target of full compliance aims us towards improving all structures, processes and outcomes. However, there may be specific situations or circumstances where the expected level of compliance is less than 100%, depending on the

Box 12.10 Example 7: Audit record, influenza vaccination

AUDIT RECORD
(Author: High Street Practice Nurses)

			Key:	Y – Yes
				N = No
Sample:	30			N/A = Not Applicable
				N/R = No Response
Time Frame:	1 month			E = Exception
Auditor (s):				
Date:				
Audit Objective		Are practice nurses able assess all patients over the age of 65 and provide information about the benefits of vaccination, to reduce risk of influenza and provide patients with information for decision making about vaccination?		

TARGET GROUP	CODE	OBSERVATION 1 2 3 4 5 6 7...30	TOTALS Obs Y N		COMPLIANCE Expected Actual		COMMENTS
Practice environment	S2	N R Y Y Y Y Y	29	29 0	100	100	
Record review	S4/04b	N N Y Y N N N	30	6 24	100	80	
Practice environment	03/04a	Y N Y Y N Y Y	30	23 7	100	76.6	No vaccination leaflets available
Patient	S3	Y Y Y N Y E Y	26	25 1	100	96.2	Several patients being cared for by a health visitor
Patient	P1	N Y Y N N N Y	30	22 8	100	73.3	
Patient	P2a	Y Y Y Y Y Y Y	30	30 0	100	100	Assessment often discussed with patient
Patient	P2b	Y N Y Y Y Y Y	30	28 2	100	93.3	Some evidence of verbal referral
Patient	P2d	N E Y Y Y N N	27	8 19	100	29.6	
Patient	P2c(a)	Y N Y N N Y Y	30	8 22	100	26.7	
Patient	P2c(b)	Y N Y Y Y Y Y	30	28 2	100	93.3	
Patient	P3	Y Y Y Y Y N Y	30	21 9	100	70	Difficult to ask about; data aggregated with diagnosis
Patient	01a	N Y Y Y Y Y Y	30	25 5	100	83.3	
Patient	01b	Y Y Y Y Y Y Y	30	30 0	100	100	
Patient	01c	N Y Y Y Y Y Y	30	25 5	100	83.3	
Patient	02a	Y Y Y Y Y Y Y	29	28 1	100	96.6	1 patient cannot remember
Patient	02b	Y Y Y Y Y Y Y	30	28 2	100	93.3	

local environment in which the standard is written, for example cases in which there is a high level of unpredictability of circumstances or where there are structural or resource constraints.

Comparing the actual with the expected level of compliance allows the auditor to see at a glance areas where achievement of the standard is good, and areas where the standard of care is lower than expected. This forms the basis for preparing the *audit summary*, the next stage in the audit process.

Summarising and interpreting audit data

Information from the data record is summarised in the audit summary, see Example 8 (Box 12.11), representing the final step within the second phase of the quality improvement cycle.

Box 12.11 Example 8: Audit summary, influenza vaccination

AUDIT SUMMARY
(Author: Practice nurses)

Reference No: PR/VAC/IN

Sub-Topic: Influenza assessment and information giving

Audit Objective: Are practice nurses able to assess all patients over the age of 65 and provide information about the benefits of vaccination , to reduce risk of influenza and provide patients with information for decision making about vaccination?

Client-Provider: 5 practice nurses for 200 patients, over a 1 month period

Sample Context:
Time-Frame: 1 month
Auditors:

Summary Date:

ACTIVITY	FINDINGS	CONCLUSIONS
	Areas that have been identified with 80–100% compliance	
1. Ensuring that all resources including vaccination leaflets are available (S2 & S3)	Average 92% compliance	
	There was 100% compliance with the majority of the resources. However, at the time this audit was conducted the leaflet for the patients requiring vaccination (12%) were still in preparation: and this would therefore account for the low average compliance score.	Once the vaccination leaflet is published, it should aim for 100% compliance in all resources.
2. Ensuring that there is evidence of patient assessment and that care plans are individualised (P2a/P2b)	Average 97% compliance	Excellent result overall. To continue to emphasise the importance of individualised care plans and assessment.
2b Ensuring that the patient knows the care goals and vaccination date has been set (P2b/c)		Patients knew what the goals were but these were often not actually set with the patient. To aim to involve patients even more.

Having compared the expected to actual compliance scores, the auditor uses the audit summary to record the key audit findings. In the first column, labelled *activity*, the auditor notes the particular issue or criterion which was studied (for example the level of patient assessments that have taken place). In the *findings* column, the auditor reports the findings of the audit in terms of the level of compliance, plus any additional data from the more detailed qualitative comments which may help to explain the findings.

This does not mean that the results for each of the audit criteria has to be reported in the audit summary. It may be that prior to conducting the audit the auditor agrees with the group to report back the exceptional scores (for example those above 90% and below 70%). The exact nature of the feedback, including the range of acceptable scores, must be negotiated at local level, depending on the expected compliance scores agreed from the outset. However, it is essential that the audit summary should provide constructive feedback by reporting on areas of both high and low achievement. The group can then discuss why some areas have been more successful, and how to extend this high achievement to the other areas considered.

Presenting audit data

Whatever type of analysis you undertake, graphically representing audit data can be helpful, especially when feeding back to a group. Possible methods include simple graphs, bar charts, pie charts and histograms.

The information from data analysis can then be recorded on the audit summary. Once the audit summary is complete, the auditor feeds back the findings to the quality improvement group for interpretation. The auditor should not complete the *conclusions* section without consulting and involving the group.

In the influenza vaccination example the levels of compliance are given as percentages. Findings can be categorised into three groups:

1. Low compliance (less than 60%)
2. Medium compliance (60–80%)
3. High compliance (80–100%).

The group can discuss and interpret the findings with the auditor and begin to clarify the key areas where action is required to improve the level of achievement. This takes them into the third phase of the quality cycle, that of *planning and implementing action to improve quality.*

CHANGING AND IMPROVING ON PRACTICE

This third phase of the audit cycle is vital for effecting change and making quality improvement happen in practice.

There are a number of key steps to take to complete the *action plan*:

- Agreeing appropriate courses of action for the problems identified
- Agreeing a named person responsible for the action
- Deciding the time-scale for action
- Re-audit and evaluation.

Agreeing the appropriate course of action

The group members interpret the key problems identified in the audit and consider each one individually, brainstorming and discussing possible ways of addressing the problem. They then select the most appropriate course of action to remedy the problem and record this in the second column of the action plan.

In the vaccination example, you will see that the group agreed to implement action in the three key areas where their level of compliance to the standard was less than 80%. For each of these problems, specific actions to be undertaken to improve quality are listed (see Example 9, Box 12.12).

Agreeing on a named person responsible for action

In the next column of the action plan, the group identifies a named individual or individuals to be responsible for leading or coordinating each of the actions specified. Different people may take responsibility for different actions, depending on the person most appropriate to deal with the problem and the type of intervention required. For example in the influenza action plan, a total of four different people have named responsibility for action.

Deciding the time-scale for action

Having agreed on the courses of action and the individual/s responsible, the group then determines how long they will need to implement each of the actions identified. This depends on the nature of the problem and the type of action required (see Example 10, Box 12.13):

1. Short term actions – those which can be remedied almost immediately, within a period of 1–4 weeks.
2. Medium term actions – these require a longer period of up to 3 months to implement.
3. Long term actions – those which will take over 3 months to achieve.

ACTION PLAN
(Author: Practice nurses)

Reference No: PR/VAC/IN

Sub-Topic: Influenza assessment and information giving

Standard Objective: Practice nurses assess all patients over the age of 65 and provide information about the benefits of vaccination, to reduce risk of influenza and provide patients with information for decision making about vaccination.

Audit Objective: Are practice nurses able assess all patients over the age of 65 and provide information about the benefits of vaccination, to reduce risk of influenza and provide patients with information for decision making about vaccination?

Plan Date:

IDENTIFIED PROBLEM	SUGGESTED ACTION	STAFF MEMBER RESPONSIBLE	TIME PERIOD
Patient records not completed with information about assessment	Records to be updated during visit in consultation with multidisciplinary team	A Jones B Smith C Brown	4 weeks (MT)
	Education sessions to be carried out to ensure everyone understands assessment documentation. Checklist to be included in the planner.		
Goals not being set with patients	Education sessions on care planning and importance of documentation.	C Brown	8 weeks (LT)
Information leaflet	Leaflet updating and availability to be carried to ensure they are always available	A Jones C Brown	4–8 weeks
	Education of staff regarding how important it is to share information with patients. Present findings at staff meetings.	D Green	

Re-audit and evaluation

Taking into account the actions to be implemented and the time-scale for these, the group sets a date to re-audit the standard. This should be after the deadline for the most long term action to be implemented. Comparing the first and second set of audit results will then enable the group to evaluate what improvements have been made and possible areas where further action is required.

On completion of the re-auditing stage the group will have moved through the whole audit cycle. Depending on the results obtained, they must then agree on their next course of action, which may involve one of several possible steps:

> **Box 12.13** Example 10: Short, medium and long term actions
>
> An audit was conducted of pain management. A number of actions needed to be taken. These included:
> **Short term actions,** ensuring that all nurses are using the pain assessment scale
> **Medium term actions,** such as undertaking a pain assessment on all patients
> **Long term actions,** which involved patient focus groups on pain management.

- If problems remain or new problems are identified, the group plan further action and re-audit as before.
- If they are achieving the standard, the group may elect to raise the expected level of achievement of the standard in order to aim for further improvement.
- If they are achieving the standard, the group may set a timetable for regular review of the standard, and then move on to address a new issue for quality improvement.

Whichever of these steps the group agrees to take, they are continuing to work their way through the dynamic process of quality improvement. In theory there is no end to this spiral of activity. However, in practice problems relating to motivation and the momentum of the system may be encountered. Ongoing support and attention are required to sustain an effective quality improvement process.

CONCLUSION

This chapter has aimed to explore the background and reasons for carrying out audit in clinical practice, and to show you how to audit. This approach to audit is a criterion based approach. Throughout the text many examples of collecting and collating audit information have been given. It is not essential to use all of these forms, although it is recommended that they are used in the first few instances so that the team can explore all the issues affecting quality of care, and pull together all aspects covered in the audit.

QUESTIONS FOR DISCUSSION

- What is the quality of the data you collect on a regular basis? Can you count on it to produce a true picture of your prescribing practice?
- How can you ensure rigour in your audit?

- How can you aim to make audit a dynamic and ongoing process?

FURTHER READING

EVIDENCE BASED PRACTICE

Greenhalgh, T. (1997) How to Read a Paper: The Basis of Evidence Based Medicine, London, BMJ Publishing.

Haynes, R.B., Sackett, D.L., Gray, J.M., Cook, D.J., & Guyatt, G.H. (1996) 'Transferring evidence from research into practice: 1. The role of clinical care research in clinical decisions.' *Evidence Based Medicine*, 1(7): 196–197.

McClarey, M. & Duff, L. (1997) 'Clinical effectiveness and evidence-based practice.' *Nursing Standard*, 52(11): 33–37.

Muir Gray, J.A. (1997) Evidence Based Healthcare: How to Make Health Policy and Management Decisions, London, Churchill Livingstone.

Sackett, D., Rosenberg, W.M., Gray, J.A., Haynes, R.B. & Richardson, W.S. (1996) 'Evidence-based medicine: what it is and what it isn't.' Editorial. *British Medical Journal*, 312(7023): 71–72.

Sackett, D.L., Richardson, W.S., Rosenberg, W. & Haynes, R.B. (1996) Evidence Based Medicine: How to Practice and Teach EBM, London, Churchill Livingstone.

CLINICAL GUIDELINES

Duff, L., Kitson, A., Seers, K. & Humphris, D. (1996) 'Clinical guidelines: an introduction to their development and implementation.' *Journal of Advanced Nursing*, 23: 887–895.

Duff, L., Kelson, M., Marriott, S. et al. (1996) 'Clinical guidelines: involving patients and users of the service.' *Journal of Clinical Effectiveness*, 1(3): 104–112.

Duff, L., Kelson, M., Marriott, S. et al. (1996) 'Involving patients and users of services in quality improvement: what are the benefits?' *Journal of Clinical Effectiveness*, 1(2): 63–67.

Field, M.J. & Lohr, K.N. (1992) Guidelines for Clinical Practice from Development to Use, Washington DC, National Academy Press.

Grimshaw, J., Freemantle, N., Wallace, S. & Russell, I. (1995) 'Developing and implementing clinical practice guidelines.' *Quality In Health Care*, 4(1): 55–64.

Grimshaw, J. & Russell, I. (1993) 'Achieving health gain through clinical guidelines. I: Developing scientifically valid guidelines.' *Quality In Health Care*, 2(4): 243–248.

Grimshaw, J. & Russell, I.T. (1994) 'Achieving health gain through clinical guidelines. II: Ensuring guidelines change medical practice.' *Quality in Health Care*, 3(1): 45–52.

McClarey, M. & Duff, L. (1997) 'Making sense of clinical guidelines.' *Nursing Standard*, 12(1): 34–36.

STANDARD SETTING

Ellis, R. & Whittington, D. (1993) Quality Assurance in Healthcare: handbook, London, Edward Arnold.

Sale, D. (1996) Quality Assurance for Nurses and Other Members of the Health Care Team, 2nd edn, London, Macmillan.

AUDIT AND EVALUATION

Baker, R. & Frazer, R.C. (1995) 'Development of review criteria: linking guidelines and assessment of quality.' *British Medical Journal*, 311: 370–373.

Balogh, R. (1996) 'Exploring the links between audit and the research process.' *Nurse Researcher*, 3: 5–16.

Bowling, A. (1991) Measuring Health. A Review of Quality of Life Measurement Scales, Buckingham, Open University Press.

Bowling, A. (1995) Measuring Disease, Buckingham, Open University Press.

Campbell, R. & Garcia, J. (eds) (1997) The Organization of Maternity Care: A Guide to Evaluation, Hale, Cheshire, Hochland & Hochland.

Cook, P. (1996) 'Audit methodology: time for a rethink?' *Network*, issue 22, pp. 6–8.

Fitzpatrick, R. & Hopkins, A. (eds) (1993) Measurement of Patients' Satisfaction with their Care, London, Royal College of Physicians of London.

Fitzpatrick, R. & Boulton, M. (1994) 'Qualitative methods for assessing health care.' *Quality in Health Care*, 3: 107–113.

Harvey, G. (1996) 'Relating quality assurance and audit to the research process in nursing.' *Nurse Researcher*, 3: 35–46.

Hearnshaw, H., Baker, R., Cooper, A., Eccles, M. & Soper, J. (1996) 'The costs and benefits of asking patients for their opinions about general practice.' *Family Practice*, 13(1): 52–58.

Jenkinson, C. (ed) (1994) Measuring Health and Medical Outcomes, London, UCL Press.

Jenkinson, C. (ed) (1997) Assessment and Evaluation of Health and Medical Care: A Methods Text, Buckingham, Open University Press.

Kelson, M., Redpath, L. (1996) 'Promoting user involvement in clinical audit: surveys of audit committees in primary and secondary care.' *Journal of Clinical Effectiveness*, 1(1): 14–18.

Parsley, K. & Corrigan, P. (1994) Quality Improvement in Nursing and Healthcare: A Practical Approach, London, Chapman and Hall.

Russell, I.T. & Wilson, B.J. (1992) 'Audit: the third clinical science?' *Quality in Health Care*, 1(1): 51–55.
Smith, R. (ed) (1992) Audit in Action, London, *British Medical Journal*.

INFORMATION ON RESEARCH METHODS

There are numerous texts on research methods, which may be useful to consult when undertaking the audit process. Some examples of these are listed below.

GENERAL

Bell J (1993) Doing your Research Project: A Guide for First-time Researchers in Education and Social Science, Buckingham, Open University Press.

Bowling, A. (1997) Research Methods in Health: Investigating Health and Health Services, Buckingham, Open University Press.

Britten, N. (1995) 'Qualitative interviews in medical research.' *British Medical Journal*, 311: 251–253.

Cox, K., Bergen, A. & Normann I.J. (1993) 'Exploring consumer views of care provided by the Macmillan nurse using the critical incident technique.' *Journal of Advanced Nursing*, 18: 408–413.

Field, P.A. & Morse, J.M. (1985) Nursing Research: The Application of Qualitative Approaches, London, Croom Helm.

Jones, J. & Hunter, D. (1995) 'Consensus methods for medical and health services research.' *British Medical Journal*, 311: 376–380.

Keen, J. & Packwood, T. (1995) 'Case study evaluation.' *British Medical Journal*, 311: 444–446.

Lamping, D.L., Rowe, P., Clark, A., Black N. & Lessof, L. (1998) 'Development and validation of the menorrhagia outcome questionnaire' *British Journal of Obstetrics and Gynaecology*, 105: 766–779.

Mann, P.H. (1985) Methods of Social Investigation, 2nd edn, Oxford, Blackwell.

Mays, N. & Pope, C. (1995) 'Observational methods in health care settings.' *British Medical Journal*, 311: 182–184.

Pope, C. & Mays, N. (1995) 'Reaching the parts other methods cannot reach: an introduction to qualitative methods in health and health services research.' *British Medical Journal*, 311: 42–45.

Lofland, J & Lofland L H (1984) Analyzing Social Settings: A Guide to Qualitative Observation and Analysis, 2nd edn, California, Wadsworth.

McIver, S. (1991) An Introduction to Obtaining the Views of Users of Health Services, London, King's Fund Centre.

Moser, C.A. & Kalton, G. (1981) Survey Methods in Social Investigation, 2nd edn, London, Heinemann.

Polit, D.F. & Hungler, B.P. (1985) Essentials of Nursing Research: Methods and Applications, Philadelphia, Lippincott.

STATISTICS AND QUANTITATIVE ANALYSIS

Altman, D.G. (1991) Practical Statistics for Medical Research, London, Chapman and Hall.

Clegg, F. (1992) Simple Statistics: A Course Book for the Social Sciences, Cambridge, Cambridge University Press.

Downie, N.M. & Heath, R.W. (1983) Basic Statistical Methods, 5th edn, New York, Harper and Row.

Kramer, H.C. & Thiemann, S. (1987) How many Subjects? Statistical Power Analysis in Research, Newbury Park, California, Sage.

Marsh, C. (1988) Exploring Data: An Introduction to Data Analysis for Social Scientists, Cambridge, Blackwell.

QUALITATIVE ANALYSIS

Donnan, P. (1996) Quantitative analysis. In: The Research Process in Nursing, ed D. Cormack, Oxford, Blackwell.

Miles, M.B. & Huberman, A.M. (1994) Qualitative Data Analysis: An Expanded Sourcebook, London, Sage.

CROSS-CULTURAL APPROPRIATENESS AND FEASIBILITY OF RESEARCH METHODS

Ahmad, W.I.U., Kernohan, E.E.M. & Baker, M.R. (1989) 'Cross-cultural use of socio-medical indicators with British Asians.' *Health Policy*, 13: 95–102.

Baider, L., Ever-Hadani, P. & Kaplan, A.D. (1995) 'The impact of culture on perceptions of patient-physician satisfaction.' *Israeli Journal of Medical Science*, 31: 179–185.

Chalmers, B. & Meyer, D. (1994) 'What women say about their birth experiences: a cross-cultural study.' *Journal of Psychomatic Obstetrics and Gynecology*, 15: 211–218.

Chen, C., Lee, S.Y. & Stevenson, H.W. (1995) 'Response style and cross-cultural comparisons of rating scales among East Asian and North American students.' Psychological Science, 6(3): 170–175.

Guillemin, F., Bombardier, C. & Beaton, D. (1993) 'Cross-cultural adaptation of health related quality of life measures: literature review and proposed guidelines.' *Journal of Clinical Epidemiology*, 46(12): 1417–1432.

Helman, C.G. (1990) Culture Health and Illness, Oxford, Butterworth Heinmann.

Herdman, M., Fox-Rushby, J. & Badia, X. (1998) 'A model of equivalence in the cultural adaptation of HRQoL instruments: the universalist approach.' *Quality of Life Research*, 7: 323–335.

Hunt, S.M (1998) Cross-cultural issues in the use of quality of life measures in randomizes controlled trials. In: Quality of Life Assessment in Clinical Trials, ed. Staquet, M.J., Hays, R.D. & Fayers, P.M., pp. 51–67, Oxford, Oxford University Press.

Kleinman, A. (1987) 'Anthropology and psychiatry: the role of culture in cross-cultural research on illness.' *British Journal of Psychiatry*, 151: 447–454.

Kitzinger, J. (1995) 'Introducing focus groups.' *British Medical Journal*, 311: 299–302.

Segall, M.H., Dasen, P.R., Berry, J.W. & Poortinga, Y.H. (1990) Human Behaviour In Global Perspective: An Introduction to Cross-Cultural Psychology, Oxford, Pergamon Press.

Smith, P.B. & Bond, M.H. (1993) Social Psychology Across Cultures: Analysis and Perspectives, London, Harvester Wheatsheaf.

Suyono, H., Piet, N., Stirling, F. & Ross, J. (1981) 'Family planing attitudes in urban Indonesia: findings from focus group research.' Studies in Family Planning, 12(12): 433–442.

Yelland, J. & Gifford, S.M. (1995) 'Problems of focus group methods in cross-cultural research: a case study of beliefs about sudden infant death syndrome.' *Australian Journal of Public Health*, 19(3): 257–263.

REFERENCES

Batstone, G. & Edwards, M. (1994) Clinical audit – how do we proceed? *Southampton Medical Journal*, 1, 13–19.

Centre for Reviews and Dissemination (1996) Influenza vaccination and older people. *Effectiveness Matters*, **2(1)**, 1–6.

Cluzeau, F., Littlejohns, P., Grimshaw, J. & Feder, G. (1997) *Appraisal instrument for clinical guidelines. Version 1*. London: St George's Hospital Medical School.

Department of Health (1989) *Working for Patients. The Health Service: Caring for the 1990s*. London, HMSO.

Department of Health (1993) *Clinical Audit – Meeting and Improving Standards in Health Care*, London: Department of Health.

Harvey, G. (1994) *The DySSSy Workbook*. Oxford: Royal College of Nursing.

Lampling, D. & Rowe, B. (1996) *Users' Manual for Purchasers and Providers: survey of women's experience of maternity services*. (Short form.) London, Health Sciences Research Unit, London School of Hygiene and Tropical Medicine.

Morrell, C. (1999) *The Audit Handbook*. London: Baillière Tindall.

13 Nurse prescribing

Can nurses manage it?

Stephen Chapman

Key issues

♦ The need to manage prescribing patterns in the face of patient demand.

♦ The influence of the pharmaceutical industry on prescribing patterns.

♦ The risk of drug cost-shifting to nurse prescriber budgets.

♦ Evidence-based nurse prescribing.

♦ Teamwork and medicines management.

INTRODUCTION
Why do we need medicines management?

Prescribing has been the focus of attention for many of the key stakeholders in the National Health Service, primarily as a result of the steadily increasing costs. Unlike many health activities, medicine costs are visible, easily measured and monitored at practice, health authority, regional and national level. During the financial year April 1996 to March 1997 over £4 billion was spent on drugs in England, of which 85% was primary care prescribing. Prescribing costs continue to increase – the annual rate of increase over the last 5 years was around 8%. The bill for medicines will continue to rise as a consequence of both socio-demographics – an increase in the age of the population will place greater demand on the service for medicines – and the introduction of novel and higher cost medicines (Fig. 13.1).

Many of these newly introduced drugs are new classes of drugs in fields

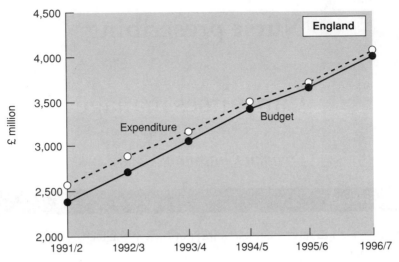

Fig. 13.1 The growing cost of medicines in England (1991–97).

such as cancer and psychotic illness, and some, such as beta interferon for multiple sclerosis and donepezil for Alzheimer's disease, are new drugs for conditions that were previously untreatable with conventional medicines. Other classes of drugs are emerging which are blurring the boundaries between medical and social care – for instance the emerging anti-obesity drugs, and treatments for male impotence. Such drugs raise interesting ethical issues around how much a cash limited, publicly funded service should be investing in, say, the treatment of obesity and how much individual responsibility patients will need to take for lifestyle adjustments.

Thus the management of medicines is more than a simple exercise in controlling costs. It is important to be able to balance the costs and benefits in order to have a clear idea of desirable outcomes and their relevance to the total clinical care of the patient. In order to do so the prescriber needs reference to an increasingly complex and diverse evidence base. It has been estimated that there are about 30 000 biomedical journals, but only about 1% of the articles in these journals are considered to be scientifically sound (Smith, 1991). Published trial findings therefore cannot always be accepted at face value. Given this huge body of evidence and a massive variation in the quality of evidence, it is a considerable task for any prescriber to keep themselves up to date with the gold standards' for prescribing. For the average doctor to keep up to date with the quality peer group reviewed articles, they would need to read about 17 articles a day, every day of the year (Evidence-based Medicine Working Group, 1992). Perhaps, in part due to this information overload, prescribers continue to base their clinical decisions on increasingly out-of-date primary training or the over-interpretation of experiences with individual patients (Haines and Jones, 1994). Even dramatically positive results from rigorous clinical studies remain largely unapplied (Faber, 1993).

Thus prescribing, as the 'end product' of the medicines management process, is the result of a complex decision-making process based on clinical evidence, correct diagnosis, personal ethics and experience, and finally – and probably to a lesser extent – cost. Given the huge challenge in identifying correct evidence alone, it seems sensible that any further delegation of the prescribing role away from those most experienced in it (i.e. in primary care the general practitioners) must be within strictly controlled guidelines and protocols. Ideally this should be accompanied by large tranches of both undergraduate and postgraduate education.

The issue of which profession is most capable of taking on the management of prescribing then becomes one of whose skills are already most closely matched to those required. In this chapter we will explore the issues around prescribing, the influences on prescribers, the tensions between the evidence base and clinical practice, and how this will fit in within the new world we find ourselves in with primary care group commissioning following the changes proposed by the White Paper (NHS Executive, 1998).

THE INFLUENCES ON PRIMARY CARE PRESCRIBING

The factors that influence general practitioners to prescribe a particular medicine, or class of medicines, are extremely diverse and as previously suggested, not always evidence based. It stands to reason therefore that the same influences will be brought to bear on whichever group of healthcare professionals takes over part of that prescribing role from the general practitioner. Indeed it may well be that because they are new to the role and enthusiastic about its potential, they may involuntarily become susceptible to less evidence-based influences. In particular, patient demand rather than patient need, and the subtle overtures of the pharmaceutical industry are likely to provide particular challenges for the new and enthusiastic nurse prescriber.

Patient demand

Following the Audit Commission's first report on prescribing in general practice in England and Wales, in which they estimated that up to £275 million could be saved on the NHS drugs bill if over-prescribing of drugs was reduced (Audit Commission, 1994), prescribers were encouraged to say no to demands from patients. The clear implication of training doctors to decline inappropriate prescriptions was that it was the patients expectations that were partly responsible for the problem (Bradley, 1994). This view, initially articulated by Marinker (1973), was that 'we may see the doctor as helpless in the face of a population of patients who have an overwhelming need to alter chemically their experience of the world in which they live'. However, Britten (1995) argues that the evidence that it is the patients that put pressure on prescribers is at best equivocal. She suggests that pragmatically between 5% and 7% of prescriptions are never dispensed (Bardon et al., 1973) and about a fifth of patients leave general practice consultations with prescriptions they did not expect (Webb and Lloyd, 1994). Britten quotes a series of studies that show inconsistent results, two that show demand had no influence on prescribing (Hepler, Clyne and Donter, 1982; Segal and Hepler, 1982), and five that showed that demand was associated with higher rates of prescribing (Webb and Lloyd, 1994; Hadsell, Freeman and Norwood, 1982; Schwartz, Soumerai and Avorn, 1989; Bradley, 1992; Virji and Britten, 1991).

Britten suggests that some doctors may justify their poor prescribing habits by blaming patients instead of recognising they sometimes misuse prescribing, for example to close a difficult consultation (Britten, 1995). It is imperative therefore that any health care professional taking on the prescribing mantle is aware of the hazards, firstly of too readily acquiescing to patient demand, but perhaps more importantly, not anticipating patient demand and enthusiastically rushing to prescribe. Patient pressure is bound to increase – new drugs continue to be announced in the national press, the recent examples of donepezil, beta interferon and montelukast being such cases. These drugs all enjoyed coverage on the TV, radio and in the national newspapers. The problem with such publicity is that comparisons are rarely made with existing products and the cost consequences of these drugs are often not considered.

Socio-demographics

Socio-demographic factors can account for up to half of the variability in prescribing. Age is a major factor – elderly people receive more prescriptions per head than any other group and Roberts's work suggests the majority of patients over 65 have one or more chronic conditions requiring long-term medication (Roberts and Harris, 1993). The Department of Health's own statistical bulletin showed that in 1995 patients over 65 received an average of 21 prescriptions per head compared with an average of six prescriptions per head for the rest of the population (DoH, 1997). As the quality of life for the elderly increases with improved social and welfare conditions and better and more sophisticated medicines available, the population who are or who will be aged over 65 is increasing, which can be expected to influence prescribing expenditure (CSO, 1995).

The pharmaceutical industry

The pharmaceutical industry over the years has developed sophisticated marketing strategies to enhance the traditional persuasive skills of their medical representatives. The conventional placing of advertisements in medical and professional journals, direct or indirect sponsorship of key consultants, provision of equipment or staff for research units and company sponsored symposia are commonplace. Although many physicians who partake in these activities will doubtless have high personal standards of integrity, it is very difficult for them to dissociate themselves from a sponsoring company, particularly when dealing around issues with specific drugs. Codes of conduct and standards are set by the Association of the British Pharmaceutical Industry (ABPI) to maintain an ethical framework for these promotional activities. However, this code of conduct is not compulsory and the only sanction truly available to the ABPI is expulsion from the ABPI, which, although it may carry some stigma for the company, is unlikely to have a profound commercial effect on the company's products.

Similarly, while the strategic lead of the company may be of the highest ethical standards, there is always the possibility that at the operational level, company employees may be tempted to push the boundaries of the ABPI code of conduct in order to obtain the sales and bonuses which enhance their salaries. The government has expressed their determination to deal with inappropriate gifts from the industry to prescribers and pharmacists and to separate sponsorship from pressure to prescribe. Recently, nurses have increasingly been drawn into the net as the pharmaceutical industry has realised they have the potential to influence general practitioners prescribing decisions, and they are much more readily accessible in general practice than the doctors themselves.

Company employed nurses have been placed in practices in order to case-find in order for doctors to prescribe. Recent examples include nurses case-finding for *H. pylori* eradication therapy, treatment with lipid lowering drugs, or ACE inhibitors for heart failure. Whilst the objective of the exercise is laudable, that is to get maximum health gain by optimal prescribing, care must be taken not to overstep the mark between prescribing the appropriate class of drugs or just prescribing a particular drug which is the product of the company sponsoring the initiative. Prescribing advisers in health authorities have been particularly concerned about the activities of some nurses involved with stoma care where they felt that either company sponsored nurses were guiding patients and prescribers towards particular stoma care products, or that brand loyalty was being generated by marketing techniques such as saving vouchers from stoma care boxes to post off in exchange for items of equipment in the practice. As with all such initiatives, the actions may be well intentioned, but they do carry an inherent degree of moral hazard and nurses partaking in such activity should be aware of the potential for compromising probity.

Nurses employed by practices have also become keenly targeted by medical representatives. This has been particularly apparent in areas where some element of prescribing responsibility has been transferred to the nurse – particularly in chronic disease areas such as the treatment of asthma. There is real benefit to a practice in having a nurse running, say, an asthma clinic to counsel patients on inhaler techniques and appropriate use of their inhalers. However, once the counselling moves onto the next stage and into recommendation of an inhaler device, the prescriber, or the healthcare professional recommending the prescription, be it nurse or general practitioner, needs to be appraised of the evidence base for making that recommendation. The final choice should be arrived at using the appropriate decision-making matrix encompassing clinical effectiveness, sound clinical evidence, ethics and cost.

As was mentioned earlier, prescribing physicians are not always this evidence based. Indeed, although the majority of general practitioners would consider themselves not to be unduly influenced by the activities of the pharmaceutical industry, there is reported evidence that they may be more influenced than they perceive. Avorn's work shows there are multitudinous factors affecting GP prescribing (Schwartz et al., 1989). A fascinating report by Heminki crystallised this dilemma beautifully (Heminki *et al.*, 1975). In this study, doctors were asked to list the things they thought influenced their prescribing; unsurprisingly, the pharmaceutical activities of medical representatives and advertising were towards the bottom of this list. Heminki then asked them to describe key drugs in free text sections at the end of the questionnaire. The majority of the prescribers described the key drugs in the language of the latest drug company advertisements. Thus although they believed themselves not to be influenced, they had inevitably absorbed the message from the pharmaceutical company and tended to perceive drugs in that light. Nurses, or indeed pharmacists, will be no exception to this. The industry will continue to be strategic and focused in its approach; as nurses take on a greater role in prescribing, they can expect to be exposed to the same battery of influences. Thus the importance of having evidence-based protocols to aid prescribing and a thorough understanding of the reasoning behind those protocols becomes paramount.

Hospitals

Up until now the drug budgets for primary and secondary care have come from different treasury votes. Hospital prescribing has been part of the trust budget which is part of the cash limited HCHS (Hospital and Community Health Services) vote. Non-fundholder prescribing has come from a separate, non cash limited treasury vote, although the fundholders are cash limited.

Hospital physicians have been swift to realise they could move the pressure off their cash limited budgets by initiating prescribing in secondary care but then referring the patient on to general practitioners to continue the prescribing. Cost pressures occasionally meant that this was not always the most clinically appropriate way of delivering health care for the patient. It also meant that it propagated a practice of 'loss leading' of drugs into hospital by pharmaceutical companies. There have been many examples of drugs that were made available at discounts to hospitals and which, when referred on to the primary care prescribing, incurred substantive costs for GPs. Hospital pharmacists are increasingly aware of the implications of such practices for the NHS and wherever possible are rejecting such offers in the interests of preserving good relationships with primary care. However, examples still exist of how strong prescribing influences from consultants can lead to peculiarly skewed prescribing patterns in primary care (Price, Heatley and Chapman, 1996). In theory, the unified budget that will arise with the changes in the White Paper will mean that any adverse cost pressures placed on primary care by just cost dumping will now come full circle back to the local hospitals and impinge directly on their budgets. Hopefully therefore, in the future, loss leading will become much less prevalent as hospital physicians have to take account of primary care expenditure to prevent any erosion of their own hospital budget.

EVIDENCE-BASED MEDICINE AND NURSE PRESCRIBERS

The new government has placed the quality of clinical care and outcomes at the heart of its agenda for the NHS. They want to encourage clinicians to prescribe effectively and to challenge ineffective therapies and inefficient prescribing. As nurses take on the prescribing role, these same criteria should be applied to the prescribing they undertake. Currently nurse prescribing is restricted to diagnostic tests, simple analgesia and dressings and wound management – an area in which nurses have traditionally had a significant input.

Wound management and other associated dressings actually now account for £11.5 million worth of expenditure for the West Midlands region, nearly 2% of the total prescribing budget – this is the fifth highest cost for a single group (Prescription Pricing Authority – PPA, 1998). Simple economies can be made even within the area of dressing prescribing. For instance, dressing packs are high cost, high waste items. They are composite packs containing items which are frequently unnecessary given the application technique needed for modern dressings. Reducing the use of dressing packs could save a typical health authority up to £180 000 based on the 1997 annual PACT figures.

The evidence base for dressings is difficult to trawl and is mainly to be found in journals not usually read by practice nurses and health visitors. For instance, a study within a major UK accident and emergency department concluded that tap water was satisfactory as a cleanser for open traumatic wounds (Rayat and Quinton, 1997). There is no evidence for the routine use of any other cleanser than tap water or saline on pressure sores or leg ulcers. If Steripot 20 ml and Sterijet 25 ml were replaced by mains water cleansing, a saving of £357 000 annually would be made within the West Midlands alone. Such evidence will become invaluable, particularly within the cost-constrained environs of the primary care groups. Knowing that such evidence exists and being able to apply it in practice would increase the value of a nurse prescriber to a primary health care team.

Currently, nurse prescribers must have a health visitor or a district nurse qualification and have undergone special training in prescribing, including passing an examination. Their current open learning pack and tuition prior to examination covers many issues including:

- How to prescribe
- Pharmacology and side-effects of the preparations prescribable by nurses
- The drug tariff
- Financial issues
- Ethical issues.

Even with this training and with a relatively restricted Nurse Prescribers' Formulary, there have still been misinterpretations by nurses, pharmacists and even the PPA! Fortunately, this was realised early on in nurse prescribing pilots and the nurse prescribing training course has been amended so more time is spent on the use of the formulary itself. However, there is still a considerable gap in training nurses in the culture of evaluating an evidence base. This raises an interesting point for nurse education and nurse trainers: do we educate nurses and inculcate them with a culture of evaluation of the evidence base for the products they prescribe? Or do we recognise that in many cases this may be too steep a learning curve and instead provide them with sets of guidelines which have themselves been drawn up and validated by the relevant experts in the field? If guidelines and protocols are the way forward, should they be national, regional, health authority or practice based? There is necessarily tension between wanting local ownership of protocols and guidelines and being able to take account of local prescribing policies, and avoiding the necessity of duplicating the evaluation of the evidence many times over across the country.

In the prescribing pilot site in the West Midlands, guidance on prescribing in a number of specific areas such as wound management, incontinence, stoma and skin is being developed. These highlight where similar products exist and where there are cost savings to be made as well as some practical issues concerning the use of specific products. This should enable more cost-effective use of the nurse prescribing budget.

The challenge of prescribing to an evidence base is not unique to nurse prescribers, however. The Audit Commission's report (Audit Commission, 1994) identifies several areas of general practitioner prescribing where changes in accordance with the database could save money with no discernible effect on the patient. For instance, they estimated that nationally £52 million extra was being spent on dry powder inhalers where metered dose inhalers could have been tried first line, £49 million extra was being spent on modified release products, and £28 million on combination drugs that had less costly and equally effective substitutes. Thus the difficulty in assimilating and acting on evidence base is not unique to one professional and is not pejorative to any group of professionals' particular education – none of us would have the time to critically review all the evidence before every prescription. This reinforces the case for guidelines, and strengthens the case for evaluating the evidence once, nationally, and finding an effective way of disseminating the evidence.

The government currently has several initiatives in place and in progress to aid GPs with evidence-based prescribing. The National Institute of Clinical Effectiveness (NICE) will be constituted to provide evidence-based guidelines on key drugs and key areas of prescribing. A computer generated decision support system, PRODIGY, is being piloted to help GPs with evidence-based prescribing. Guidelines are held on the computer, and when GPs key in certain diagnoses they get a 'drop screen'. This screen guides them on appropriate treatment steps, the first, second and third line choice of drug, and also generates, where appropriate, a patient information leaflet to help with the patient consultation. One possible solution to keeping nurse prescribers up to date with evidence-based guidelines may be to provide such an electronic support system. This is likely to be some time off yet as PRODIGY for general practitioners is still some way from full roll out.

Having generated guidelines, in order for them to have credibility they still require a certain degree of local ownership and input. In the West Midlands, we have MTRAC (Midlands Therapeutics Review and Advisory Committee), which is a committee of GPs, chaired by a general practitioner and supported by a team of non voting specialist experts. The specialist team includes a drug information pharmacist, clinical pharmacologist, medical ethicist and health economist. MTRAC is highly regarded by general practitioners and exists to ensure they are supported in their decision making on the safety and appropriateness of using new and sometimes high cost drugs in primary care. General practitioners or professional advisers can request that any drug be reviewed by MTRAC. For each product, a critical appraisal of all the appropriate published evidence is produced which evaluates the findings of these studies and makes a first analysis. A representative local specialist is then given the opportunity to enhance this analysis with their practical experience of the drug. At this stage the committee debates the value of the product, its anticipated safety in primary care, resources available and monitoring requirements. The committee's final recommendation is then sent to all general practitioners in the region. While the committee appreciates the economic issues, its remit is to make decisions on the grounds of clinical evidence and safety within primary care. Such an MTRAC model might well be very useful in the near future in helping nurses develop their prescribing guidelines.

PRIMARY CARE GROUPS: THE CHALLENGES FOR NURSE PRESCRIBERS

Opportunities presented by the White Paper

'The New NHS' White Paper provides six important principles underlining the proposed changes. Of these, at least three will be directly applicable to nurse prescribers:

1. To make the delivery of health care against new national standards a matter of local responsibility. Local doctors and nurses are in the best position to know what patients need and will be in the driving seat in shaping patient services.

2. To get the NHS to work in partnership. By breaking down organisational barriers and forging stronger links with local authorities the needs of the patient will be put at the centre of the care process.

3. To shift the focus onto quality of care so that excellence is guaranteed to all patients and quality becomes the driving force for decision making at every level of the service.

The White Paper goes on to reinforce the principles of a system based on partnership driven by performance with the emphasis on the pursuit of quality and efficiency. Theoretically, traditional professional barriers should be eroded. This presents both opportunities and challenges for nurse prescribers.

The level of responsibility for the overall management of the primary care group and the strategic steer alters significantly as primary care group levels progress from level 1 to level 4 (Fig 13.2). The move to primary care groups represents a very fundamental change for prescribers, be they general practitioners or nurses. It could be considered to be almost the end of Hippocratic decision making; prescribers will no longer have to consider just the patient in front of them, but will also have to consider:

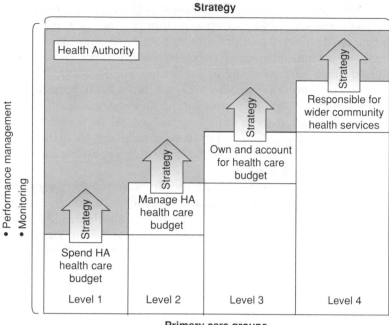

Fig. 13.2   Primary care group/health authority needs.

- The needs of the other patients on their list
- The patients of their partners in the practice
- The patients of the other practices within the primary care group.

The unified budget of the primary care group will place peer group pressure on prescribers within the group; as with any group of professionals, there are bound to be outliers either under- or over-prescribing. It is likely this will also apply to nurse prescribers.

Once the primary care groups develop to level 2 and beyond, the performance management of these outliers will no longer be the responsibility of the health authority, rather that of their peers within the primary care group. This peer group performance management is bound to initially feel uncomfortable both to those being performance managed and those doing the performance managing.

This brings us to the next challenge for primary care groups: how will the management structure be organised and how will the relevant professionals ensure they are properly represented on the management board?

Changing traditional relationships

The nurse's role has achieved increasing importance and significance in the last few years, both in terms of prescribing recommendations and in taking on the prescribing role, but the relationship between the nurse and the doctor has been, with a few exceptions, that of employer and employee. There will need to be a paradigm shift by both parties if nurses are to have an equal and recognised voice on the management board, and an equal and recognised voice on prescribing issues. Unlike fundholding, the practices involved in primary care groups will not have been brought together voluntarily, rather it will be a function of their geographical location. In order to be successful, there are going to have to be sound networking systems and a real willingness by nurse prescribers to work towards a 'corporate agenda' and not let practice loyalties jeopardise the success of the locality group as a whole.

There is, however, a wonderful opportunity to revisit the prescribing role in a creative and open-minded way, and to structure primary care teams to optimise the skills of all the key health professionals. Figure 13.3 shows the traditional primary care roles as they exist at the moment. The doctor still diagnoses and in most cases still prescribes. There is still an element of

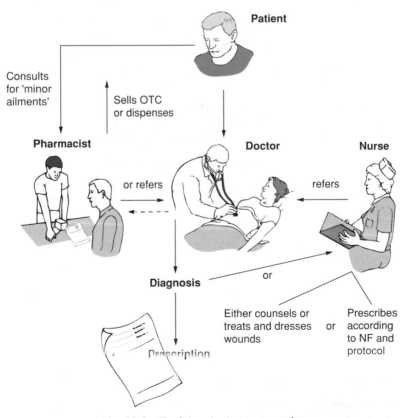

Fig. 13.3 Traditional primary care roles.

referral for specific areas of treatment such as wound dressings or asthma inhaler technique training and in some cases the possibility of nurse prescribing.

The pharmacist is still very much in the supplier role, dispensing the medicine according to either nurse or doctor prescriptions and accompanying this with advice where appropriate. Pharmacists may on occasion refer patients who are repeatedly coming in for minor ailments on to the doctor if they consider a condition to be more serious – for instance repeated and cluster headaches. However, such arrangements are still quite informal and rely on goodwill, mutual trust and cooperation between community pharmacists and their local practice.

Working with pharmacists

New roles can be created within a primary care group for both pharmacists and nurses that should empower both professions to work to their strengths. As the traditional compounding and dispensing roles of pharmacists have become de-skilled, the emphasis has shifted to patient centred advice on medicines. Undergraduate training, and the shift to the new 4-year degree course reflect this need, and place the emphasis firmly on medicines knowledge, literature evaluation and clinical skills. Initiatives such as the Centre for Pharmacy Postgraduate Education (CPPE) continue the same focus by providing voluntary postgraduate education for community pharmacists. The trained clinical pharmacist's drug knowledge is recognised and readily utilised in the hospital environment; pharmacists are included and consulted on consultant ward rounds; they check patient charts and intervene with the consent of the prescriber; in some cases they take responsibility for discharge prescribing.

Within the profession there is some debate as to whether hospital or community pharmacists would be most appropriate for recruitment for practice based work in primary care groups. In fact, both groups would be equally suitable – they just have different training needs. Hospital pharmacists need to be trained in the workings of primary care and the realities of primary care prescribing issues; community pharmacists are already familiar with the general practice population, but they need to get their clinical knowledge up to date. Time alone will tell which turns out to be more appropriate.

Extending the boundaries

Nurses and pharmacists continue to push at their respective professional boundaries. The White Paper encourages them to further break down these artificial barriers. The challenge for both professions, if they want the respect of government and the medical profession, is to do so in the best interests of the patient. It is unrealistic to pretend that there are no potential areas of conflict. Pharmacists believe their drug knowledge best equips them for the delegated prescribing role; nurses believe that their direct patient contact and close working relationships with doctors in general practice makes them the logical choice. Pharmacists believe they are best equipped to advise patients on issues such as asthma inhaler technique; nurses would argue this is best done by them during asthma clinics in the practice.

The advent of the nurse prescribing pilots indicates that nurses have to an extent won the first part of the argument – they can prescribe from a limited formulary. Inevitably they will want to expand the range of medicines they can prescribe; their best chance of achieving this may be to consider the component parts of the prescribing process and work with pharmacists in an enhanced system of medicines management. Equally, the pharmacists should recognise the nurses' skills and move away from practices such as blood pressure measurement in their pharmacies.

The nurse's skills are focused on direct patient contact and a history of caring for and supporting a patient's physical and emotional needs – changing dressings, providing encouragement. The pharmacist, although certainly not uncaring, tends to be more technically focused on the specific attributes of medicines and dressings, and has training in their independent evaluation. Pharmacists can help generate the protocols and guidelines that nurses could work to, and can monitor and give them constructive feedback on how their practice is matching the protocols. Both can discuss the clinical outcomes of their work and refine their guidelines appropriately.

Figure 13.4 illustrates one such idealised model. Receptionists direct patients to either the nurse or the doctor, according to an agreed protocol. The nurse or doctor diagnoses and decides whether to prescribe; if they do prescribe, they recommend a drug by class rather than name and leave the practice based pharmacist to make the final drug choice. Such symbiosis, although utopian, does make a powerful case for further enhancement of the nurse prescriber's role, and frees general practitioners' time for the many challenges facing them with the advent of primary care groups.

QUESTIONS FOR DISCUSSION

* Are nurses able and prepared to accept the responsibilities of medicines management?
* Will nurse prescribing escalate the cost of the NHS drugs bill?
* How will allowing nurses to prescribe contribute to the medicines management process?

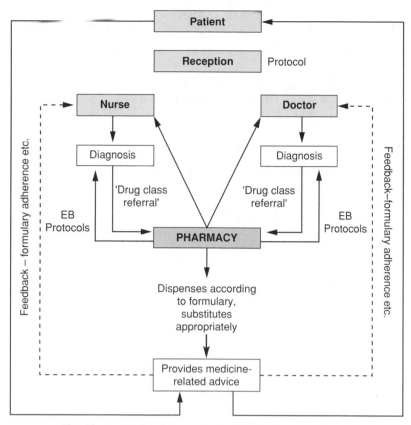

Fig. 13.4   Possible future roles for PCG primary care team.

REFERENCES

Audit Commission (1994) *A Prescription for Improvement: towards more rational prescribing in general practice*. London: HMSO.

Bardon, P.H.G., McGilchrist, M.M., McKendrick, A.D., McDevitt, D.G. & MacDonald, T.M. (1973) Primary care non-compliance of prescribed medication in primary care. *British Medical Journal*, **307**, 846–848.

Bradley, C. (1994) Learning to say 'no': an exercise in learning to decline inappropriate prescription requests. *Education for General Practice*, **5**, 112–119.

Bradley, C.P. (1992) Uncomfortable prescribing decisions: a critical incidence study. *British Medical Journal*, **304**, 294–296.

Britten, N. (1995) Patients' demands for prescriptions in primary care. *British Medical Journal*, **310**, 1084–1085.

Central Statistical Office (1995) *Social Trends*. London: HMSO.

Department of Health (1997) Statistics of prescriptions dispensed in the community: England 1986–1996. *Statistical Bulletin*, **15**, 1–37.

Evidence-Based Medicine Working Group (1992) Evidence-based medicine. A new approach to the teaching of medicine. *Journal of the American Medical Association*, **268**, 2420–2425.

Faber, R.G. (1993) Information overload. *British Medical Journal*, **307**, 383.

Hadsell, R.S., Freeman, R.A. & Norwood J.G. (1982) Factors related to the prescribing of selected psychotropic drug by primary care physicians. *Social Science and Medicine*, **16**, 1747–1756.

Haines, A. & Jones, R. (1994) Implementing findings of research. *British Medical Journal*, **308**, 1488–1492.

Heminki, F. *et al.* (1975) *Social Science and Medicine*, **9**, 111–115.

Hepler, C.D., Clyne, K. & Dunter, S.T. (1982) Rationale as expressed by empiric antibiotic prescribers. *American Journal of Hospital Pharmacy*, **39**, 1647–1655.

Marinker, M. (1973) The doctor's role in prescribing. *Journal of the Royal College of General Practitioners*, **23(Suppl.2)**, 26–29.

NHS Executive (1998) *The New NHS: modern and dependable*. London: NHS Executive.

Prescription Pricing Authority (1998) PACT data 1998.

Price, A.J., Heatley, H.F. & Chapman, S.R. (1996) Buccalling under the pressure: do secondary care establishments influence primary care prescribing? *British Medical Journal*, **313**, 1621–1624.

Rayat, M.S. & Quinton, D.N. (1997) Tap water as a wound cleansing agent in accident and emergency. *Journal of Accident and Emergency Medicine*, **14**, 165–166.

Roberts, S.J. & Harris, C.M. (1993) Age, sex and temporary residents' originated prescribing units (ASTRO PUs): new weightings for analysing prescribing of general practices in England. *British Medical Journal*, **307**, 485–488.

Schwartz, R.K., Soumeraim S.B. & Avorn, J. (1989) Physician motivations for non-scientific drug prescribing. *Social Science and Medicine*, **28(6)**, 577–582.

Segal, R. & Hepler, C.D. (1982) Prescribers beliefs and values as predictors of drug choices. *American Journal of Hospital Pharmacy*, **39**, 1891–1897.

Smith, R. (1991) Where is the wisdom? The poverty of medical evidence. *British Medical Journal*, **303**, 798–799.

Virji, A. & Britten, N. (1991) A study of the relationship between patients attitudes and doctors prescribing. *Family Practice*, **8**, 3014–3019.

Webb, S. & Lloyd, M. (1994) Prescribing and referral in general practice: a study of patients expectations and doctors actions. *British Journal of General Practice*, **44**, 165–169.

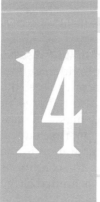

14 Nurse prescribing

Lessons from America

Jan Towers

Key issues

♦ An overview of the development of nurse prescribing in the USA.

♦ Lobbying tactics used to promote nurse prescribing.

♦ Nurse prescribing and level of practice – advanced practice nursing/the nurse practitioner role.

♦ Educational programmes for nurse prescribing.

♦ Nurse prescribing as a key asset in improving patient care.

INTRODUCTION

The expanded role of the professional nurse now known as the nurse practitioner in the USA had its roots in two areas of health care need in the 1960s. One of these was the lack of preventive and primary care in under-served populations and the other was a perceived shortage of physicians in the country at that time. Early nurse practitioner programmes were sanctioned more by the medical community, who initially prepared these providers, than by the nursing community, who felt that nurses who chose to expand their role in this way were abandoning nursing and stepping back into a role of dependency within the traditional medical domain.

As a result, many programmes preparing nurse practitioners were initiated in a variety of settings such as hospitals, medical schools and family planning agencies, with a limited number established in traditional professional schools of nursing. The first highly recognised nurse practitioner was Loretta Ford, who along with Mark Silver, a paediatrician, established a paediatric nurse practitioner programme in Colorado in the early 1960s. Her priorities were to prepare nurses to expand their role to meet the needs of children in the area of health promotion and disease prevention. This required the preparation of nurses to provide services within primary care settings. While primary care encompasses the activities of health promotion and disease prevention, it also requires an ability to conduct comprehensive health assessments, make clinical diagnoses and prescribe treatments, many of which are pharmaceutical preparations. This meant that nurses needed advanced preparation in the areas of clinical diagnosis and prescribing of medications for conditions seen in the primary care setting. Initially this preparation was limited to the primary care of children, but as the role began to be exended to other specialties, the need for preparation in the primary care of adults grew, first in women's health and later in family practice, adult internal medicine and gerontology.

EDUCATION

Creating education programmes to prepare for prescribing

While nurses were well grounded in pharmaceutical knowledge, the need for increased clinical diagnostic skills and an understanding of drug selection based on clinical diagnoses became evident. Programmes were initiated that built on the nurses' basic knowledge of anatomy, physiology, pathophysiology and pharmacology. Initially, the emphasis was placed on diagnosing and managing common acute episodic conditions such as infections, and managing stable chronic diseases such as hypertension and diabetes. However, it soon became clear that patients walking into primary care settings were not limited to these disorders and that nurse practitioners needed to be prepared to recognise and treat a much broader scope of conditions. Programmes expanded to provide nurses with additional knowledge and skill in the area of clinical diagnosis and treatment. They were subsequently constructed to include multiple didactic courses that included pathophysiology, pharmacology, physical diagnosis and clinical decision making, in addition to courses in the clinical management of primary care illnesses for the populations encompassed in their specialty. Such courses included extensive clinical practicums where nurse practitioner students gained 'hands on' experience in diagnosing and managing all problems seen in primary care settings. The end result was – and is – a combination of health promotion, disease prevention and management skills achieved in professional nursing education and physical assessment, clinical diagnostic and pharmalogical and nonpharmacologic management skills learnt in the nurse practitioner graduate education programme.

As the role of the nurse practitioner became established and successful, the federal government saw that preparing nurse practitioners might alleviate the shortages of medical providers in primary care. Such preparation would be more cost-effective than preparing physicians, and would provide primary care to patients in a more efficient manner. As a result, discretionary funds were allotted by Congress for the preparation of nurse practitioners. This funding was overseen by the division of nursing in the health resources services administration of the Department of Health and Human Services of the federal government. Legitimising the role in this manner drew mainstream graduate nurse education programmes into the business of preparing nurse practitioners. In addition, it facilitated the standardisation of educational programmes preparing nurse practitioners and changed the direction of oversight from the medical profession to the nursing profession.

THE LAW

Legalising prescriptive authority in the USA

Initially the role of the nurse practitioner focused on increased skill in recognising disease states. Prescribing was delegated by physicians through formularies similar to standing orders. Such methods had traditionally been utilised to delegate certain treatment decisions to nurses providing care to patients in acute care institutions or long term care facilities. As the role developed, the need to protect the authority of the nurse practitioner to participate in defined expanded activities under law became evident, and steps began to be taken to carry this out.

In the USA, all health care professionals practice under state statute and regulation. Each state has its own Medical Practice Act, Nurse Practice Act and Pharmacy Act, all of which have some oversight regarding the provision of medical care in the state. While these acts are similar, none are exactly alike, so that altering statute and regulation to allow nurse practitioners to function in their advanced role required amending the laws in each state, based on the way the statutes were originally written in that state. Not all states recognised nurse practitioners initially. In fact, one state, Illinois, continues to provide no title protection to nurse practitioners. (See map of prescriptive authorities in Fig. 14.1.)

Initially, in those states where nurse practitioners began to be prepared and function, statutes were altered to allow nurse practitioners to prescribe medications under rules and regulations, generally promulgated by both the Boards of Medicine and the Boards of Nursing. The first rules and regulations limited prescribing to physician delegation or to prescriptive power under the signature of the physician. Later, in one or two states, over-the-counter drugs and a limited number of prescriptive drugs were placed on a formulary that could be prescribed by nurse practitioners

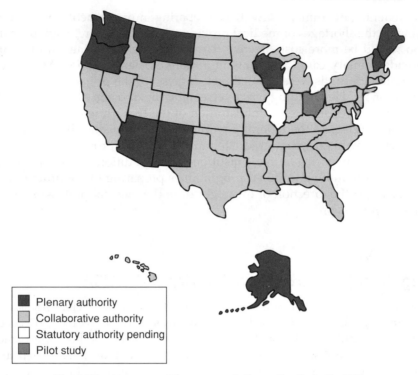

Fig. 14.1 Nurse practitioner prescriptive authority in the USA.

under their own signatures. As nurse practitioners began to increase activity in the states, statutes and regulations were altered to allow nurse practitioners to prescribe a broader array of drugs under their own signature.

The first regulations were written utilising statewide formularies; then states began to allow for more flexibility in nurse practitioner prescribing activities by creating 'negative formularies' (creating a list of drugs the nurse practitioner was *not* allowed to prescribe). Generally these regulations allowed a nurse practitioner and a supervising physician (later this became a collaborating physician) to create their own formulary or protocols for use in the nurse practitioner's practice. In some states these were submitted to the Boards of Nursing or Medicine or both for approval. Sometimes this approval process was delegated to a committee comprising representatives from both boards and occasionally from the Board of Pharmacy. The makeup of those committees greatly influenced the extent to which nurse practitioners were allowed to prescribe within that state. As new states changed their statutes and regulations, statewide formularies were abandoned and replaced by the requirements for written agreements between physicians and nurse practitioners outlining the prescriptive activities of the nurse practitioner. In some states these were submitted to one or more of the boards or their designated committees for approval. In others they were required to be kept in the files of the practice for review if so requested. In a number of rural states, statutes were changed to allow nurse practitioners to prescribe solely by virtue of their own licenses based on educational preparation and in some cases national certification. They made no requirements for protocols or written agreements to be established with physicians in order to prescribe drugs in that state.

As was stated, initially, nurse practitioners were permitted only to prescribe over-the-counter medications, certain antibiotics and oral contraceptives. As their skill became recognised, these limitations have been expanded to nearly all legend drugs and subsequently to controlled substances (narcotics). Currently, nurse practitioners are able to prescribe legend drugs under their own name in 45 states and in the District of Columbia. They have plenary authority in 10 states and are able to prescribe controlled substances in 32 states. Many states that have had very limiting statutes and regulations have, more recently, made statutory or regulatory amendments that further liberalise the nurse practitioner's ability to prescribe. Although attempts have been made by certain elements of the medical community to stop this forward movement, or to reinstate restrictions on nurse practitioner prescribing authority, they have not been successful.

Changing statutes and regulations

The statutory and regulatory authority for nurse practitioners to prescribe in the USA was not conferred solely by independent and insightful leaders in state government. The proactive activity of nurse practitioners who organised and campaigned for statutory title recognition and authorisation that legalised their prescriptive authority was crucial to the passage of legislation and regulation that legitimised and supported their prescribing activities. Armed with research outcomes that proved their safety, nurse practitioners began meeting with regulators and subsequently legislators to initiate statutory changes that supported the activities nurse practitioners were successfully undertaking in the provision of primary care.

Initially members of Boards of Nursing and Medicine were approached by nurse practitioners in each state to negotiate the regulatory changes that would be necessary to protect nurse practitioner prescribing activities in the state. In most states, it was discovered that statutory changes would need to be made in order to authorise the promulgation of regulations for nurse practitioners, since most Nurse Practice Acts had either prohibitory language or no language supporting the independent prescribing of medication without a physician's order. To do so in some states would have been construed as practising medicine without a license. Statutory change required state legislatures to pass new legislation or amend Nurse Practice Acts, Medical Practice Acts and, in some instances, Pharmacy Acts in the state, in order to give nurse practitioners prescriptive authority.

Most state legislatures are designed in a fashion similar to the United States Congress, that is a two party legislature made up of a larger House of Representatives and a smaller Senate. A few states have a one chamber legislature, but these are clearly in the minority. In order for laws to be changed in the state, new legislation or amendments to existing statutes must be introduced by a legislator or group of legislators into the House or the Senate or both in the state legislature. Once introduced, the legislation is referred to a committee or committees of jurisdiction for consideration. Since the chairs of those committees control the agenda for the committee, it is important to have the support of the chair of the committee in order for it to be approved by the committee to be presented to the floor of its particular legislative chamber (House or Senate). The chairs of the committees are always members of the majority party in the House or the Senate, therefore it is also very important to have the support of the legislators (particularly on the committees of jurisdiction) who are members of the majority party in each chamber. The same party may not be the majority party in both chambers.

Once legislation is voted out of committee it can be brought to the floor of its legislative chamber for a vote. Such legislation can itself be amended at any time in committee and on the chamber floor by a majority vote of the committee or the chamber. After the legislation is approved in one chamber it must be sent to the other chamber, where it is again referred to a committee or committees of jurisdiction for approval before being taken to the floor of the chamber for its vote. The factors influencing the original committee and chamber also influence this chamber, which may or may not be led by the same majority party.

Sometimes Bills are introduced in both chambers simultaneously (called Companion Bills). In this case, once the Bills are voted upon in each of the chambers, they are referred to a conference committee made up of leadership from both chambers to work out compromise language suitable to both. This new language is taken back to the two chambers for a final approval before being sent to the governor of the state for signature, making the Bill law. The governor may or may not be a member of the majority party of either or both the House and the Senate of the state.

In some states the legislatures meet for only a small portion of the year, or only once in 2 years. This limits the windows of opportunity for change within that state and requires well thought-out strategic planning to implement desired legislation in reasonable time frames.

Once new legislation is passed or current law is amended, then regulations guided by the stipulations of the passed legislation can be written by the designated entities (preferably the Board of Nursing). In most states such regulations are also subject to some kind of legislative approval, whether it be a committee of a particular chamber or the full membership of a given chamber of the state legislative body.

This obviously is a very slow and tedious process, which becomes slower and more tedious if there is opposition to the proposed legislation. Passage of legislation such as that required for nurse practitioner prescriptive authority could not take place without intense advocacy and dedicated proactive activity on the part of the parties involved (i.e. nurse practitioners). Tenacity has perhaps been the characteristic most likely to help nurse practitioners achieve their goals for title recognition and prescriptive authority in the USA.

NURSE PRACTITIONER ACTIVISM
Influencing legislators

In order to initiate statutory changes in the states, nurse practitioners and organisations representing nurse practitioners began by meeting together to determine goals and develop strategies for making statutory changes in their states. In most states sympathetic legislators were identified to serve as mentors or, if members of the majority party of committees of jurisdiction, as sponsors of the proposed legislation. The statutory goals were shared and where possible nurse practitioners participated in the development of the language of the new legislation or the statutory change.

The first step to find and bring legislators into an arena of support for prescriptive authority for nurse practitioners was to educate them about nurse practitioners and their role. In many states regular legislative days were organised; nurse practitioners made appointments with their representatives and senators and visited them as constituents, explaining the need and educating the legislators about themselves and their practices. In others legislators were visited in their home districts by their nurse practitioner constituents.

Initially, few legislators knew much about nurse practitioners. They attributed prescribing to the practice of medicine and did not understand why nurse practitioners needed statutory authorisation to carry out their role. While title recognition was not as big a problem, because of changes in reimbursement laws at the federal level the need for prescriptive authority was often a hard message to impart to the legislators.

Occasionally there would be a legislator who was also a nurse, who would mentor and facilitate, if not initiate legislation on behalf of nurse practitioners in the state. In a number of states legislators who were physicians would also mentor; however, the converse was sometimes likely to be true. Nurse practitioners discovered in this process that often legislators were not convinced with one visit, but that as they continued to meet and talk, they would begin to see the need and the worth and begin to be responsive to requests for support, even agreeing to co-sponsor, if not be the primary sponsor of a Bill on their behalf.

Fact sheets and brochures, comprehensive and long enough to cover the subject but short enough to guarantee that they would be read, were developed. The fact sheets stated the issues and made statements quoting national and state figures about the number, qualifications and effectiveness of nurse practitioners and the results of research regarding the skills and acceptance of nurse practitioners in practice. Professional Scope of Practice statements (see Figs. 14.2a, 14.2b) were distributed to legislators and their staffs.

Scope of practice for nurse practitioners
(Academy of Nurse Practitioners, 1993)

PROFESSIONAL ROLE

Nurse practitioners are primary health care providers. As advanced practice nurses they provide nursing and medical services to individuals, families and groups, emphasizing health promotion and disease prevention, as well as the diagnosis and management of acute and chronic diseases. Services include but are not limited to ordering, conducting and interpreting appropriate diagnostic and laboratory tests, prescription of pharmacologic agents and treatments and non-pharmacologic therapies. Teaching and counseling individuals, families and groups are a major part of nurse practitioners' activities.

Nurse practitioners work autonomously as well as in collaboration with a variety of individuals to diagnose and manage clients' health care problems. They serve as health care resources, interdisciplinary consultants and patient advocates.

EDUCATION

Educational preparation is defined by guidelines established by the profession to assure appropriate knowledge and clinical competency necessary for the delivery of primary health care. This is accomplished through a program of formal advanced education encompassing both knowledge and clinical practice. The importance of self-direct continued learning and professional development beyond the formal advanced education is emphasized.

ACCOUNTABILITY

The autonomous nature of advanced clinical practice of nurse practitioners requires accountability for outcomes in health care. Insuring the highest quality of care requires certification, periodic peer review, clinical outcome evaluations, a code for ethical practice, evidence of continuing professional development and maintenance of clinical skills. Nurse practitioners are committed to seeking and sharing knowledge that will promote quality health care and improve clinical outcomes by conducting research or applying the research findings of others.

RESPONSIBILITY

The role of the nurse practitioner continues to evolve in response to changing societal and health care needs. As leaders in primary health care, nurse practitioners combine the roles of provider, mentor, educator, researcher and administrator. Members of the profession are responsible for advancing the role of the nurse practitioner as well as ensuring that the standards of the profession are maintained. This may be done through involvement in professional organizations and through participation in health policy activities at the local, state, national and international levels.

Have you talked with your legislator recently?

If you have not yet spoken with your federal legislators about nurse practitioners (NPs), now is the time to do so. This November, every member of the House of Representatives and one third of the members of the Senate are up for reelection. As a result, legislators will be more sensitive to the wishes and needs of their constituents during the next few months.

If you have never talked with your legislator, you will want to make an appointment the next time he or she comes home. Most legislators have offices in a centrally located town in their districts or, in the case of senators, in the capital and in the larger metropolitan areas of the states they represent. A call to 'Telephone Information' in those locations should help you to locate their offices and local phone numbers. If you have difficulty finding them, the League of Women Voters or your local Republican and Democratic headquarters should have the information you need. If you have visited your legislator, let them know that you have spoken before, that you appreciated the assistance you had received, and that you would like to talk again. If you had a previous successful interaction the legislator may remember you with pleasure and will want to meet with you again.

If possible, when visiting your congressperson, take a group of NPs with you. Be sure to let the staff know that you are a constituent. Legislators are elected to represent the people in their electoral district in government. As a result, they are particularly interested in the concerns of the population responsible for putting them in office.

TALKING WITH YOUR LEGISLATOR

When you speak with your legislators, what should you talk about? First introduce yourself and tell briefly what you do. Ask if they are familiar with NPs. If there is hesitation, or you are told, 'Well my wife's sister is a nurse,' then you know you need to educate. Discuss what NPs are and what they do. Describe a typical day to them. It is often useful to give them brochures such as the *Nurse Practitioner*[1] to examine after you leave. Describe the patients or clients you serve and why they need you. Invite them to your practice to see you in action.

If you are discussing third-party reimbursement, you need to be frank about the medical activities NPs undertake. Conclude by discussing the specific issues needing the legislators help. Ask for assistance and advice. Follow up with a letter of thanks for taking time to speak with you. In that letter, you can restate the issues you discussed. Let the legislator know that you will be in contact with his or her office in a few weeks, in case more information or help is needed.

CONTENT OF DISCUSSION

If you are discussing specific legislation, limit yourself to one or two bills. Frame your issue in the light of larger issues of concern in the area of health and health care so that your legislator will see the importance of your concern. They are especially concerned about access to care, particularly primary care, and guaranteeing quality health care in cost-effective ways to the medically underserved. If your issue relates to these concerns, you will have their ear.

Tell them about the bills in which you are interested. Bill numbers are useful to help staff identify and locate the pieces of legislation you are discussing. However, don't be afraid to discuss pending legislation without bill numbers, if they are not available. If you wish specific support such as becoming a cosponsor of the bill, tell the staff and ask them to contact the legislator who introduced the bill to 'sign on' as a cosponsor. Your postvisit thank-you letter should reiterate your request for assistance. A follow-up call a few weeks later to see if any action has taken place is appropriate. Let the staff know that you will be doing this, so they will be prepared for your call.

---

[1]American Academy of Nurse Practitioners, Capitol Station, LBJ Bldg., P.O. Box 12846, Austin, TX 17811.

It is important to realize that you don't need to be an expert to discuss the legislation with your legislators. If you don't know the answer to questions, inform them that you will try to find the answer or have someone with the answer get in touch. Call resources such as the Academy to obtain answers or assistance.

If you are unable to obtain an appointment with your legislators, visits with staff members who have the ear of your legislators are appropriate. Your approach should be the same. Find out how familiar they are with NPs and what NPs do. Educate the uninformed and offer to supply them with additional information and materials if they are needed. Such resources are available through the Academy. Discuss your issue in the context of the larger issues with which the legislator is concerned and follow-up as previously described.

WRITING LETTERS

In addition to visiting your legislators in their home offices, writing letters to their Washington offices regarding specific issues is important. Letters should be addressed as follows:

The Honorable (name of senator)
United States Senate
Washington, DC 20510

Dear Senator (last name of senator)

or

The Honorable (name of representative)
United States House of Representatives
Washington, DC 20515

Dear Mr./Ms. (name of representative)

Letters do not need to be long, but they should be in your own words. Form letters are not as well received as those that are individualized. Briefly state your issue, ask for support and, if possible, address some good reasons why your legislator should support you. The statement of your issue should appear early in the letter. The action you desire your legislator to take should be clearly stated. Ask for a specific reply to your request, offer help if further information is needed, and thank them for their assistance.

TELEPHONE CALLS

Although person-to-person contact with legislators or their staffs produces the best results, telephone conversations can be productive. They are particularly helpful when legislative votes are pending in committee or on the floor of the House or the Senate, or when you are paving the way for a professional representative in Washington to make contact with specific legislators or staff.

When you call, ask for the legislator's 'Health LA (legislative assistant).' Sometimes there is more than one; in that case, briefly describe your issue to the receptionist. If that individual is not available, leave a message for your call to be returned and obtain the name of the person with whom you should be speaking. If your call is not returned in a reasonable length of time, call again. (Reasonable should be measured by the urgency of the issue, i.e., if you are calling to ask for support of a vote pending that day, calling back the same day is not unreasonable. However, if you are calling to discuss an issue and to educate, a few days wait is not unreasonable.) You want to be able to speak with the person when they have time to really hear what you have to say.

It is important to be professional and courteous during these calls regardless of how the legislative representative behaves on the phone. Abruptness or curtness on their part often has more to do with stresses 'on the hill' than with the issue you are discussing. When initiating the conversation, again, introduce yourself and identify your issue. If your agenda is not urgent, tell them you would like to talk with them for a few minutes and offer to set another time for the call if they sound harried or abrupt. Calls should be followed by a letter thanking the LA for spending time with you and reiterating the issues you discussed. File the name of the Health LA in a safe place so that you will know who to contact in the future regarding NP issues.

CONCLUSION

Generally, legislators and their staffs are very interested in hearing and gathering information from constituents, particularly when they provide answers to dilemmas they are facing in the legislative arena. Nurse practitioners have those answers, but they need to be communicated. So don't hesitate to make those contacts. After all, you are the expert when it comes to your patients and practice and their needs. Then, let us know how it turned out.

Jan Towers, PhD, RN, C, CRNP
Carole Jennings, PhD, RN
American Academy of Nurse Practitioners
Washington, DC

Fig. 14.2a, 14.2b (a) Scope of practice for nurse practitioners (American Academy of Nurse Practitioners, 1993) (b) Suggestions for discussing legislation with your legislators (Towers and Jennings, 1992).

Many legislators were invited to visit nurse practitioners in their practice to see what they did and to meet the patients who came to them for care. Such activity contributed significantly to legislator support.

In addition to meeting directly with their legislators, meetings were also arranged with legislative staff, educating them and keeping them informed of nurse practitioner issues. It was soon found that supportive staff had the ear of the legislators and would often see to it that nurse practitioner issues were kept on the table when necessary in the presence of the many other demands of the state legislative agenda.

Once significant interest had been raised, an appropriate sponsor or co-sponsors for a Bill were found, a final draft of the Bill would be agreed upon and the Bill introduced. Depending on how much committee support was present, the Bill moved on through committee and to the chamber floor for a vote. Again depending on how much support there was among chamber leadership, the Bill would be brought to the floor of the chamber for a vote, passed and sent to the other chamber of the legislature for consideration.

In most cases Bills had to be introduced in more than one legislative session before enough momentum could be engendered to attain passage of the Bill in one chamber, let alone two. Nurse practitioners learnt early that it was important to educate legislators in both chambers of the legislature about nurse practitioners, even if the Bill was introduced in only one chamber. It was not always easy to predict how fast a Bill would move, and if it did move quickly in one chamber and nurse practitioners had not prepared members of the other chamber about the issues and did not have support for the legislation already established in the second chamber, the Bill could die before it could be passed.

In addition, nurse practitioners learnt that it was important to continue meeting with legislators and their staffs to keep proposed legislation in the forefront and moving. The busy agendas of very short legislative session could allow an issue of importance to nurse practitioners to be over-shadowed by major political and/or economic issues affecting the state. Likewise, if there was opposition to the legislation, individuals and groups participating in the opposition would also be meeting with legislators to have the proposed legislation defeated or amended more to their liking. It was important for nurse practitioners and their representatives to be aware of the agendas of opposing forces and to continue to meet with legislators regarding the issue.

In a number of states nurse practitioners and organisations representing nurse practitioners hired professional lobbyists to assist with the passage of their legislation. While such action generally proved to be helpful, it was found that lobbyists needed to be chosen carefully to assure appropriate and knowledgeable representation of the position of nurse practitioners. In addition, it was found that lobbyists alone cannot accomplish passage of legislation of this nature. If nurse practitioner constituents did not continue to keep the issue before the legislators, the lobbyists would face a losing battle in the attempts to get their legislation passed. The most successful lobbyists have been those who informed themselves thoroughly about the issues, who met with nurse practitioners regularly and involved them in their lobbying activities surrounding prescriptive authority for nurse practitioners.

Utilisation of nurse practitioner allies helped in many states. Organ-isations representing rural health, certain patient constituencies such as organisations for the elderly, children and certain aspects of health care assisted by expressing their support for the nurse practitioner legislation. Likewise in many states, patients of nurse practitioners were able to convince legislators of the worth of the proposed legislation, not just by seeing them in clinic visits, but also by writing letters and placing calls in support of the proposed legislation for nurse practitioners.

Dealing with the opposition

Unfortunately, as worthy as such legislation is, nurse practitioners did have to deal with opposition to passage of statutory changes that would give them the authority to prescribe medications for their patients. While many physicians and nurses supported nurse practitioners and the authority to prescribe medications, others did not. Most opposition came from organ-ised professional groups representing medicine and, in a few instances, pharmacy.

Often ground was gained by meeting with representatives of these groups and working out language that would satisfy the needs of all groups, while still allowing nurse practitioners to have authority to prescribe in the state, hence the variety of collaborative arrangements and initially the limitations on drugs that could be prescribed by nurse practitioners. In some instances, proposed legislation was amended in committee or on the chamber floor so as to limit nurse practitioners' ability to function, even though prescriptions could be written. In those cases the Bills often were pulled at the request of the nurse practitioners and the groups representing them. In most instances, the Bills were again introduced in the next legislative session after nurse practitioners had had an opportunity to meet and discuss the issues with their legislators and their staffs. Often a reconfiguration of legislators or committee members would be enough to keep such negative movements from happening again. At other times continuing to educate legislators helped. Sometimes it would take several legislative sessions before appropriate legislation would finally be passed out of committee and both chambers in a way that was not harmful to nurse practitioner practice.

Occasionally other members of the nursing profession would not be supportive of one segment of the profession moving forward in the area of prescriptive authority without other segments. Such attitudes could effectively sabotage the forward movement of legislation because it appeared that the nursing community could not agree about which nurses, if any, should be able to prescribe medications. States where successes were most easily attained were those where the nursing community supported nurse practitioner prescriptive authority, even though most of them would not also be able to prescribe.

It has been pointed out that most legislators either know or are related to at least one nurse; what more powerful influence could be desired than that? The number of voters represented by the nursing community is quite high in most communities, and it was soon found that nurses, if they worked together, could have a strong impact.

It's not over until the governor signs the Bill into law (Fig. 14.3)

Once legislation is passed though both the House and the Senate of the state legislature, it is sent to the governor for signature into state law. Occasionally, a governor has refused to sign such legislation, either because of personal conviction or as a result of outside lobbying efforts by opposing groups. While this has happened only infrequently, it has pointed out to nurse practitioners the need to educate and stay in communication with members of the executive branch as well as the legislative branch of the state government.

Having the governor on the side of nurse practitioners, has helped with the passage of legislation in some states. Often legislators will support legislation endorsed by the governor, particularly if they are members of

Legislative Process

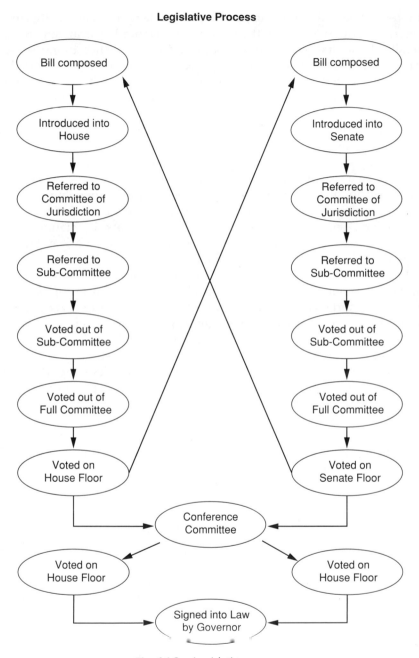

Fig. 14.3 Legislative process.

the same political party. Such support can contribute significantly to passage of legislation such as this. Thus it was important for nurse practitioners to meet with representatives of the governor, if not with the governor, to educate, discuss needs and issues of concern regarding prescriptive authority in the state. If the governor was supportive, having the legislation signed in a press conference where nurse practitioners could be present to thank him and to publicise the event had far reaching endorsing effects.

Influencing the development of regulation

Once statutory changes have been made to authorise the development of regulations for nurse practitioners, regulatory bodies then proceeded to develop regulations to facilitate the authorisation of nurse practitioners to prescribe in the state. In most states advisory committees of nurse practitioners were created and utilised by the regulating bodies, most of which are Boards of Nursing whose members are appointed by the governors of the state for an established period of time. The majority of the members of the Board of Nursing are registered nurses. Their role is to protect the public by regulating the profession of nursing. This is done through the establishment of educational and testing requirements, practice parameters and disciplinary procedures and actions for nurses practicing in their state.

In the early days, Boards of Nursing did not always understand, and sometimes did not accept the role of the nurse practitioner. In those cases, just as with the legislators, it was important for nurse practitioners to meet with members of the boards and their staffs to educate them about nurse practitioners and their roles, so that appropriate regulations could be drawn up for title recognition and prescriptive authority for nurse practitioners. Again the provision of documents, fact sheets and research outcomes was helpful in updating members of these boards regarding the practice of nurse practitioners.

In some instances nurse practitioners were appointed to Boards of Nursing; this provided an avenue of direct input into the actions of the board. In others the actions of the advisory committees were important in assisting the board with its development of regulation. In both instances, and even more importantly in the absence of such direct input into the boards' deliberations, it was important for nurse practitioners to attend all public sessions of the board to monitor its activities and to request opportunities to address the board in public comment sessions, as well as meet with them to discuss the development of regulations regarding nurse practitioner prescriptive authority.

In cases where regulations had to be approved by an identified legislative body it often became necessary for nurse practitioners to meet with legislators and their staffs again to educate them regarding the role and

activities of nurse practitioners as well as the regulatory needs in authorising prescriptive authority. Provision of documentation regarding the role
and activities of nurse practitioners was again necessary in these instances.

Where more than one board (usually the State Board of Nursing and the
State Board of Medicine) or an interdisciplinary committee was appointed
or assigned the task of developing regulations for nurse practitioner prescriptive authority, it became important for nurse practitioners to stay
visible and to work with the members of those boards and/or inter-
disciplinary committees regarding the development of those regulations.
This again necessitated monitoring all public meetings and requesting
opportunities to meet with the boards or committee regarding the regulatory issues.

AFTER 35 YEARS

As one looks back over the last 35 years, it is clear that nurse practitioners
have succeeded in successfully undertaking a very formidable task. While
the needs of patients and the skills of nurse practitioners have certainly
driven the worth of nurse practitioners to its present status, the activities
undertaken by the nurse practitioner community and its allies to assure
title recognition, the ability to practice and the authority to prescribe have
clearly guaranteed, through statute and regulation, that nurse practitioners
are here to stay. Without such authority, the ability of nurse practitioners to
function within the scope of their preparation and training would have
been severely curtailed. While nurse practitioners still have a number of
barriers to overcome in an ever changing health care system in this country,
the proactive steps they have taken have helped to assure their presence
and their ability to care for their patients.

CONCLUSION

As the result of the efforts discussed in this chapter, nurse practitioners are
prescribing in all 50 states and the District of Columbia. The need to prescribe under the signature of a physician as well as the nurse practitioner
exists now only in four of the 50 states. The authority to prescribe
controlled substances is continuing to expand as the role of the nurse
practitioner has been recognised in each state. The 50 000 plus nurse
practitioners in the USA have become high-quality, mainstream health care
providers, particularly in the primary care arena.

Nurse practitioners are currently involved in achieving recognition by
new medical insurance entities in the USA in both fee for service and
managed care systems. Attaining prescriptive authority has been helpful in
these domains. As nurse practitioners in the USA continue to move into the
mainstream of health care in the next decade, it is anticipated that the

quality of primary care will grow and remain high through their efforts. While the evolution of the discipline will not reach closure for some time, it is clear that actions such as those of nurse practitioners on behalf of their patients and their own practices described above, have – and will continue to have – an impact on the quality of future health care provision in the USA.

QUESTIONS FOR DISCUSSION

- Does the connection between prescribing rights and the nurse practitioner role in the USA have any relevance to the scope and level of practice of nurse prescribers in the UK?

- How might we learn from developments in the USA so far as promoting nurse prescribing in the UK is concerned?

- Are the lobbying tactics employed by would-be nurse prescribers in the USA any more effective than those used in the UK?

REFERENCES

American Academy of Nurse Practitioners (1993) *Scope of Practice for Nurse Practitioners*. Austin, Texas: American Academy of Nurse Practitioners.
Towers, J. & Jennings, C. (1992) Have you talked with your legislator recently? *Journal of the American Academy of Nurse Practitioners*, **4(2)**, 79–80.

QUESTIONS FOR DISCUSSION

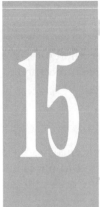

Nurse prescribing

The future

Mark Jones

Key issues

♦ Recommendations of the second Crown review into prescribing.

♦ Analysis of Crown recommendations as relevant to nursing.

♦ Suggestions for moving the nurse prescribing agenda forward.

INTRODUCTION

This final chapter of the book is but the beginning of the reality of nurse prescribing. The publishers have been driven to distraction waiting for this chapter to be written, just as the nursing profession has been driven to distraction waiting for the publication of the Crown Report. Anyone with any interest at all in the extension of prescribing rights for nurses will appreciate the significance of this report and why it would have been futile to speculate on the future of nurse prescribing without some idea of its content. So, this last minute contribution is being compiled in the second week of March 1999, just as the Crown Report is published. There has as yet been little debate on the content of the report and what follows is the first analysis of its recommendations and implications.

THE CROWN RECOMMENDATIONS

Before we embark upon an analysis of the Crown Report recommendations, it is worth remembering that they concern the extension of prescribing rights to those health care professionals who do not currently have them. So while we will necessarily focus upon nursing, we have to bear in mind that Crown is suggesting a whole new future for a range of professional groups, and the report's recommendations are therefore worded in such a way as to be appropriate to that range. When discussing the extension of prescribing rights to nurses in this chapter therefore, the 'generic' application of the Crown recommendations has been interpreted as far as possible to the specifics of that profession.

The main recommendations

Having considered the not insignificant 700 plus items of evidence received during the consultation process, in its final report, submitted to ministers in October 1998 and published in March 1999, the Crown review team make three main recommendations towards a:

> *proposed new framework for prescribing, supply and administration of medicines inside and outside the NHS in which:*
> * *the majority of patients continue to receive medicines on an individual patient basis;*
> * *the current prescribing authority of doctors, dentists, and certain nurses (in respect of a limited list of medicines) continues;*
> * *new groups of professionals would be able to apply for authority to prescribe in specific clinical areas, where this would improve patient care and patient safety could be assured.* (DoH, 1999, p. 3)

The first recommendation addresses the issue of supply and administration of medicines using group protocol arrangements as detailed in the first report from the Crown review (DoH, 1998). Although several authors in this book have alluded to the usefulness of group protocol arrangements, the essential rationale for this has been that they provide a way around the current restrictions on prescribing (i.e. a doctor having to do this) whereby nurses can select the appropriate medicines to be supplied or administered to patients. It is logical, given the recommendations in the second part of Crown, that the new prescribing mechanisms should be utilised to provide patients with medicines on an individual basis wherever possible, and group protocol systems used where patients fit into tightly defined categories (for example those requiring immunisation).

The second recommendation also makes sense, although it could cause concern, depending upon specific interpretation. There may well be certain aspects of medical prescribing worthy of review, but this was not Crown's remit; it makes sense therefore to suggest that doctors should continue to prescribe as at present. Note, however, the second part of this recommendation, which suggests that 'certain nurses' already prescribing from a limited list should continue to do so. These nurses are of course the health visitors and district nurses who have completed a prescribing course and who are utilising the Nurse Formulary either in a nurse prescribing pilot site or in the additional locations where this mode of prescribing rights for nurses is being rolled out. So long as Crown is suggesting that this should continue *in addition* to further extension of prescribing powers there is not a problem, but if it is envisaged that *only* this model should be allowed to continue, this would clearly be unacceptable to organisations such as the RCN who have campaigned for far wider prescribing powers for nurses. (This point is discussed further below.)

It is the third recommendation, that 'new groups of professionals' who currently do not have prescribing rights might apply for this authority to be extended to them, which contains the 'good news'. Crown envisages two ways in which this might happen:

Independent prescribing

Crown suggests that an independent prescriber be identified as someone:

> *who is responsible for the assessment of patients with undiagnosed conditions and for decisions about the clinical management required, including prescribing.* (DoH, 1999, p. 39, para. 6.19)

It is pointed out that at present only doctors and dentists and those nurses prescribing from the Nurse Formulary are legally authorised prescribers. As stated above, they fulfil the criteria of being able to assess patients with undiagnosed conditions and make a prescribing decision, and they should continue to do so. However, Crown states that 'certain other health professionals may also become newly legally authorised independent prescribers'.

Dependent prescribing

Crown defines the dependent prescriber as someone:

> *who is responsible for the continuing care of patients who have been clinically assessed by an independent prescriber. This continuing care may include prescribing, which will usually be informed by clinical guidelines and will be consistent with individual treatment plans; or continuing established treatments by issuing repeat prescriptions, with the authority to adjust the dose or dosage form according to the patients' needs. There should be provision for regular review by the assessing clinician.* (DoH, 1999, p. 39, para. 6.19)

The essential difference here is that a dependent prescriber will not have the diagnostic and assessment ability to make a decision about an initial prescription, but will have sufficient knowledge to determine whether that prescription should be continued, or whether to alter the dosage. Furthermore, a dependent prescriber may still be able to prescribe a drug for the first time, but this would be within the parameters of clinical guidelines for a given condition, and the care plan of a patient. This system differs from the supply and administration of medicines using group protocols in that the dependent prescriber will be able to provide patients with a prescription form which they can take to a pharmacy to have their medicines dispensed. This cannot happen with protocol arrangements.

There is a certain irony in learning of these recommendations as they are almost identical to those made in the first Crown Report considering the possibility of nurse prescribing a decade ago (DoH, 1989). In her first report, Crown suggested three modes of prescribing for nurses: initial, time and dose, and protocol. The latter option – protocols – was addressed by the first report of the second Crown review (DoH, 1998). In the second report of the second review we see independent prescribing embracing the original concept of 'initial' prescribing, and dependent prescribing clearly including the idea of 'time and dose' prescribing. Although this second Crown review is far more wide ranging than just the nursing profession, one has to wonder why it has taken over a decade for Dr June Crown's original review group's thinking to be accepted and reiterated once again in a very similar way. Nursing could have got on with the whole concept 10 years ago, and no doubt by now the other professional groups considering prescribing would have learned from the experience and be well on their way to developing their own practice.

HOW WILL IT WORK?
General principles

The Crown review team put forward 11 key principles for the extension of prescribing rights:

a. *All health professionals authorised to prescribe must be fully qualified and registered with a recognised regulatory body.*
b. *All health professionals authorised to prescribe should have appropriate post qualification training.*
c. *All health professionals authorised to prescribe should undertake continuing professional education relevant to their prescribing role.*
d. *All health professionals authorised to prescribe should be so identified on the register of the relevant regulatory body and this information should be updated at specific intervals.*
e. *Health professionals should only prescribe in circumstances where they are competent to assess all relevant aspects of the a patient's clinical condition, to decide on an appropriate programme of clinical management and to take responsibility for prescribing and related decisions.*
f. *No health professional should undertake any aspect of patient care for which they are not trained and which is beyond their professional competence.*
g. *Overall responsibility for the co-ordination of care will normally remain with the general practitioner or, during episodes of hospital care, with a named lead consultant.*

h. *All health professionals authorised to prescribe should have access to the patient's clinical records and schedules of medication. Wherever possible there should be integrated clinical records, with full regard to confidentiality.*

i. *When responsibility for all or part of a patient's care is transferred from one professional to another, there should be transfer of full information on clinical status and medication, and the doctor with overall responsibility for the patient should be informed.*

j. *There should normally be a separation of responsibilities for prescribing and for dispensing.*

k. *Arrangements for prescribing should take into account communications and other factors in the relationship between patient and practitioner which might affect the patient's willingness to follow the prescribed treatment.*
(DoH, 1999, pp. 23–24, para. 4.4)

All of these principles make sense, and encompass the points put forward by organisations lobbying for prescribing rights (the RCN, for example) in that they acknowledge the need for appropriate training, regulation and updating, and acknowledge that prescribing should take place within a framework of professional accountability and competency. The next step is to establish some form of mechanism to ensure that these principles are implemented and maintained. For this purpose the Crown review team suggest the setting up of a new body independent of those currently governing and monitoring the provisos of the Medicines Act and of the various professional bodies. The 'New Prescribers Advisory Committee' (NPAC, see below) will be responsible for promulgating clear criteria for extensions to prescribing and is expected to advise on the following aspects of individual applications:

- *the clinical need for the proposed extension of prescribing;*
- *the definition and registration arrangements of the professional group concerned, ensuring that there are clear criteria for determining which individuals may be included in the group. They may include consideration of the education and training requirements of the group;*
- *the need for additional prescribing to be 'independent' or 'dependent' in the senses defined above;*
- *the broad category(ies) of the medicines that might be prescribed;*
- *the need for prescribing by the new group to be funded by the NHS.* (DoH, 1999, p. 44, para. 6.28)

New Prescribers Advisory Committee

As medicines legislation applies across the whole of the UK, the review team recommend the establishment of a new advisory body with a UK remit – the 'New Prescribers Advisory Committee' (NPAC) (DoH, 1999, p. 44, para. 6.27).

Crown envisages that the membership of NPAC would be made up as follows:

Members of NPAC should be chosen for personal expertise, and not as representatives of any particular interest or body. Nevertheless, a wide range of perspectives will be needed. These include:
i. *current prescribers*
ii. *other relevant health care professions*
iii. *professional regulatory bodies*
iv. *education and training accrediting bodies (currently the National Boards for Nursing, Midwifery and Health Visiting; the Medical Royal Colleges and Faculties; the Royal Pharmaceutical Society of Great Britain; and the professional Boards of the Council for Professions Supplementary to Medicine)*
v. *NHS commissioners and provider units*
vi. *patient groups.* (DoH, 1999, p. 47, para. 6.31)

NPAC would consider applications from professional organisations seeking powers for suitably trained members to become independent or dependent prescribers. These applications would be considered according to a predetermined checklist prior to a recommendation being made to ministers for the extension of prescribing rights (see Fig. 15.1).

The good news is that nursing will have access to NPAC through its own membership organisations. Crown expects that proposals for new professional groups to be considered as potential prescribers by NPAC will come from 'nationally recognised organisations' (DoH, 1999, pp. 47–48, para. 6.33). As such, it would seem that nursing organisations such as the RCN, Community Practitioner and Health Visitors Association (CPHVA), Community and District Nursing Association (CDNA), and others would be able to put proposals to NPAC as to why groups of their members should have dependent or independent prescribing rights. The review team suggest a number of criteria NPAC would apply to their consideration of applications:

i. *What clinical benefits are expected to be derived from the proposed extension of the authority to prescribe? Could these benefits be secured in a different way, for example through use of supply or administration under group protocol, or through amendments to the POM Order, by removing prescription status of particular medicines?*
ii. *What impact would the change have on patient convenience and patient choice?*
iii. *Does the proposed process ensure that only professionals with appropriate specialist qualifications, recorded or registered with the approriate regulatory body, would be allowed to apply for prescribing authority?*
iv. *Are there adequate arrangements for ensuring that all new prescribers will:*
• *undergo satisfactory training in all relevant aspects of prescribing?*

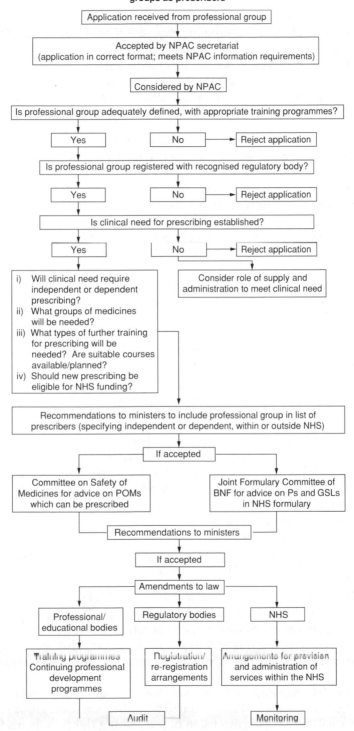

Fig. 15.1 Summary of proposed arrangements for authorisation of professional groups as prescribers (DOH, 1999, p. 45).

- *undertake regular continuing professional development related to their prescribing, approved by the appropriate professional body?*
- *participate in professional audit or other quality assurance activities?*

v. *What would be the benefits from allowing prescribing at public expense, and are these sufficient to justify any additional costs which might be incurred?* (DoH, 1999, p. 48, para. 6.34)

These criteria are entirely reasonable, and any professional group – including nursing – seeking the extension of prescribing rights to themselves should accept their responsibility in meeting them. With this in mind, it would make enormous sense if the national nursing membership organisations could in some way coordinate their efforts so as to make the most effective application to NPAC. A range of proposals from different organisations suggesting different criteria for inclusion of the same group of nurses would only serve to illustrate that the nursing profession was not cohesive and that it would be difficult to determine common standards. Without unity in nursing, the chance of prescribing rights being extended as fast as possible will be jeopardised as NPAC either rejects proposals or seeks for the lowest common denominator.

The UKCC would of course have a role in identifying future nurse prescribers. Crown suggests (DoH, 1999, para. 6.33) that the appropriate regulatory body for new groups seeking prescribing rights must be satisfied with proposals for training and for registration of prescribers. In tandem with whichever nursing organisation were putting forward a proposal to NPAC, the UKCC would be required to:

ensure that adequate arrangements would be established for:
i.   *accrediting training programmes for prescribing;*
ii. *maintaining a register of individuals who have acquired and are maintaining competency as prescribers;*
iii. *reviewing the results of clinical audit programmes and ensuring that any general lessons are fed back into the content of training;*
iv. *keeping the content of the prescribing formulary under review and submitting proposals for change to the Medicines Control Agency.* (DoH, 1999, p. 67, para. 8.12)

Significant responsibility beyond making the initial submission to NPAC is therefore placed upon the nursing profession, in that it would be responsible for establishing its own system of education for prescribing nurses together with a monitoring and registration system. This is exactly the way forward envisaged by the RCN in its evidence to the second Crown review (Fig. 15.2).

The model proposed by the review team is not too dissimilar to that of the college, although as it has a 'generic' application to all groups of health professionals seeking the extension of prescribing rights to themselves, it is

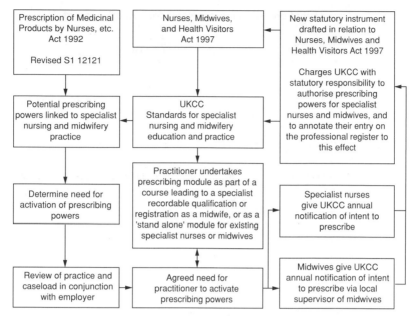

Fig. 15.2 Proposed professional and legal regulatory system for nurse and midwife prescribing (RCN, 1997).

not quite so specific as the RCN model which addresses the needs of nursing in particular. Nevertheless, the Crown model (Fig. 15.3) contains the core principles proposed by the college: recognised training and competence, completion of a prescribing course, activation of prescribing powers, and a system of continuing education, periodic assessment and notification of prescriber status.

Who should prescribe?

As discussed above, Crown charges professional organisations with the responsibility to identify new prescribing groups and to put a proposal to NPAC describing why they should be allowed to prescribe. This sounds fine in principle, but the practice may well be quite difficult. For example, the RCN believes that prescribing rights should be linked to specialist practice status (RCN, 1997). This is all well and good when a group of practitioners can easily be identified as specialists, as for instance where a particular qualification is mandatory to practice. However, there are many areas of nursing practice where practitioners would consider themselves to be working at specialist level but for which their is no uniformity of definition of prerequisite education and/or experience. Any professional organisation wishing to propose a new group of prescribers to NPAC will

Summary of proposed arrangements for authorisation of individual prescribers

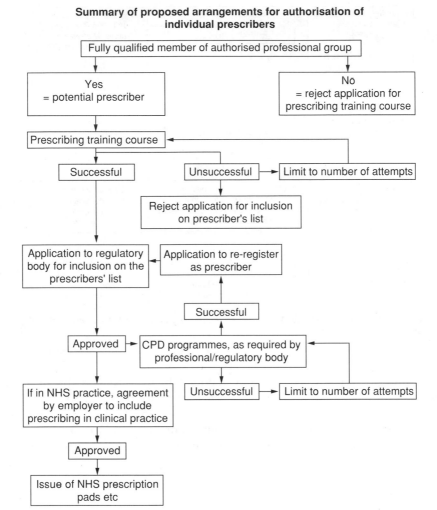

Fig. 15.3 Summary of proposed arrangements for authorisation of individual prescribers (DOH, 1999, p. 52).

first have to identify competency criteria for that particular group so as to be able to convince the committee of its homogeneity. Inevitably some groups of specialist practitioners may be split if a proportion of their members do not have skills and competencies which correlate with what the professional organisation putting forward the proposal believes to be the competencies required to prescribe in their particular field of practice. Again it is imperative that nursing organisations adopt a common approach to this issue, presenting the most cohesive and cogent proposals possible to NPAC.

Further difficulty may lie in the Crown recommendation that new groups of prescribers proposed by a national organisation are 'formally recognised by the appropriate regulatory body'. Take the issue of nurse practitioners for example. The RCN has a clear view of what a nurse practitioner is (RCN, 1996) and could feasibly present NPAC with a proposal including what it believes to be the essential educational underpinning for the role in general and specifically for prescribing rights to be extended. Yet the UKCC has consistently refused to acknowledge that it is possible to identify the role of nurse practitioner, and has not instructed the National Boards for Nursing to determine and implement any national standards for an appropriate educational qualification, possession of which would lead to a recordable qualification on the professional register. It is possible therefore that while Crown would envisage a great deal of power being given to national organisations so far as bringing forward proposals for new prescribing groups are concerned, the UKCC will act as final arbiter; if they are not convinced of the merits of such a proposal they will not go ahead. Once more it will be crucial that all national nursing organisations work together with the UKCC and agree a common framework for the submission of proposals to NPAC.

Dependent or independent?

In addition to determining which groups of nurses they will propose to NPAC as new prescribers, national nursing organisations and the UKCC will have to agree as to what type of prescriber these groups of nurses will be. It is clear from the descriptions of the two prescriber groups recommended by Crown (DoH, 1999, para. 6.19) that the competency base of each is distinct.

The independent prescriber possesses a diagnostic ability and is able to assess the prescribing needs of a previously undiagnosed patient. Clearly these are 'high level' skills which not every nurse will possess, but no doubt some will. Many nurse experts will possess sufficient knowledge to make a diagnosis – for example the asthma specialist would be able to make a diagnosis of that condition, and even today, in the absence of prescribing rights, be able to determine the optimum medicine required to assist the patient. Independent prescriber status for such a nurse would seem reasonable. Once again, nursing organisations will have to work to identify the specific skill base which is required to provide a would-be independent prescribing nurse with the ability to diagnose and assess without necessarily referring to another independent prescriber (i.e. a doctor).

A key development associated with independent prescriber status for nurses is that such prescribers would be able to draft care plan arrangements in order to facilitate dependent prescribers in their work. We should be able to develop the situation in nursing practice whereby an expert independent nurse prescriber is able to make an assessment of the patient, derive a diagnosis, make an initial prescription and determine a plan of care for that patient which can subsequently be amended by a dependent prescriber. Even more useful is that the dependent prescriber need not be a nurse. Crown is of course making recommendations about all health care professionals who currently do not have prescriber status. As such, an independent nurse prescriber could well facilitate other dependent pre-scribers (for example pharmacists, physiotherapists, occupational thera-pists, or others) as they seek to determine the most appropriate medicines for any given patient as their care plan is fulfilled. Although not strictly legally necessary, the independent nurse prescriber could also draft treatment and care plans to be followed by less experienced medical colleagues who could prescribe in a dependent way. All of these interactions were foreseen by the nursing profession as it lobbied the Crown review team (e.g. RCN, 1997).

Determining eligibility for dependent prescriber status may well prove a little easier, given that the nurse would be working from an existing diagnosis and care plan, with a prescription already having been decided. The dependent prescriber will, by and large, be limited to repeating a prescription or making minor alterations, in addition to tailoring dosage to a particular patient's needs. Again these skills are not exhibited by every nurse, and specialist practitioner level is probably where they will be identified, but far more nurses should be able to prove eligibility for dependent prescriber status. This level of prescribing should prove invaluable in situations such as the delivery of family planning care, where for example specialist nurses will be able to use their expertise to determine whether more oral contraceptive pills should be issued, or whether the prescription needs to be altered. All clinical situations in which dosage and drug variation would come within the ability of the specialist nurse will see benefits to patients from dependent prescribing to, for example, the diabetic person requiring insulin, the asthmatic requiring a bronchodilator, the patient with blood pressure management problems requiring oral hypertensives, and so on.

Aside from determining which nurses would be able to access indepen-dent or dependent prescriber rights, we still need to remember the highly useful facility of group protocol arrangements. Although nurses obviously need to have a sufficient level of expertise to select drugs for supply or administration under group protocols, many more should be able to practice in this way than would be in the two de facto prescriber options. The exciting development is, however, that independent prescriber nurses could establish group protocols through which nurses without any form of prescriber status could provide appropriate medication for patients.

Professional organisations for nurses wishing to bring forward proposals to NPAC should immediately begin a scoping exercise within their mem-bership in order to determine how patients might benefit from certain groups of their members being eligible for independent or dependent prescriber status. The necessary education and competencies required must then be determined, and agreement gained from the UKCC that a good case has been made for the proposal. Even if the Crown recommendations were implemented tomorrow, this process could take many months, if not years. Those nursing groups which have had the foresight to begin this exercise in the absence of the Crown report should have an advantage and will hopefully assist their colleagues in other specialist areas.

EDUCATION

As rather worryingly emphasised by Banning in Chapter 6, educational provision for prescribing nurses – and in particular for those who will be independent prescribers – will require urgent review if the full potential of the Crown recommendations are to be realised. It is clear that the content of the current nurse prescribing course approved by the National Boards for Nursing for England and Scotland, underpinning the current developments in prescribing by health visitors and district nurses (NHS Executive, 1998), is a long way from being sufficiently comprehensive to support independent prescriber status.

Again Crown puts the responsibility for extending prescribing – in this instance ensuring appropriate education is available – firmly back into the hands of the profession:

> *Professional organisations, in putting forward proposals for new groups of professionals to have the authority to prescribe certain medicines, should ensure that all necessary training aspects are covered in their proposals.* (DoH, 1999, p. 59, para. 6.62)

and:

> *Professional groups putting forward proposals for extended prescribing should liaise with education providers and bodies responsible for approving training courses to develop suitable training programmes in the required prescribing competencies. All training should include a period of supervised practice, and professional and regulatory bodies should take firm action against supervisors who fail to discharge their responsibilities.* (DoH, 1999, p. 66, para. 8.9)

Professional nursing organisations putting forward groups of their members for prescribing status will therefore not only have to consider means of identifying the appropriate level of practice, but will also have to determine the educational requirements in terms of the various competencies they have identified as being necessary. For nursing, professional organisations are again in quite a strong position so far as determining the future for extension of prescribing rights to nurses. The RCN, for example, could determine which nurses they would see as independent and dependent prescribers, and design and provide appropriate education through their own academic institute, either just for their own membership or in partnership with other national nursing organisations. Crown does, however, recommend that such developments should be:

> in conjunction with the appropriate professional regulatory organisations ... [and that the] ... appropriate regulatory body ... has seen and is content with the proposed arrangements for training in prescribing. (DoH, 1999, para. 6.33)

For nursing this will necessitate any professional organisation wishing to put a prescribing extension proposal to NPAC working in partnership with the appropriate National Board for Nursing and the UKCC if the current model of professional regulation and validation of educational provision is still in operation at that time.

Given the points raised by Banning, and the obvious need for some commonality in the knowledge base of independent prescribers (including doctors and nurses), the nature of educational provision is set to be one of the main agenda issues so far as expanding prescribing rights is concerned. For example, in order to justify their ability to make a diagnostic decision, subsequent assessment of patient need, then write a prescription, an independent prescriber nurse will need sufficient expertise in both pharmacology and physical assessment skill.

It is worth noting that major proponents of the extension of prescribing rights to nurses – such as the RCN – have always argued for the ability of suitably qualified and competent nurses to prescribe in order to meet their patients *nursing* care needs. As such, competency and underpinning educational provision for any given nurse prescriber will depend on the nature of the 'nursing' they perform in their own particular practice. If their nursing encompasses physical assessment and diagnosis of a physical condition for which they intend to prescribe, the educational base may well be different from that of a nurse who exhibits sufficient expertise to be a prescriber of wound care products or surgical appliances. In its evidence to Crown the RCN proposed that nurses with prescribing powers would self-limit those powers on the basis of individual professional accountability (RCN, 1997). What this means in practice is that although nurses may be recognised as independent prescribers, they would only exercise those prescribing rights for therapeutic interventions of which they had sufficient knowledge and experience to be competent prescribers; educational provision will have to reflect this (see below for more detailed discussion of scope of prescribing by nurses).

LEGAL PARAMETERS

In Chapter 5, Caulfield describes the complexities of the current legislation governing prescribing, which is clearly both confusing and anachronistic.

Primary legislation such as the 1968 Medicines Act is far behind current nursing practice, to name but one of the health care professions Crown is trying to provide with an essential tool for the next millennium. If the extension of prescribing rights is to go ahead smoothly and without unnecessary delay, it would be impossible to rely on an outdated legal framework or expect major legislative change to be enacted each time some new aspect of prescribing practice is considered, whether this be a new group of prescribers to be recognised or some adjustment to the formulary they might use. Crown recognises this need for a more rapid legislative response and recommends that all that is required to allow expansion of prescribing is for the government to take 'general powers' in primary legislation, enabling ministers through regulations to designate new categories of dependent and independent prescribers (DoH, 1999, p. 66, para 8.7). Such an arrangement would allow alterations to be made to the law much more quickly than would be the case if primary legislation had to be revisited each time a change was required.

Nursing should be at an advantage here, given that the primary legislation is already on the statute book in the form of the Prescription of Medicinal Products by Nurses etc. Act 1992. All NPAC will have to do is suggest regulatory amendments along the lines described by Caulfield in order to allow a wider group of nurses to prescribe from a much more comprehensive formulary. Alternatively, government may believe that primary legislation needs to be laid which would give general powers allowing a wider group of health care professionals access to prescribing rights, which would encompass nurses also. This would require the repeal of the 1992 nursing legislation which seems a little unnecessary, but at least this Act could provide a good template for legislation relevant to other professional groups.

One would assume that once primary legislation – in whatever form – is enacted which permits new prescriber categories to be added and which describes the way in which the formulary from which they prescribe might be extended, then NPAC would make additional ad hoc recommendations to ministers as to what specific secondary regulations needed to be brought forward in order to legalise prescribing by those groups of professionals proposed by their national organisations with whom the committee concur. In principle this would appear to be a flexible and much more expedient system than the current prescribing legislation, although whether anything so obvious and simple will be accepted remains to be seen.

PRESCRIBE WHAT?

Crown's proposals to extend prescribing rights, so creating potential categories of independent and dependent nurse prescribers, are widely welcomed, but what most nurses will want to know is the extent of the formulary to which they will have access. Uniquely so far as those professional organisations who responded to the Crown consultation exercise were concerned, the RCN suggested that all specialist nurses with proven competence and appropriate educational underpinning should have access to the whole of the BNF, and that their prescribing patterns should not be restricted by complex legal regulation. The rationale for this suggestion was that nursing was a self-regulating profession, with its members being individually accountable to their governing body – the UKCC. Being aware of their *Code of Professional Conduct*, and *Scope of Professional Practice* (UKCC, 1992a, 1992b), nurses only practice in a manner in which they consider themselves to be competent. Any extension of their role must be accompanied by appropriate education and the willingness to be accountable and accept sanction from the regulatory body if their practice exceeds their competence. This connection between personal accountability, competence and prescribing patterns is acknowledged within the Crown report:

> *All legally authorised prescribers should take personal responsibility for maintaining and updating their knowledge and practice related to prescribing, including taking part in clinical audit, and should never prescribe in situations beyond their professional competence.* (DoH, 1999, p. 68, para. 8.14)

This principle of prescribing scope linked to competency would mean that if nurses with independent prescriber status had access to a wide formulary – say the majority of the BNF – they would not prescribe medicines or other products if their knowledge base was insufficient for them to make a competent decision (see the RCN proposal to the Crown review team, Fig. 15.4). Thus an expert independent nurse prescriber working in a respiratory speciality might prescribe a bronchodilator, but would not think of prescribing pain control for a terminally ill child. Nurses might technically have the legal authority to do the latter, but the limits of their competence and awareness of their scope of practice and professional accountability criteria would stop them doing so. This model does of course rely on nurse prescribers being aware of the limits of their competence and some form of review of prescribing patterns being put in place.

Specific restrictions

Crown does not offer any emphatic view as to the scope of formulary any new group of prescribers will have access to, presumably this would be the remit of NPAC. The report does, however, contain some definitive and suggestive guidance. First, it is suggested that:

> *newly authorised prescribers should not normally be allowed to prescribe medicines in the following categories:*

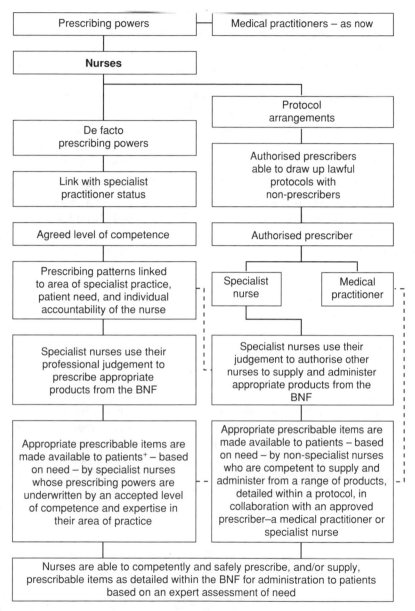

Fig. 15.4 Prescribing powers linked to professional accountability and competence (RCN, 1997).

*Patient is a term of convenience, used here to refer to all people receiving care of assistance from nurses, midwives, or health visitors.

i. *controlled drugs which are drugs subject to the Misuse of Drugs Act (1971)*
ii. *unlicensed drugs, or drugs used outside their licensed indications, including drugs undergoing pre-licensing clinical trials, and certain medicines which are commonly used for children but have never been licensed for paediatric use;*
iii. *'black triangle' drugs; which are newly-introduced drugs, still subject to special monitoring for potential side-effects by the MCA*
iv. *drugs over which there is continuing professional concern, for instance drugs used to treat children and young people with mental health problems;*
v. *drugs which on public health grounds should be subject to particular care, for instance antibacterial antibiotics. (DoH, 1999, p. 55, para. 6.53)*

For the most part these exclusions to the formulary of any new prescriber seem reasonable, and one may well believe that they should also exist for current prescribers (i.e. doctors), although they were outside the remit of the Crown team. Unlicensed drugs and those drugs which are being closely scrutinised ('black triangle' drugs) clearly demand a strict review system and involvement of medical personnel in their prescription, as do those drugs for which there is already a medical concern. It is also reasonable that Crown now takes the opportunity to restrict access to antibiotics and other drugs which have been subject to inappropriate prescribing. The review cannot affect the prescribing habits of existing independent prescribers, but it is right to use its recommendations to make sure new prescribers do not continue this practice. The inability of new prescribers to prescribe controlled drugs is rather more contentious. It is certainly possible that an expert palliative care nurse working, for example, in a primary care based pain control team could today make an effective and competent judgement involving the prescription of a controlled drug. This is certainly common-place, and without adverse incidents, among nurse prescribers in many states in the USA (see Towers, Ch. 14). Hopefully, Crown's suggestion that new prescribers should not *normally* prescribe such drugs as detailed above will give professional groups proposing new prescribers and NPAC some latitude in deciding just what drugs will be accessible to which prescribers.

Broad or limited formularies?

Aside from these specific restrictions, Crown also intimates further limits to the formulary of any new prescriber. Paragraph 6.8 acknowledges the case made by the RCN that that practitioners bound by a professional code of conduct and adequately trained should be given access to a wide formulary, as their prescribing decisions would be based upon a recognition of the limits of their own competence. Any practitioner prescribing outside of those limits would be acting unprofessionally (DoH, 1999, p. 36). However, the review team believes that such a wide extension of prescribing authority is not necessary to achieve benefits in patient care and suggests that:

> *Legal authority for new professional groups to prescribe or authorise NHS expenditure should normally be limited to medicines in specific therapeutic areas related to the particular competence and expertise of the group and may include prescription only medicines ...*

and:

> *The Team believes that doctors and dentists will continue to form the majority of independent prescribers for POMs. Any extensions, beyond district nurses and health visitors who are already legally entitled to prescribe from a limited list of medicines, are likely to be limited to specific therapeutic areas.* (DoH, 1999, pp. 37–38, paras. 6.10 and 6.15)

We can interpret this statement as meaning that an independent nurse prescriber would normally only be able to prescribe drugs relevant to their specific clinical area of practice, because this is all they would be competent to do. On the face of it this might seem reasonable, endorsing the principle that independent nurse prescribers should only prescribe within the limits of their competence. In practice, however, the situation could be quite complicated, and attempting to define the formulary for any particular specialist could be difficult – for example the stoma care nurse whose formulary contains the appliances needed for patient care may well need access to treatments for skin breakdown and analgesia. Crown offers a possible solution: it is suggested that some professionals may gain additional qualifications in two or more specialist areas within their profession, all of which confer prescribing authority (DoH, 1999, p. 37, para. 6.11). We can see a situation developing whereby specialist nurses with independent prescriber status undertake a range of assessments underpinning prescribing practice utilising a number of specialist formularies. Problems could occur with independent nurse prescribers who have a wide remit of care (such as nurse practitioners in primary care) and who need access to a broad formulary. Perhaps a generic formulary could exist to which all independent prescribers have access once proven competent, with specialist formularies acting as a top-up?

These proposals fall short of the idea that a nurse prescriber would self-regulate prescribing patterns from a broad formulary, although they do allow specialist nurses to prescribe to meet the immediate care needs of their patients in the most part, albeit having completed a series of assessments and competency tests if they wish to access a range of formularies.

The real problems will be those around the implementation and regulation of such a system of ring-fenced specialist formularies. If ministers choose to restrict nurse prescribers' access to medicines and products within the BNF by some regulatory mechanism which makes it 'legally' impossible to prescribe drugs outside of the therapeutic area one works in, rather than 'professionally irresponsible' to do so, the complexity of managing a professional register delineating the prescribing permissions of a range of nurse specialists would be without precedent. Similarly, what kind of system would need to be put into place to allow a pharmacist dispensing a nurse prescriber's prescription to know exactly which range of medicines that nurse was permitted to prescribe from? It makes far greater sense to allow the professions themselves, in conjunction with their regulatory body, to draw up a system based on professional accountability which meets the approval of NPAC in order to ensure that nurse prescribers only prescribe drugs for which they have a proven competency.

THE TREASURY

Although the Crown Report has seemingly by and large met with ministerial approval, we have learnt elsewhere in this text that cost issues associated with the expansion of prescribing will be the main determining factor so far as any future developments are concerned. Crown readily acknowledges this point and pre-empts potential Treasury disquiet in saying that:

> *In assessing applications for new prescribing involving NHS reimbursement, the NPAC will need to form a judgement on whether the benefits would justify any net costs to the NHS. Where these costs could be significant or there appears to be a large degree of uncertainty these judgements should be tested through piloting and evaluation.* (DoH, 1999, p. 64, para. 7.9)

Yet again it would seem that the whole notion of cost and benefit analysis could delay the introduction of further prescribing rights for nurses and others. There is some hope though, in that Crown adds the caveat that such cost benefit evaluation 'should not be allowed to result in unnecessary delays in improving care' (DoH, 1999, p. 64, para. 7.9). Of course what is deemed unnecessary by the nursing profession and what is deemed unnecessary by the Treasury may well be different, but at least Crown is willing to fire a shot across the bows of those who would delay implementation just for the sake of cash savings. The onus will be well and truly on individual nurses and the profession as a whole to be aware of the need for excellence not only in medicines management (see Chapman, Ch. 13) but also in the ability to audit and justify their prescribing practice (see Fennessy, Ch. 12). As Crown emphasises, based on 'more detailed recent analysis of prescribing data' from the pilot sites which is yet unpublished:

> *there should be no overall increase in prescribing costs as a result of introducing nurse prescribing, if properly managed.* (DoH, 1999, p. 31, para. 5.10, vi)

At every stage in the extension of prescribing rights to nurses – from the compilation of the initial bid to NPAC right through to implementation and roll out on the ground – nursing will have continually to justify and account for its ability to prescribe effectively, whether or not we consider this to be reasonable. Nurse prescribers are not going to be issued with a blank cheque and it is imperative that we should be able to demonstrate that we can keep a balance sheet of positive clinical outcome against any increased cost. If we do not have the skills and wherewithal to do this today, we must begin to acquire them without delay.

CONCLUSION

The Crown review team itself gives an excellent summary of the likely impact of implementing its recommendations:

> *We believe that our recommendations will bring clear benefits to patients in three main areas:*
>
> i.   *Our proposals will make more effective use of the skills and experience of groups of professionals who are not at present authorised to prescribe. In particular:*
>
> - *in many clinical situations, we foresee an end to the artificial separation of the prescribing decision from other aspects of the patient's clinical management, creating clearer accountability and increasing the patient's confidence in the consultation;*
> - *the prescribing choice can be made by the professional with particular specialist skills and experience, resulting on occasions in more clinically appropriate and sympathetic prescribing and reducing the potential for wasteful use of resources;*
> - *dependent prescribing, in particular, opens up the possibility of making more effective use of the expert knowledge of a wider range of professionals, allowing the clinician responsible for the assessment to concentrate on the broad management of the patients.*
>
> ii. *We expect in some important instances to see an improvement in patients' access to advice and treatment, resulting in better uptake of services and better concordance between the perceptions of patients and professionals:*
>
> - *in some situations, improved access to the prescriber will result in more timely initiation of treatment with, in some cases, reduced duration of illness, better control of chronic disease, and fewer complications;*
> - *some vulnerable groups of people who find it difficult to access care at present may be more easily contacted by prescribers who will be able to initiate treatment immediately, reducing the risk of loss of contact with care services;*
> - *some new prescribers may in the course of their duties already be spending significant time with patients, resulting in better communication and thus adherence to treatment programmes.* (DoH, 1999, pp. 61–62, para. 7.2)

The publication of the Crown Report, reviewing for the second time the future of nurse prescribing, is at one and the same time the end of a 20-year fight to have this principle recognised as being of benefit to nurses and patients, and the beginning of a bright future for the way in which health care is delivered in the UK. In recommending the extension of prescribing rights to nurses and other health care professionals, Crown has demolished the supposition that only doctors have the skills and need to prescribe for patients, and has recognised that the future of health care delivery is about teamwork and having the right professional, sufficiently skilled and sufficiently equipped, to deliver the right care at the right time. It is true that the quest for prescribing rights for nurses has at times been single-minded and, as shown by Rafferty and colleagues (Ch. 7), has sometimes perhaps sprung as much from a desire to make a professional point as from the wish to improve patient care. However, nursing must accept the principles laid down by Crown and begin to work with colleagues right across the field of health care delivery. Prescribing by nurses will not work unless it is developed in association with colleagues in the medical and pharmacy professions in particular, and also in conjunction with other colleagues seeking to acquire prescribing rights for themselves.

Within nursing specifically, professional organisations must be ready and willing to work together and combine their expertise in preparing their submissions to the New Prescribers Advisory Committee. It will not help if NPAC receives a myriad of individual submissions all suggesting different reference points as markers of competence, level of practice, and education to be associated with the extension of prescribing rights to nurses. Furthermore, the separation of professional organisations representing members' interests and regulatory body defending the public must cease in the case of nurse prescribing. By working together to achieve the legalisation of prescribing rights for nurses, professional organisations and the UKCC can meet their own agendas by ensuring that nurses acquire a right which has been long overdue to them – a right which will bring with it great improvements in patient care.

On many occasions the diversity within nursing has been something to celebrate, but on the occasion of convincing NPAC of the form of prescribing rights we desire, a unity and common purpose within the profession, perhaps as we have never seen before, will be crucial if nurse prescribing politics are to be translated into actual nurse prescribing practice.

QUESTIONS FOR DISCUSSION

- Do the Crown proposals satisfy the current demands for prescribing rights for nurses?

- How can nurses make an effective case for prescribing rights to be extended to themselves?

- What mechanism should be put in place so as to ensure the best results from nurse prescribing?

- Is nursing really ready to accept the challenge?

REFERENCES

Department of Health (1989) *Report of the Advisory Group on Nurse Prescribing.* Chair Dr June Crown. London: Department of Health.
Department of Health (1998) *Review of Prescribing, Supply and Administration of Medicines. A report on the supply and administration of medicines.* Chair Dr June Crown. London: Department of Health.
Department of Health (1999) *Review of Prescribing, Supply and Administration of Medicines. Final report.* Chair Dr June Crown. London: Department of Health.
National Health Service Executive (1998) *Nurse Prescribing: a guide for implementation.* Leeds: NHSE.
Royal College of Nursing (1996) *Nurse Practitioners: your questions answered.* London: RCN.
Royal College of Nursing (1997) *Review of Prescribing, Supply and Administration of Medicines. Evidence submitted by the Royal College of Nursing.* London: RCN.
United Kingdom Central Council for Nursing, Midwifery and Health Visiting (1992a) *Code of Professional Conduct.* London: UKCC.
United Kingdom Central Council for Nursing, Midwifery and Health Visiting (1992b) *Scope of Professional Practice.* London: UKCC.

Index

Page numbers in **bold** type refer to illustrations and tables.